The
Running Injury
Recovery Program
WORKBOOK

The
Running Injury
Recovery Program
WORKBOOK

Bruce R. Wilk, P.T., O.C.S.

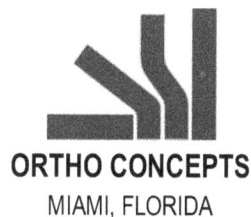

ORTHO CONCEPTS
MIAMI, FLORIDA

The Running Injury Recovery Program Workbook
First Edition (paperbound)
Published by Ortho Concepts, Inc.

ISBN-13 (paperbound) 978-0-9883603-1-0

Workbook Contents

INDEX OF TECHNIQUE FIGURES

Basic and Regional Closed-Chain

Fitness Walking, Glides, and Glide Drills

Accelerations and Hills

Plyometrics

Introduction

The Running Injury Recovery Program Workbook is a continuation of *The Running Injury Recovery Program.* Before starting this *Workbook*, you must read *The Running Injury Recovery Program* to acquire certain skills and knowledge, and you'll need to refer to it as you complete the *Workbook*.

This *Workbook* contains the step-by-step instructions you will follow to treat your own running injuries. In this book you become your own physical therapist. You will explore the causes of your running injury, develop your individualized recovery plan, determine your exercise schedule, and select your exercises. Your recovery program will include manual therapy, stretching exercises, closed-chain exercises for strength and balance, and training in post-injury running. You'll keep records, fill out self-assessments, and monitor your progress through the recovery program.

The *Workbook* begins with a general *Course Map* that covers the entire *Running Injury Recovery Program* from education to treatment and evaluation. The program is divided into four recovery phases, each with specific goals and clearance checkpoints. Each phase begins with a *Guidelines* table that summarizes the goals of that phase for different treatment groups.

The central part of your recovery program is a series of step-by-step *Self-Assessments* that contain all of the *Worksheets* that will help you determine your treatment group, monitor your progress, and clear you through the checkpoints on your *Course Map*. The *Self-Assessments* will also refer you to the Appendices in the back of the book which you'll use as you fill in your *Worksheets*.

In each recovery phase, the *Self-Assessments* will lead you to an individualized set of treatments or exercises for your specific injury, and to the *Log Forms* that you'll need to fill out. You will see examples of how each of these forms is filled out in the *Case Studies* section of this book.

Each section of the Workbook is described below in more detail. If you have questions, or need more help in following the instructions, see the *FAQs* at the end of this book, or visit our website at postinjuryrunning.com.

The Course Map

The first step of your *Running Injury Recovery Program* begins on line 1.1 of the *Course Map*. Just as everyone in a race follows the same course, the *Course Map* for this book is the master checklist for everyone's recovery program. The *Course Map* will guide you through the *Self-Assessments*, *Worksheets*, and *Log Forms*, and keep you on track from start to finish.

Each line of the *Course Map* is numbered for the chapter in *The Running Injury Recovery Program* where that material is explained. It follows the *Program* book, chapter by chapter, and lets you check off each of your accomplishments as you complete them.

The *Course Map* has three levels of checklists. Educational goals are found in white boxes. The lighter-shaded boxes require you to take a specific action. The darker-shaded boxes are checkpoints for moving through the phases. As you read through *The Running Injury Recovery Program*, you can start checking off the lines in white boxes related to education. When you start your *Workbook*, it's important to check off all of the lighter-shaded boxes (action lines) and darker-shaded boxes (checkpoints) in order.

There are always checkpoints between phases, and there are also some checkpoints within phases. You must check off all of the lines above each checkpoint, and all of the lines within each checkpoint, before continuing to the next section on your *Course Map*.

Although everyone will follow the same general *Course Map*, there are some additional checkpoints for Group 2 in Phases One, Two, and Three. There is also one section of the *Course Map* where Group 1 and Group 2 take entirely separate lines. In lines 15.13A through 15.26A, Group 1 takes the faster track, which will save them some time. Group 2 detours to lines 15.13B through 15.34B, which is a longer track but will get them to the same place (completion of Phase Three) more safely. All groups will merge together at the *Checkpoint to Enter Phase Four* and continue to the *Checkpoint to*

Return to Running, which is the finish line of your *Course Map*.

The Guidelines

The *Guidelines* are tables that summarize the treatment groups, exercise assignments, and clearance goals for Phase One, Phase Two, Phase Three Part One, Phase Three Part Two, and Phase Four. Each table appears first in the chapter of *The Running Injury Recovery Program* where that particular phase is introduced, and is numbered for that chapter. For example, *Table 5-1: Guidelines for Phase One Treatment Groups* first appears in Chapter 5 of *The Running Injury Recovery Program*. The *Guidelines* for each phase are repeated here in the *Workbook*, at the beginning of the Self-Assessments for each phase.

In Phase Three Part One, and again in Phase Four, everyone will be in the same treatment group, and there is one set of *Guidelines*. In all other phases, the *Guidelines* tables are divided by group, and sometimes by subgroup.

Each *Guidelines* table begins with a group definition and a reference to a *Self-Assessment*. You will not be able to follow these *Guidelines* until you have completed the *Self-Assessment* that determines which treatment group you are in for that particular phase. Complete all your *Self-Assessments* in order, and they will tell you which *Guidelines* to follow.

The second part of each *Guidelines* table contains specific instructions for different treatment groups. Follow the instructions for your group as determined by your *Self-Assessments*.

Each *Guidelines* table ends with a summary of the clearance requirements for that phase, and a reference to another *Self-Assessment.* However, remember that the full requirements for clearance are found in the *Self-Assessments* and *Course Map*, not in the *Guidelines*.

The Self-Assessments and Worksheets

There are twenty separate *Self-Assessments* that will guide you, step-by-step, through the day-to-day work of your recovery program. The *Self-Assessments* are numbered by Phase and must be completed in order: 1A, 1B, 1C etc.

Each *Self-Assessment* begins with one or more *"Course Map References."* Before starting any *Self-Assessment*, you should check off all of the previous lines on your *Course Map*.

The *"Instructions"* section lists the goals of the *Self-Assessment.*

In the *"Self-Assessment"* section, you will fill in *Worksheets* that may be used to determine your treatment group, your exercise schedule, or which exercises you will be doing. Some *Self-Assessments* will instruct you to prepare personalized *Log Forms*, or to evaluate your *Log Forms* for clearance to the next level.

Each *Self-Assessment* ends with a *"What to do now"* section that will guide you to your next step. It may guide you to another *Self-Assessment*, or it may guide you to the next line on your *Course Map*. To complete your *Running Injury Recovery Program Workbook*, you must follow the instructions and complete all of the *Self-Assessments.*

The Log Forms

The *Log Forms* are blank forms that you will use to record the results of your daily exercises for P.T. Time and your Base Schedule. The *Log Forms* for P.T. Time include forms for ICE (**Log Form I**), for stretch/mobilization cycles (**Log Form C** or **Log Form M**); and for closed-chain exercises (**Log Form B** or **Log Form R**). The forms for your Base Schedule consist of a series of **Log Forms S**, starting at Level 0 or higher (depending upon your treatment group) and ending at Level 8.

Each *Log Form* has its own set of instructions for preparing and filling out that form, which must be followed carefully. Some instructions include their own Self-Assessments to help you prepare or revise that form for different stages in your recovery program. For example, Line 8 of the *Instructions for Log Form R* contains the *Initial Assessment* for Phase Three Part Two (Stage 1).

The results that you fill in on each *Log Form* will be evaluated in a daily *Self-Assessment* which is identified in the instructions for that form. Most *Log Forms* will be evaluated for clearance to the next higher level. One exception is **Log Form M: Maintain Mobility**, which is used to monitor your flexibility after you have cleared **Log Form C: Stretch/Mobilization Cycles**. The other exception is Stage 2 (the *Final Target* level) of **Log Form R: Regional Closed Chain**. Once you have cleared the requirements for Regional Closed-Chain and Hill Closed-Chain Exercises in Stage 1 (the *Symmetry Target* level), you will be working to improve your strength and balance, but there is no further clearance requirement.

Different *Log Forms* are introduced in different Phases (*see Tables W1A and W1B*). **Log Form I** is used only by those who need to ICE in Phases One and Two. **Log Form C** is introduced in Phase Two, and is used only until you have achieved the degree of symmetry required for your group and subgroup (*Self-Assessment 2C*). **Log Form M** then replaces **Log Form C** for the remainder of your *Running Injury Recovery Program.*

Log Form B: Basic Closed-Chain is introduced in Phase Three Part One. Everyone will progress to **Log Form R: Regional Closed Chain** in Phase Three Part Two, but different groups will progress at different times.

Log Form S: Base Schedule is also introduced at the start of Phase Three Part Two, but different groups will start at different levels, and follow different time schedules.

Time Management

As you move through the phases of recovery, you'll need to coordinate and schedule the various elements of your individualized *Running Injury Recovery Program.* Some tasks (such as Basic Closed-Chain Exercises) are performed only during one specific time period. Other tasks (such as ICE, or fitness walking your Base Schedule), are performed only by certain groups. Some elements of your recovery plan (such as Stretch/Mobilization Cycles and Regional Closed-Chain Exercises) are introduced, and you will continue with them until the end of your recovery program. Other elements (such as glide drills and acceleration drills) will come and go at specific times in your schedule. In Phase Three, you'll also have to coordinate your P.T. Time and Base Schedule with certain clearance requirements in your *Self-Assessments.*

Table W-1: Time Management Schedules by Group will help you keep tack of what you should be doing during any particular phase. There are four possible Time Management Schedules for the different treatment groups and subgroups. In Phases One and Two, you will be assigned to either Group 1 or Group 2. In Phase Three Part Two, you will be sorted into subgroup A or B, depending upon how long it takes you to clear Basic Closed-Chain Exercises.

Note that the *Time Management Schedule* for Group 1B ends in Phase Three because, when this group completes Basic Closed-Chain Exercises in Phase Three Part Two, they will follow the Guidelines for *Group 1B Reassessment* and will be reassigned to either Group 1A or Group 2A.

Table W-1A: Group 1 Log Forms and Schedules

C   Stretch/Mobilization Cycles
M   Maintain Mobility
B   Basic Closed-Chain
R   Regional and Hill Closed Chain
S0   Base Schedule Level 0: Fitness Walking (Groups 1B, 2A and 2B Only)
S1-5   Base Schedule Walk/Glide Sets, Levels 1 through 5
S6   Base Schedule Level 6 with Acceleration Drills
S7   Base Schedule Level 7 with Hill Drills
S8   Base Schedule Level 8 with Plyometrics and Glide Drills

Group 1A: No Red Flags, *Able* to clear Basic Closed-Chain

PHASE		One	Two	Three		Four		
Part→				1	2	Accel.	Hills	Plyo.
PT Time	Stretches/Self-Mobs		C	M	M	M	M	M
	Basic Closed-Chain			B				
	Regional Closed-Chain				R	R	R	R
	Hills Closed-Chain					R	R	R
Base Schedule	Walk/Glide sets*			S1-5		S6	S7	S8
	Glide Drills			S1-5				S8
	Phase Four Drills					S6	S7	S8

*Self-Paced Plan

Group 1B: No Red Flags, *Unable* to clear Basic Closed-Chain
(Move to Group 1A or Group 2A after *Group 1B Reassessment*)

PHASE		One	Two	Three	
Part→				1	2
PT Time	Stretch/Mob Cycles		C	M	M
	Basic Closed-Chain			B	B
	Regional Closed-Chain				R
	Hill Closed-Chain				
Base Schedule	Fitness Walking *			S0	
	Walk/Glide Sets*				S1-5
	Glide Drills				S1-5
	Phase Four Drills				

*Self-Paced Plan

Table W-1B: Group 2 Log Forms and Schedules

I	ICE
C	Stretch/Mobilization Cycles
M	Maintain Mobility
B	Basic Closed-Chain
R	Regional and Hill Closed Chain
S0	Base Schedule Level 0: Fitness Walking (Groups 1B, 2A and 2B Only)
S1-5	Base Schedule Walk/Glide Sets, Levels 1 through 5
S6	Base Schedule Level 6 with Acceleration Drills
S7	Base Schedule Level 7 with Hill Drills
S8	Base Schedule Level 8 with Plyometrics and Glide Drills

Group 2A: Red Flags, *Able* to clear Basic Closed-Chain

PHASE		One	Two	Three		Four		
Part→				1	2	Accel.	Hills	Plyo.
PT Time	ICE	I	I					
	Stretches/Self-Mobs		C	M	M	M	M	M
	Basic Closed-Chain			B				
	Regional Closed-Chain				R	R	R	R
	Hills Closed-Chain					R	R	R
Base Schedule	Fitness walking **			S0				
	Walk/Glide sets **				S1-5	S6	S7	S8
	Glide Drills				S1-5			S8
	Phase Four Drills					S6	S7	S8

** 2-Week-Interval Plan

Group 2B: Red Flags, *Unable* to clear Basic Closed-Chain

PHASE		One	Two	Three		Four		
Part→				1	2	Accel.	Hills	Plyo.
PT Time	ICE	I	I					
	Stretches/Self-Mobs		C	M	M	M	M	M
	Basic Closed-Chain			B	B			
	Regional Closed-Chain				R	R	R	R
	Hills Closed-Chain					R	R	R
Base Schedule	Fitness walking **			S0				
	Walk/Glide sets **				S1-5	S6	S7	S8
	Glide Drills				S1-5			S8
	Phase Four Drills					S6	S7	S8

** 2-Week-Interval Plan

Start With a Positive Attitude

The *Running Injury Recovery Program* and *Workbook* seem complicated because we try to cover just about every possible combination of circumstances for every runner and every type of running injury. However, your actual course as you work through your individualized recovery program will not be that difficult.

Getting started is simple. The first step is to read all of the chapters in *The Running Injury Recovery Program* and make the mental commitment to follow the program. It's really important to keep a positive attitude and strong mental focus so that you can stick with your schedule, do your exercises correctly, and complete all the requirements in each phase before moving ahead. I know it's tempting to try to rush through your recovery and get back to running as quickly as possible but believe me, trying to do too much too soon will only slow down your recovery. That's exactly why we have clearance checkpoints in each phase – to set the correct pace and make sure you are fully prepared for each new challenge.

When you have read all the chapters in the *Program* book and are ready to start the *Workbook*, check line 1.1 on your Course Map, and proceed to line 1.2, which will send you to *Self-Assessment 1A*. Follow the *Course Map* and the *Guidelines* for your group, and they'll keep you on track.

A word of encouragement: Don't let all the Worksheets and Log Forms in the Self-Assessments intimidate you. I've designed these forms and instructions for the most detail-oriented and compulsive of readers. Anyone who follows these instructions to the letter will get the same level of treatment they would receive if they were a patient at my own P.T. clinic. However, I understand the frustrations that many people have with following detailed instructions and filling out complex forms, because I myself fall into that category. If a certain form really bothers you, then don't worry about it. Even if you don't fill in every single form, you will still benefit from doing the exercises and improving your running habits.

That said, try to do your best. The closer you follow the *Running Injury Recovery Program*, the faster you will recover and the better you will run. If you need help timing the exercises, or filling out the forms, or seeing whether you are able to exactly match the positions shown in the photographs, then it's okay to ask someone to help you. If a running companion, or coach, or physical therapist helps you through this program, then they might be inspired to explore some of these techniques as well.

I personally use all of the techniques described in this program in my P.T. clinic every day to treat injured runners, and I see how well they work. I know that, if you follow your individualized *Running Injury Recovery Program*, you can overcome your running injury, correct the underlying causes, and improve your running habits – and you will become a better runner.

SECTION 1: COURSE MAP

KEY

Educational Goals	White boxes contain educational goals from the *Running Injury Recovery Program*.	X
Action Required	Light-shaded boxes require you to take a specific action in the *Running Injury Recovery Program WORKBOOK*.	X
Checkpoints	Dark-shaded boxes are Checkpoints for moving through phases in the *Running Injury Recovery Program WORKBOOK*.	X

NOTE: Read all of the chapters in the *Running Injury Recovery Program* before starting your *Running Injury Recovery Program WORKBOOK*.

PHASE ONE:
Education and Self-Help

Section I: History and Self-Assessment (Chapters 1 -4)

CH 1: Do I Really Have a Running Injury?

1.1	I have read Chapter 1 in *The Running Injury Recovery Program*.	
1.2	I have determined that I have an injury caused by running (*Self-Assessment* **1A**).	
1.3	I have completed my *Running History* (*Self-Assessment 1B*) and entered the last day I ran on **Worksheet 1D**.	
1.4	I have made a list of *intrinsic* and *extrinsic factors* that might affect my running (**Worksheet 1B1**) and I am taking steps to correct them.	
1.5	I have completed my *Medical History* (*Self-Assessment* 1C) and recorded any relevant pre-existing medical conditions (**Worksheet 1C1**).	

CH 2: Introduction to the Four Phases of Recovery

2.1	I have read Chapter 2. in *The Running Injury Recovery Program*.	
2.2	I have decided to undertake a phased recovery plan for my running injury.	

CH 3: How Bad is my Injury?

3.1	I have read Chapter 3 in *The Running Injury Recovery Program*..	
3.2	I have documented my pain pattern and any visible swelling associated with my running injury (*Self-Assessments* **1D1 and 1D2**).	
3.3	I have determined the severity of my injury on the Running Injury Stage Scale, and whether or not I have any Red Flag symptoms (*Self-Assessment* **1D3**).	
3.4	I have summarized my original injury by *possible affected region* (*Self-Assessment* **1D4**).	
3.5	I have determined which treatment group I am in for Phase One (*Self-Assessment* **1D5**).	

CH 4: What Type of Injury Do I Have?

4.1	I have read Chapter 4 in *The Running Injury Recovery Program*.	
4.2	I understand the difficulties in the diagnosis of running injuries, and why we focus on injury regions in running-injury management.	
4.3	I understand the differences between *simple* running injuries and *complex* running injuries, and why they are treated differently.	
4.4	I will assess my running injury and begin self-management for all affected regions.	

Section II: Education and Self-Help (Chapters 5 - 9)

CH 5: Entering Phase One, Self-Help

5.1	I have read Chapter 5 in *The Running Injury Recovery Program*..	
5.2	I understand the goals of Phase One.	
5.3	I understand PRICE and how it applies to me.	
5.4	I have followed the instructions for Protection and Recovery.	
5.5	I have determined that I do not need to ICE (Group 1). **OR** I have begun to ICE and I am filling out my *Log Form I* (Group 2).	

CH 6: The Right Recovery Plan

6.1	I have read chapter 6 in *The Running Injury Recovery Program*..	
6.2	I understand when to seek professional help [**Box 6-1**].	
6.3	I understand how to evaluate professional help [**Box 6-2**].	
6.4	I understand that my management program must include both active treatment and education.	
6.5	I have obtained medical clearance to self-manage my running injury. **OR** I am following medical advice to resolve any medical issues before starting self-management.	

CH 7: What to Watch out For

7.1	I have read chapter 7 in *The Running Injury Recovery Program*.	
7.2	I understand the importance of not running while taking medication for pain or inflammation.	
7.3	I understand the importance of active treatment and weight-bearing exercise in running-injury management.	
7.4	I can distinguish between effective treatments and "tricks" for running-injury management.	
7.5	I will undertake an active recovery program, without medication for my running injury.	

CH 8: Running Shoes and Running Injuries

8.1	I have read chapter 8. in *The Running Injury Recovery Program*.	
8.2	I understand the relationship between running shoes and running injuries.	
8.3	I understand the importance of wearing a well-fitted, supportive training shoe for running-injury management.	
8.4	I will do my post-injury training in a proper training shoe.	

CH 9: Choosing the Right Shoe

9.1	I have read chapter 9. in *The Running Injury Recovery Program*.	
9.2	I have undergone a professional *gait analysis* to determine what type of functional support I need. **OR** I understand what type of functional support I need.	
9.3	I have chosen a new pair of *post-injury training shoes* based on function, fit, and feel [**Box 9-1**].	
9.4	I have inspected my shoes for defects [**Box 9-2**].	

CHECKPOINT TO ENTER PHASE TWO:

I am taking steps to protect and recover from my running injury.	
Group 2 ONLY: I am icing and filling out Log Form I.	
I have completed all of my *Phase One Self-Assessments*.	

PHASE TWO:
Regaining Mobility (Chapters 10 through 12)

CH 10: Phase Two, Manual Therapy and Self-Mobilization

10.1	I have read chapter 10. in *The Running Injury Recovery Program*.	
10.2	I understand the goals for Phase Two.	
10.3	I understand the Goals, Techniques, and Guidelines for Self-Mobilization.	
10.4	I understand how to perform *Self-Mobilizations by Region* [**Box 10-2**].	
10.5	I have obtained the necessary *Tools for Self-Mobilization* [***Table 10-1***].	
10.6	I will find the tenderness and restricted regions that affect my running, and improve my mobility.	

CH 11: Keep it Moving

11.1	I have read chapter 11. in *The Running Injury Recovery Program*.	
11.2	I understand the concept of P.T. Time.	
11.3	I understand how to perform a *Mobility Self-Assessment* [**Box 11-1**], and how each self-mobilization is associated with one specific injury region [***Table 11-3***].	
11.4	I understand *Stretch/Mobilization Cycles* for affected and unaffected regions [**Box 11-2**].	
11.5	I understand how to perform *Stretching Exercises* [**Box 11-3**], and how each exercise is associated with one or more specific injury regions.	
11.6	I have obtained all the equipment I need to perform *Stretching Exercises* [***Table 11-4***].	
11.7	I have completed my *Mobility Self-Assessment* (***Self-Assessment 2A* and Worksheet 2A1**).	
11.8	I have determined my affected and unaffected region(s) for this injury, and the order in which I will do my stretches and self-mobilizations in Phase Two (***Self-Assessment 2A***).	
11.9	I have recorded my program of Stretch/Mobilization Cycles for Phase Two on my first *Log Form C: Stretch/Mobilization Cycles*.	
11.10	I have determined my treatment group for Phase Two, and whether I will follow guidelines for *simple* or *complex* injuries (***Self-Assessment 2B***).	

11.11	I have started a daily schedule of Phase Two P.T. Time, following the instructions for my treatment group (**Table 11-1**) and my complexity subgroup (**Table 11-2**); I am recording the results on *Log Form C*; and I am evaluating my daily *Log Form C* for symmetry requirements for my complexity subgroup (**Self-Assessment 2C**).	
11.12	I have cleared Phase Two symmetry requirements for my complexity subgroup (**Self-Assessment 2C**), and I will now use *Log form M: Maintaining Mobility* to record my stretch/mobilization cycles during P.T. Time.	✓
11.13	I have evaluated my *Log Form C* for regional tenderness (**Self-Assessment 2D**).	

CH 12: The Psychology of Running Injuries

12.1	I have read chapter 12. in *The Running Injury Recovery Program.*	
12. 2	I understand the mental challenges of running-injury management.	
12. 3	I understand the importance of focusing on the instructions in this book while self-managing my running injury.	
12. 4	I will follow my post-injury training program with proper mental focus.	

CHECKPOINT TO ENTER PHASE THREE PART ONE:

I have achieved the degree of symmetry and range of motion required for my (simple or complex) injury.	
(Group 2 only) I have completed two weeks of icing and all inflammation is cleared.	
I have completed *Phase Two Self-Assessment*.	
I am continuing with my individualized list of self-mobilizations and stretches, and I am recording the results on *Log form M: Maintaining Mobility*.	
I am now following the Guidelines for Phase Three Part One in *Table 13-1*.	

PHASE THREE:
Improving Strength and Balance (Chapters 13 through 15)

CH 13: Entering Phase Three, Training Plans and Habits

13.1	I have read chapter 13 in *The Running Injury Recovery Program.*.	
13.2	I understand the goals for Phase Three.	
13.3	I understand the importance of an individualized *Regional Training Plan*.	
13.4	I understand how *Basic Closed-Chain Exercises* are used for self-assessment in Phase Three Part One.	
13.5	I understand how *Regional Closed-Chain Exercises* are used to improve strength and balance, and how they fit into P.T. Time in Phase Three Part Two.	
13.6	I understand all of the factors used to determine which treatment group I will enter in Phase Three Part Two **[Table 13-2]**.	
13.7	I understand the concept of the *Base Schedule*, and its division by groups into *self-paced plans* and *two-week-interval plans*.	
13.9	I have determined the amount of time that I will commit to my Base Schedule.	

CH 14: Closed-Chain Exercises

14.1	I have read chapter 14 in *The Running Injury Recovery Program*..	
14.2	I understand how different *Basic Closed-Chain Exercises* are used to assess basic balance requirements in Phase Three Part One.	
14.3	I understand how my specific *Regional Closed-Chain Exercises* are used to improve strength and balance in Phase Three Part Two.	
14.4	I understand the correct techniques for performing all Basic and Regional Closed-Chain Exercises **[BOX 14-2]**.	
14.5	I have assembled the exercise equipment required for closed-chain exercises **[*Table 14-3*]**.	
14.6	I am continuing with my individualized list of self-mobilizations and stretches, and I am recording the results on *Log form M: Maintaining Mobility*.	
14.7	I have added Basic Closed-Chain Exercises to my daily P.T. Time, and I am recording the results on *Log Form B: Basic Closed-Chain*.	
14.8	I am monitoring my progress to make sure my symptoms do not increase higher than Stage 2.	
14.9	I have completed ***Self-Assessment 3A: Basic Closed-Chain Clearance***.	
14.10	I have completed my *Regions and Stress Fracture Self-Assessment* (***Self-Assessment 3B***).	
14.11	I have determined my Regional Closed-Chain Exercise plan for my Injury Regions (***Self-Assessment 3C***) and prepared my first *Log Form R: Regional Closed-Chain*.	
14.12	I have written my Impairment Statements (***Self-Assessment 3D part 1***) and understand the weaknesses that I need to work on throughout my recovery program.	
14.13	I have determined my treatment group for Phase Three Part Two (***Self-Assessment 3D part 2***).	

CHECKPOINT TO ENTER PHASE THREE PART TWO:

I am able to perform all *Basic Closed-Chain Exercises* correctly and symmetrically, with no increase in pain. OR I have completed one week of *Basic Closed-Chain Exercises*, but I am still *unable* to perform all eight *Basic Closed-Chain Exercises* correctly, symmetrically, or with no increase in pain.	
I have completed *Self-Assessments 3A* through *3E*.	
I am now following the Guidelines for Group 1A or 1B (Table 13-2) or Group 2A or 2B (Table 13-3).	

CH 15: Fitness Walking and Glides

15.1	I have read chapter 15 in *The Running Injury Recovery Program*..	
15.2	I understand the importance of gradually building a running base to prepare for post-recovery running, and using a Base Schedule to maintain the correct level and consistency of effort during post-injury training.	
15.3	I understand the importance of working at a submaximal level to keep my symptoms below Stage 3.	
15.4	I understand the importance of maintaining erect posture to load body weight through my injury.	

15.5	I understand the *Three Basic Running Strides* [**Table 15-1**] and the importance of pushing off correctly through the big toe.	
15.6	I understand the importance of fitness walking for warmup and cooldown, and the correct technique for fitness walking [**BOX 15-2**].	
15.7	I understand the importance of glides to strengthen my injury for running, and the correct technique for glides [**BOX 15-3**].	
15.8	I understand the importance of glide drills for balance, and the correct techniques for glide drills [**BOX 15-2**].	
15.9	I understand the use of progressive walk/glide sets, and how to build my individualized walk/glide program [**BOX 15-1**].	
15.10	I understand the importance of mental focus to maintain correct form.	
15.11	I have established a *Base Schedule* based on my running experience and goals, and I have reduced my P.T. Time to two times per week (*Self-Assessment 3E*).	
15.12	I have completed my **Worksheet T: Training Plan for Phase Three Part Two**.	
15.13	I will now follow the *Course Map* below for **Group 1 (A or B)** or **Group 2 (A or B)**	

GROUP 1 (A and B) ONLY

15.13A	I understand the goals of the *Self-Paced Plan*.		
15.14A	I am continuing with Stretch/Mobilization Cycles during P.T. Time, and recording the results on *Log Form M: Maintaining Mobility*.		
15.15A	**Group 1A:** 1. I have cleared all *Basic Closed-Chain Exercises* in 7 days or less. 2. I am following the guidelines for **Group 1A** in **Table 13-2**.	**Group 1B:** 1. I have **not** cleared all *Basic Closed-Chain Exercises* in 7 days or less. 2. I am continuing with *Basic Closed-Chain Exercises* during P.T. Time, and I am recording the results on *Log Form B: Basic Closed-Chain*. 3. I am following the guidelines for **Group 1B** in **Table 13-2**. 4. I have completed **Group 1B Reassessment**.	
15.16A	I have progressed to *Regional Closed-Chain Exercises* during P.T. Time; I am recording the results on *Log Form R: Regional Closed-Chain;* and I am evaluating my *Log Form R* for Stage 1 clearance (*Self-Assessment 3F*).		
15.17A	I have started my walk/glide program at the level determined in *Self-Assessment 3E*; I am following the Self-Paced Plan; and I am recording the results at the correct level in my *Log form S: Base Schedule*.		
15.18A	I am using *Self-Assessment 3G1 for Self-Paced Plan* to evaluate *Log Form S*.		
15.19A	I have successfully incorporated the glide drills for my level into the glide portion of my walk/glide program [*Table 15-4*].		
15.20A	I am focusing on correct form for fitness walking, glides, and glide drills [**BOX 15-2, Box 15-3,** and **Box 15-4**].		
15.21A	I am increasing my pace and distance gradually to prevent my symptoms from going above Stage 2.		
15.22A	I have progressed through each level of walk/glide sets with correct form and with no increase in symptoms [*Table 15-4*]		
15.23A	I have progressed to Base Schedule Level 5 (50-minute glides) [*Table 15-4E*].		
15.24A	**P.T. Time: I am able to perform all of my *Regional Closed-Chain Exercises* with symmetry and no increase in symptoms (*Self-Assessment 3F*).**		

15.25A	Base Schedule: I have completed my Base Schedule at Level 5 for one week with no increase in symptoms (*Self-Assessment 3G1*).	
15.26A	I have Cleared Phase Three P.T. Time and Base Schedule, and prepared my log forms for Phase Four (*Self-Assessment 3H*).	

GROUP 2 (A and B) ONLY

15.13B	I understand the goals of the *Two-Week-Interval Plan*.		
15.14B	I am continuing with Stretch/Mobilization Cycles during P.T. Time, and recording the results on my *Log Form M: Maintaining Mobility*.		
15.15B	**Group 2A:** 1. I have cleared Basic *Closed-Chain Exercises* in 7 days or less. 2. I have progressed to *Regional Closed-Chain Exercises* during P.T. Time, recording the results on *Log Form R: Regional Closed-Chain*, and evaluating *Log Form R* for Stage 1 clearance (*Self-Assessment 3F*). 3. I am following the guidelines for **Group 2A** in **Table 13-3**.	**Group 2B:** 1. I have **not** cleared *Basic Closed-Chain Exercises* in 7 days or less. 2. I am continuing *Basic Closed-Chain Exercises* during P.T. Time, and recording the results on my *Log Form B: Basic Closed-Chain*. 3. I am following the guidelines for **Group 2B** in **Table 13-3**.	
15.16B	I have started fitness walking my Base Schedule, following the Two-Week-Interval Plan, and I am recording the results on Level 0 of *Log form S*.		
15.17B	I am using **Self-Assessment 3G2 for Two-Week-Interval Plan** to evaluate my Log Form S.		
15.18B	I am focusing on correct form for fitness walking **[BOX 15-2]**.		
15.19B	I am increasing my pace and distance gradually to prevent my symptoms from going above Stage 2.		
15.20B	**I have completed fitness-walking my Base Schedule for at least two weeks.**		
15.21B	**I can fitness walk my Base Schedule with no increase in symptoms, and I am cleared to begin the walk/glide program (*Self-Assessment 3G2*)**		
15.22B	**Group 2B ONLY: I've progressed to *Regional Closed-Chain Exercises* during P.T. Time, I am recording the results on *Log Form R: Regional Closed-Chain*, and I am evaluating *Log Form R* for Stage 1 clearance (*Self-Assessment 3F*).**		
15.23B	I have started my walk/glide program at Level 1, following the Two-Week-Interval plan, and I am recording the results on *Log Form S, Level 1*.		
15.24B	I have successfully incorporated the glide drills for Level 1 into the glide portion of my walk/glide program **[Table 15-4A]**.		
15.25B	I am focusing on correct form for fitness walking, glides, and glide drills **[BOX 15-2, Box 15-3,** and **Box 15-4]**.		
15.26B	I am increasing my pace and distance gradually to prevent my symptoms from going above Stage 2.		
15.27B	I have completed my Base Schedule, Level 1, for at least two weeks, with correct form and no increase in symptoms **[Table 15-4A]**.		
15.28B	I have completed my Base Schedule, Level 2, for at least two weeks, with correct form and no increase in symptoms **[Table 15-4B]**.		
15.29B	I have completed my Base Schedule, Level 3, for at least two weeks, with correct form and no increase in symptoms **[Table 15-4C]**.		

15.30B	I have completed my Base Schedule, Level 4, for at least two weeks, with correct form and no increase in symptoms [*Table 15-4D*].	
15.31B	I have completed my Base Schedule, Level 5 (50-minute glides) for two weeks with correct form and no increase in symptoms [*Table 15-4E*].	
15.32B	**P.T. Time: I am able to perform all my *Regional Closed-Chain Exercises* with symmetry and no increase in symptoms (*Self-Assessment 3F*).**	
15.33B	**Base Schedule: I am able to complete my Base Schedule with 50-minute glides for two weeks with no increase in symptoms (*Self-Assessment 3G2*).**	
15.34B	**I have cleared Phase Three P.T. Time and Base Schedule, and prepared my log forms for Phase Four (*Self-Assessment 3H*).**	

CHECKPOINT TO ENTER PHASE FOUR (all Groups)

I have achieved symmetry in *Basic Form Requirements:*	

1. I can balance on one leg with my foot pointed straight forward.
    2. I can use my arms to balance my body.
    3. I can keep my body balanced while pushing off through the big toe.
    4. I can keep balanced while kicking straight back.	

I have completed all Phase Three Self-Assessments.	

PHASE FOUR: Return to Functional Running
(Chapters 16 - 18)

CH 16: Entering Phase Four, Accelerations and Hills

16.1	I have read chapter 16 in *The Running Injury Recovery Program.*.	
16.2	I understand the goals of acceleration drills and hill training.	
16.3	I understand the use of the forefooted stride in accelerations and plyometrics.	
16.4	I understand the techniques for three types of Acceleration Drills [BOX 16-1]	
16.5	I am continuing with Stretch/Mobilization Cycles during P.T. Time, and I am recording the results on my *Log Form M*.	
16.6	I am continuing with my *Regional Closed-Chain Exercises* during P.T. Time; I am increasing the difficulty and time per exercise according to my running goals [*Table 16-1*]; and I am recording the results on my *Log Form R*.	
16.7	I have added *Hill Closed-Chain Exercises* to my P.T. Time [*Box 16-2*], and I am recording the results on my *Log Form R*.	
16.8	I have added *Acceleration Drills* to my Base Schedule [*Table 16-2*], and I am recording the results on my *Log Form S, Level 6*.	
16.9	I am using my Specific Mental Focus Statement and focusing on straight posture and balance points in acceleration drills.	
16.10	I am increasing the time per acceleration drill according to my running goals [*Table 16-1*].	
16.11	I am monitoring my progress to make sure my symptoms do not go higher than Stage 2.	
16.12	**I have cleared Base Schedule Level 6 *Acceleration Drills* and *Hill Closed-Chain Exercises* (*Self-Assessment 4A*).**	
16.13	I understand the *Techniques for Hill Training*, either on the street or on a treadmill.	

16.14	I have added *Hill Training Drills* to my Base Schedule **[Table 16-3]**, and I am recording the results on my *Log Form S, Level 7*.	
16.15	I am focusing on straight posture and balance points in hill training.	
16.16	I am increasing the time per hill drill according to my running goals **[Table 16-1]**.	
16.17	I am monitoring my progress to make sure my symptoms do not go higher than Stage 2.	
16.18	**I have cleared Base Schedule Level 7 *Hill Training Drills (Self-Assessment 4B)***	

CH 17: Plyometrics

17.1	I have read chapter 17 in *The Running Injury Recovery Program*..	
17.2	I understand the goals of plyometric drills.	
17.3	I understand the techniques for the four types of plyometric drills **[BOX 17-1]**.	
17.4	I understand that plyometric exercises must be done on a level surface ONLY, never on a treadmill.	
17.5	I have added plyometric drills and glide drills to my Base Schedule **[Table 17-1A]**, and I am recording the results on my *Log Form S, Level 8*.	
17.6	I am focusing on straight posture and balance points in plyometric drills.	
17.7	I am increasing the amount of time per plyometric exercise as determined by my group (Fitness Runner or Racer) **[Table 16-1, Table 17-2B]**.	
17.8	I am gradually increasing the force exerted in each plyometric exercise, but I am still working *submaximally*.	
17.9	I am monitoring my progress to make sure my symptoms do not go higher than Stage 2.	
17.10	**I have cleared Base Schedule Level 8 *Plyometrics (Self-Assessment 4C)*.**	

CH 18: Life Decisions and Lifelong Running

18.1	I have read chapter 18 in *The Running Injury Recovery Program*.	
18.2	I understand the importance of a careful transition from *post-injury running* to *post-recovery running*.	
18.3	In *post-recovery running*, I will monitor my Injury Stage and avoid Red Flags.	
18.4	I will mix up my running activities as part of my regular training.	
18.5	I will maintain symmetry in my flexibility and watch for early warning signs of injury.	
18.6	While running, I will focus to maintain my balance and control my stride.	
18.7	I will maintain a proper Base Schedule in my regular training.	
18.8	**I have completed *Self-Assessment 4D: Clearance for Post-Recovery Running*.**	

CHECKPOINT TO RETURN TO RUNNING:

I am able to perform all of my P.T. Time exercises correctly for the specified amount of time with no increase in symptoms.	
I am able to complete my Base Schedule with plyometric exercises and glide drills with correct form and no increase in symptoms.	
I have completed all of my *Phase Four Self-Assessments*.	
I have learned running habits that will help me become a smarter and safer runner.	
I am ready to return to functional *post-recovery* running.	

SECTION 2: THE RUNNING INJURY RECOVERY PROGRAM

Phase One Workbook: Education and Self-Help

Phase Two Workbook: Regaining Mobility

Phase Three Workbook: Improving Strength and Balance

Phase Four Workbook: Return to Functional Running

This section contains the Guidelines and Instructions for all of the Self-Assessments, Worksheets, and Log Forms that make up the Workbook for each of the four phases of recovery. The Instructions for each Log Form are included at the end of the Phase where it is first introduced. You'll find an index of the complete contents of each section of the Workbook at the beginning of each phase.

You do not have to write on the Worksheets and Log Forms that are in this section of the Workbook. You will find blank Worksheets and Log Forms that you can fill in at the back of the Workbook (*see Section 6*).

All of the Self-Assessments should be completed in order. As you complete each Self-Assessment, check off the appropriate lines on your Course Map to keep track of your progress.

PHASE ONE WORKBOOK

Phase One Guidelines

Phase One of *The Running Injury Recovery Program* consists of Education and Self-Help. The *Program* book teaches you what you need to learn, and describes how to use the PRICE method (protect, recover, ice, compression and elevation) to treat your injury.

In Phase One Self-Assessments, you will document your original injury, determine the severity of your injury on the Running Injury Stage Scale, and reduce any inflammation or swelling that you might have.

If your Self-Assessments show no Red Flags and/or visible swelling, then you are in Group 1 and Phase One will consist only of reading the *Program* book and making appropriate changes for protection and recovery (PR).

If you have any signs of inflammation and/or Red Flag symptoms as determined by your Self-Assessments, you will be in Group 2. This group makes the appropriate changes for protection and recovery (PR) and will also ICE, following the instructions for Log Form I.

Table 5-1
Guidelines: Phase One

	Group 1	Group 2
Phase One Groups *(Self-Assessment 1D)*	*No* Red Flag symptoms or visible swelling within the past 2 weeks.	*With* Red Flag symptoms or visible swelling within the past 2 weeks.
P.T. Time	Progress directly to *Phase One Clearance.*	Begin ICE 20 minutes per day until symptoms improve (**Log Form I**).
Phase One Clearance *(Self-Assessment 1E)*	1. Take steps for Protection and Recovery of your running injury. 2. The symptoms of your running injury have improved. 3. Complete *Self-Assessment 1E*.	

Phase One Self-Assessments

Self-Assessment 1A: Identifying a running injury

Course Map reference: 1.2

Instructions: Follow the guidelines in Chapter 1 of *The Running Injury Recovery Program* to determine whether or not you have an injury that is caused by running.

Self-Assessment: Complete **Worksheet 1A1** below:

Worksheet 1A1: Identifying a Running Injury		
1. Do you think you might have a running injury?	No	Yes
2. Do you have pain that only appears or gets worse *while* you are running OR that only appears in a regular pattern some time *after* you run?	No	Yes
3. Do your symptoms always lessen when you *stop* running (either immediately or after not running for up to two weeks)?	No	Yes

What to do now:
• If you answered NO to one or more questions, **STOP**. You may not have a running injury. See your healthcare professional.
• If you answered YES to *all three* questions, you may have a running injury. Check line 1.2 on your Course Map and continue.

Self-Assessment 1B: Running History

Course Map references: 1.3, 1.4

Instructions:
1. Document your running habits at the time you were injured.
2. List the *intrinsic* and *extrinsic* factors that affect your running, and work to correct or optimize them.

Self-Assessment: Complete **Worksheet 1B1** below:

Worksheet 1B1: Running History

1. Write the exact day and date of the *last day you ran* (your last regular training session):

_____.

2. How many years have you been running on a regular basis?
      a. Less than 1 year
      b. 1 to 3 years
      c. More than 3 years

3. Which type of runner are you?
      a. My primary goal is to improve my fitness (**Fitness Runner**).
      b. My primary goal is to run faster in competitions (**Racer**).

4. Before your injury, how many *days* per week were you running on a regular basis?
      a. 2 days or less per week
      b. 3 to 5 days per week
      c. More than 5 days per week

5. Before your injury, how many *miles* per week were you running on a regular basis?
      a. Less than 10 miles per week
      b. 10 to 25 miles per week
      c. More than 25 miles per week

6. With this injury, how long could you run before the pain started?
      a. Less than 10 minutes or 1 mile
      b. 10 to 20 minutes, or 1 to 2 miles
      c. 20 to 30 minutes, or 2 to 3 miles
      d. 30 to 40 minutes, or 3 to 4 miles
      e. 40 to 50 minutes, or 4 to 5 miles
      f. More than 50 minutes or 5 miles

7. Based on the examples in Chapter 1 of *The Running Injury Recovery Program*, list any *intrinsic* or *extrinsic* factors that you need to work on:

What to do now:
• Use this information when you prepare your *Base Schedule* in **Self-Assessment 3E.**
• Enter the *last day you ran* at the top of **Worksheet 1D: Document Your Injury.**
• As you progress through the phases of recovery, keep track of the number of days that have passed since the *last day you ran*.
• Check lines 1.3 and 1.4 on your Course Map and continue.

Self-Assessment 1C: Medical History

Course Map reference: 1.5

Instructions:
1. Document any injuries or medical conditions that existed at the time of your injury, and that may affect your running.
2. Follow the instructions for defining traumatic versus nontraumatic injuries in Chapter 1 of *The Running Injury Recovery Program.*

Self-Assessment: Complete **Worksheet 1C1** below:

Worksheet 1C1: Medical History		
1. Have you had any previous running injuries that are not completely resolved and may still affect your running?	Yes	No
2. Have you had any traumatic injuries such as a fall, twist, sprain, or other accident within the past 12 months that affect your running?	Yes	No
3. Have you ever had surgery on any body part that might affect your running?	Yes	No
4. Do you have any pre-existing medical condition that affects your ability to run, such as osteoarthritis?	Yes	No
5. Do you take any medication for a medical condition which affects your ability to feel pain, such as a steroid or anti-inflammatory medication?	Yes	No
If you answered "Yes" to any question, list your conditions and/or medications here:		

What to do now:
• If you answered YES to *any* question, you have a *complex* injury due to medical factors.
• If you answered NO to *all* questions, you may still have a *complex* injury due to other factors, or you may have a simple running injury.
• Use this information in *Self-Assessment 2B* when you determine the complexity of your injury.
• Check line 1.5 on your Course Map and continue.

Self-Assessment 1D:
Document Your Injury and Phase One Treatment Group

Course Map references: *3.2, 3.3, 3.4, and 3.5*

Instructions:
1. Make a record of the pain pattern and the swelling pattern of your original injury.
2. Determine the *severity* (Injury Stage and Red Flags) of your injury.
3. Prepare a summary of your injury.

Self-Assessment:

1. Complete **Worksheet 1D1: Pain Pattern** and **Worksheet 1D2: Swelling Within Past 2 Weeks**.

2. Compare your patterns of pain and swelling to the illustrations in **Appendix A: Index of Affected Regions** to identify your *possible affected regions*.

3. Complete **Worksheet 1D3: Injury Stage**. Note your Injury Stage and Red Flags for each *possible affected region* (left or right).

4. Complete **Worksheet 1D4: Summary of Original Injury** to summarize the signs and symptoms of your original injury.

5. Evaluate your **Worksheet 1D4** and determine your Phase One Treatment Group (**Worksheet 1D5**):

    A. If you have had NO swelling and NO Red Flags in any region during the past 2 weeks, you will enter Phase One in Group 1.

    B. If you have had Swelling or Red Flags in any region during the past 2 weeks, you will enter Phase One in Group 2.

INSTRUCTIONS for Worksheets 1D1 through 1D5:
Document Your Injury and Phase One Treatment Group

Worksheet 1D1: Pain Pattern

1. On the chart provided, shade in all the areas of your body (left or right) where you have **pain** associated with this running injury. If your pain has subsided, shade in all the areas where you *had* pain associated with this injury.

2. Compare your shaded areas of pain to the figures in **Appendix A: Index of Affected Regions**. Next to your diagram, write the names and numbers of all the regions where you have any shading (it doesn't have to be completely shaded), and the side (left or right). These are your *possible affected regions*.

3. Go to **Worksheet 1D4: Summary of Original Injury (Left or Right)**. In the first column, *circle or highlight the number* of each *possible affected region* you wrote on your diagram.

4. Determine the **worst** pain you have experienced since your original injury, in each *possible affected region*, on a scale of 0 to 10 (where 0 = no pain, and 10 = the worst possible pain that you can imagine), and enter those numbers in the appropriate columns in **Worksheet 1D4 Left** or **1D4 Right.**). If you have two or more *possible affected regions* for the same pain, enter the same information for all regions.

Worksheet 1D2: Swelling Within Past 2 Weeks

1. On the chart provided, shade in all the areas where you have **visible swelling** associated with this running injury. If your swelling has subsided, shade in all the areas where you have had swelling *within the past two weeks*.

2. Compare your shaded areas of swelling to **Appendix A: Index of Affected Regions.** Next to your diagram, write the names and numbers of all the regions where you have any shading (it doesn't have to be completely shaded), and the side (left to right). These are also *possible affected regions*.

3. If you have swelling in any region that you did not already identify in **Worksheet 1D1: Pain Pattern**, then circle or highlight that region now in the first column of **Worksheet 1D4 Left** or **1D4 Right.**

4. For each region in which you have or had swelling *within the past two weeks*, write "Yes" in the appropriate column in **Worksheet 1D4 Left** or **1D4 Right.**

Worksheet 1D3: Injury Stage

1. On the top line of **Worksheet 1D3**, enter the side (left or right) and *possible affected regions* (from **Worksheets 1D1** and **1D2**) that you are evaluating.

2. Follow the instructions in Chapter 3 for evaluating running-injury stages.

3. Under *Emerging Symptoms* and *Red Flags* in **Table A**, circle the *maximum* symptoms that you have experienced *within the past 2 weeks*. If you have different symptoms in different regions, note the region(s) in the column for *Which Region(s)?*.

4. Enter your Injury Stages and Red Flags from **Table A** in the appropriate columns in **Worksheet 1D4 Left** or **1D4 Right.** If your symptoms might apply to more than one region, enter the same information for each *possible affected region.*

5. If your injury occurred more than 2 weeks ago, and your symptoms have changed, also fill in **Table B** to record your original symptoms for this injury.

Worksheet 1D4: Summary of Original Injury

1. Refer to Worksheets 1D1, 1D2, and 1D3 (Table A), and fill in the appropriate boxes in **Worksheet 1D4**.

2. For each region you have circled, make sure to fill out all of the boxes on that line.

3. Leave the boxes for the *unaffected* side or regions blank.

Worksheet 1D5: Phase One Treatment Group

1. Evaluate your **Worksheet 1D4** (*Self-Assessment 1D,* part 5).

2. Record which treatment group you are in for Phase One, and whether or not you need to ICE, in **Worksheet 1D5.**

Worksheet 1D:
Document Your Injury and Phase One Treatment Group

Last day you ran: _____   **Today's date:** _____

Worksheet 1D1: Pain Pattern

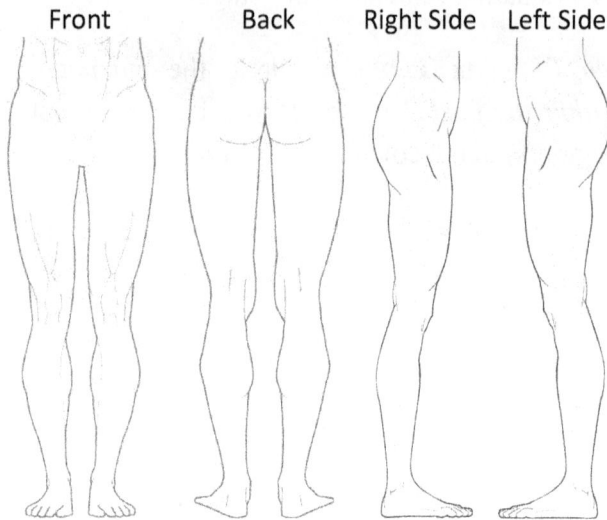

Front   Back   Right Side   Left Side

Compare to *Appendix A* and list your *possible affected regions* and side here:

_____

_____

_____

_____

_____

_____

Worksheet 1D2: Swelling Within Past 2 Weeks

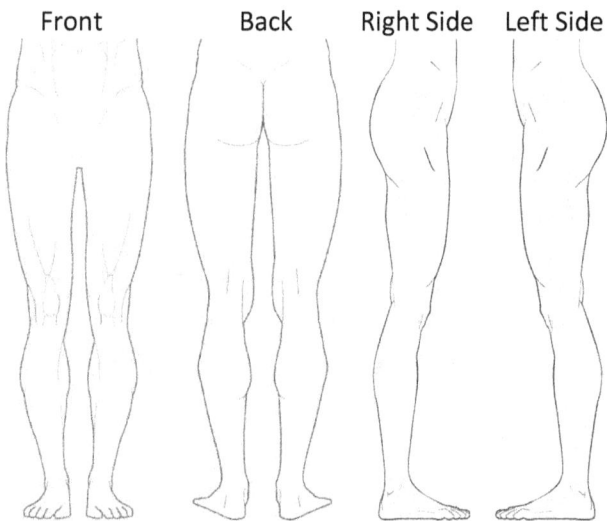

Front   Back   Right Side   Left Side

Compare to *Appendix A* and list your *possible affected regions* and side here:

_____

_____

_____

_____

_____

_____

Worksheet 1D3: Injury Stage

Injury Side and *possible affected region(s)*: _____

Table A: Maximum Symptoms *within the past 2 weeks*

Injury Stages	Emerging Symptoms	Red Flags	Which region(s)?
Stage 1	Pain while running	Pain that alters your stride	
Stage 2	Pain at rest (after running)	Pain that disturbs your rest	
Stage 3	Pain during your normal daily activities	Pain that interferes with or makes you avoid ADLs	
Stage 4	Running injury pain that you take medication for	Being in Stage 4	
Stage 5	Pain that cripples you	Being in Stage 5	

Table B: Maximum Symptoms *from more than 2 weeks ago*

Injury Stages	Emerging Symptoms	Red Flags	Which region(s)?
Stage 1	Pain while running	Pain that alters your stride	
Stage 2	Pain at rest (after running)	Pain that disturbs your rest	
Stage 3	Pain during your normal daily activities	Pain that interferes with or makes you avoid ADLs	
Stage 4	Running injury pain that you take medication for	Being in Stage 4	
Stage 5	Pain that cripples you	Being in Stage 5	

Worksheet 1D4: Summary of Original Injury

Refer to →	Worksheet 1D1: Pain Pattern	Worksheet 1D2: Swelling	Worksheet 1D3: Table A Injury Stage in Past 2 Weeks	
Left Leg Circle *Possible Affected Regions*	**Pain Severity (1-10)**	**Swelling in past 2 weeks (yes/no)**	**Injury Stage Scale (1-5)**	**Red Flag (yes/no)**
1 Toe				
2 Arch				
3 Heel				
4 Shin				
5 Calf				
6 Knee				
7 Band				
8 Hamstring				
9 Hip				
10 Buttock				

Refer to →	Worksheet 1D1: Pain Pattern	Worksheet 1D2: Swelling	Worksheet 1D3: Table A Injury Stage in Past 2 Weeks	
Right Leg Circle *Possible Affected Regions*	**Pain Severity (1-10)**	**Swelling in past 2 weeks (yes/no)**	**Injury Stage Scale (1-5)**	**Red Flag (yes/no)**
1 Toe				
2 Arch				
3 Heel				
4 Shin				
5 Calf				
6 Knee				
7 Band				
8 Hamstring				
9 Hip				
10 Buttock				

Worksheet 1D5: Phase One Treatment Group	
Circle ONE of the two statements below:	
I will enter Phase One injury management in treatment Group 1, and I do not have to ICE.	I will enter Phase One injury management in treatment Group 2, and I will now begin to ICE (**Log Form I**).

What to do now:

• Start Recovery Phase One. Follow the guidelines for Group 1 or Group 2 in *Table 5-1.*

• **If you are in Group 2, start icing your affected region(s) now**. Follow the instructions for ICE in Chapter 5, and record your icing sessions in **Log Form I** (see **Instructions for Log Form I**).

• Check lines 3.2, 3.3, and 3.4 on your Course Map and continue.

Self-Assessment 1E: Phase One Clearance

Course Map references: 5.1 through 9.4

Instructions: Determine whether you have completed Phase One and can progress to Phase Two.

Self-Assessment: Complete **Worksheet 1E1** below:

Worksheet 1E1: Phase One Clearance		
I have *no* Red Flag symptoms or visible swelling.	No	Yes
All of the emerging symptoms I recorded in Worksheets 1D1 through 1D4 have improved.	No	Yes
My sleep is not disturbed by pain due to this injury.	No	Yes
I can perform my activities of daily living (ADLs) normally, with less pain.	No	Yes
I do not need to take medication for pain and inflammation due to my running injury.	No	Yes
I have checked lines 5.1 through 9.4 on my Course Map.	No	Yes
I have followed all of the instructions in *The Running Injury Recovery Program* chapters 5 through 9 to implement protection and recovery for my running injury.	No	Yes
Group 2 ONLY: I have Iced 3 times a day, and the symptoms I have recorded on **Log Form I** have improved.	No	Yes

What to do now:
• When you can answer "yes" to all the questions in **Worksheet 1E1**, continue to the **Checkpoint to enter Phase Two** on your Course Map.

Instructions for Log Form I: Group 2 ICE Log

1. Enter the day, date, and phase on your ICE Log (**Log Form I**).

2. Rate your maximum symptoms (pain and visible swelling) in the injured region(s) *before* each icing.

3. Follow ICE instructions in *The Running Injury Recovery Program*, Chapter 5, **[Box 5-1]** and **[Box 5-2].**

4. Check the number of ICE sessions completed on each day.
   • Phase One: ICE the injured region(s) for 20 minutes, three times each day, until symptoms subside.
   • Phase Two: ICE *after* PT Time, for 20 minutes (at least one time each day). Continue ICE for a minimum of two weeks in Phase Two, or until your symptoms subside.

Log Form I: Group 2 ICE Log

Phase #	Starting DAY/DATE:		Number of ICE Days:	

Week 1 (Day/Date/Phase)	ICE#	Symptoms (0 to 10)	Week 2 (Day/Date/Phase)	ICE#	Symptoms (0 to 10)
Day:	1		Day:	1	
Date:	2		Date:	2	
Phase:	3		Phase:	3	
Day:	1		Day:	1	
Date:	2		Date:	2	
Phase:	3		Phase:	3	
Day:	1		Day:	1	
Date:	2		Date:	2	
Phase:	3		Phase:	3	
Day:	1		Day:	1	
Date:	2		Date:	2	
Phase:	3		Phase:	3	
Day:	1		Day:	1	
Date:	2		Date:	2	
Phase:	3		Phase:	3	
Day:	1		Day:	1	
Date:	2		Date:	2	
Phase:	3		Phase:	3	
Day:	1		Day:	1	
Date:	2		Date:	2	
Phase:	3		Phase:	3	

Phase Two Guidelines

The goal of Phase Two is to restore you to correct and symmetrical mobility. Running requires a greater degree of mobility than walking, and all injuries cause a certain amount of stiffness and loss of flexibility.

In Phase Two, you will do flexibility training, including self-mobilizations to improve your mobility to the appropriate level as determined by your Mobility Self-Assessment and by the severity and complexity of your original injury. There is one set of general *Guidelines* for Groups 1 and 2 (*Table 11-1*) which is based on severity, and a second set of *Guidelines* for subgroups which are based on whether your injury is simple or complex (*Table 11-2*).

Table 11-1
Guidelines: Phase Two

	Group 1	Group 2
Phase Two Groups (*Self-Assessment 2B*)	Group 1 in Phase One **AND** *No* Red Flags or visible swelling	Group 2 in Phase One **AND** *No* Red Flags or visible swelling
Phase Two PT Time	*Stretch/Mobilization Cycles* for affected and unaffected regions, 60 minutes per day (**Log Form C**).	1. *Stretch/Mobilization Cycles* for affected and unaffected regions, 40 minutes per day (**Log Form C**). 2. Continue ICE 20 minutes per day for a total of two weeks in Phase Two (**Log Form I**).
Phase Two Clearance (*Self-Assessment 2C*)	Cleared self-mobilizations and stretches as required for simple or complex injuries [*Table 11-2*].	1. All inflammation is cleared. 2. Completed 2 weeks of ICE in Phase Two. 3. Cleared all self-mobilizations and stretches as required for simple or complex injuries [*Table 11-2*].

Table 11-2 A

Guidelines for Simple Injuries

Phase Two Subgroup *(Self-Assessment 2B)*	One nontraumatic running injury, in one region. **AND** No pre-existing injury or medical condition that affects your running.
Focus	Identify one region to focus on.
Goal	Limber up the affected leg and achieve *symmetrical* range of motion with the unaffected leg.
Guidelines	1. Go directly to the tenderest spots in the affected region that correlate with the greatest restriction and loss of movement. 2. As you clear the greatest restriction, progress to other tender spots in the affected region that correlate with other loss of movement. 3. Explore all stretches, but focus on one injury region.

Table 11-2 B

Guidelines for Complex Injuries

Phase Two Subgroup *(Self-Assessment 2B)*	Injuries in 2 or more regions **OR** Pre-existing injuries **OR** Pre-existing medical condition that affects your running.
Focus	Explore all regions to find multiple areas of restriction.
Goal	Achieve *full* range of motion on both sides of the body, in all regions.
Guidelines	1. Go directly to the region that is the most tender and restricted. 2. Start with the area of greatest tenderness and tightest restriction in that region, then progress to other affected regions. 3. Progress from the most severe to the least severe tenderness in each affected region and stretch all restrictions in all regions. 4. Must be able to master all stretches and clear all regions.

Self-Assessment 2A:
Mobility Self-Assessment and Phase Two Recovery Plan

Course Map References: 11.7, 11.8, 11.9

Instructions:

1. *Part 1*: Mobility Self-Assessment
   - Read the **Instructions for Worksheet 2A1** and complete **Worksheet 2A1: Mobility Self-Assessment** to evaluate your flexibility and symmetry in *all regions*, both affected and unaffected.
   - Determine the order of stretching exercises for affected and unaffected regions for Phase Two PT Time, and enter them on **Log Form C: Stretch/Mobilization Cycles.**

2. *Part 2*: Self-Mobilizations
   - Complete **Worksheet 2A2: Ranking Affected Regions.**
   - Use **Worksheet 2A2: Ranking Affected Regions** to rank your *possible affected regions* in order of severity, and determine the appropriate self-mobilizations to be used with each stretching exercise.
   - Enter your self-mobilizations on **Log Form C: Stretch/Mobilization Cycles** to complete your Phase Two recovery plan.

Self-Assessment 2A Part 1: **Mobility Self-Assessment:** Complete Worksheet 2A1 below:

Instructions for Worksheet 2A1: Mobility Self-Assessment

1. At the top of **Worksheet 2A1**, circle or highlight your affected side (left/right) and *possible affected region(s)* from **Worksheet 1D4**.

2. For each *possible affected region* you have circled at the top of **Worksheet 2A1**, read down the column and locate pairs of shaded boxes (left/right) for stretches that are associated with that particular region. Go to the left-hand column and circle or highlight the numbers of those stretches. Each region is associated with 2 to 5 different stretches.

3. Note *all* the regions (shaded boxes) on the line for each stretch that you circled or highlighted on **Worksheet 2A1**. Locate the diagrams for those regions in **Appendix A: Affected Regions**, and refer to them as you do your Mobility Self-Assessment.

4. Read and follow the instructions for *Stretch/Mobilization Cycles for Affected Regions* [**Box 11-2A**], and the instructions for *Stretching Exercises* in [**BOX 11-3**].

5. Carefully follow the specific instructions for each stretching exercise. Do each of the 13 stretching exercises for 30 seconds on each side (left and right), and compare your flexibility with the illustrations in the book [**BOX 11-3**]. For every shaded box (region) in each stretch, assess your mobility in that region on both sides, using *Table 2A1:* **Mobility Scale for Stretches** below:

Table 2A1: Mobility Scale for Stretches		
Scale	**Flexibility**	**Guidelines**
0	No stiffness	Able to reach exact position shown in book, with no pain.
1	Almost no stiffness	Able to reach exact position shown in book, with slight pain.
2	Slight stiffness	Can almost reach exact position shown in book, with slight pain.
3	Moderate stiffness	Can't get very close to position shown in book, with moderate pain.
4	Very stiff	Can't get very close to position shown in book, with severe pain.
5	Extreme stiffness	Can't do the stretch at all, with severe pain.

6. As you complete each exercise, enter your results (0 to 5) in the shaded boxes in **Worksheet 2A1** (see *Sample* Worksheets in *Case Studies*). Make sure you have filled in *all* of the shaded boxes for every region, left and right, associated with each stretch. You can leave the unshaded boxes blank.

***

When you have completed Worksheet 2A1, use the information in Chapter 11 of *The Running Injury Recovery Program* to complete the following four sections. (See *Sample* Worksheets and Log Forms in *Case Studies*.)

1. **Evaluate Symmetry:**

A. On **Worksheet 2A1**, circle or highlight each left/right pair that has *two different numbers*, such as left = 2 and right = 3.

B. Look at the vertical column directly under each region. If *all* of the left/right pairs in a vertical column have matching numbers (no circles or highlights), then you have *symmetry* in that region.

C. You have *asymmetry* in any region where you have circled or highlighted one or more left/right pairs. The greater the difference between the higher and lower number, the greater the asymmetry.

2. Order Stretches for Affected Regions:

A. Looking ONLY at the *possible affected regions* you circled or highlighted at the top of **Worksheet 2A1**, find the circled or highlighted left/right pair in each column that has the *largest difference* between the two numbers (the greatest amount of asymmetry between left and right sides) AND has the *greatest stiffness on the affected side.*

B. Go to the identification number for that stretch (in the first column), and circle or highlight that number. In the second column for that stretch, circle or highlight the *affected side* (left or right) under *"Side,"* and write in the number "1" under *"Rank #."*

C. Continue numbering all of the stretches for your *affected side and region(s)* in order of stiffness and asymmetry. Check that the stretch number and affected side is circled or highlighted for each stretch for your *possible affected region(s)*.

3. Order Stretches for Unaffected Regions:

A. Begin ranking your list of stretches for *unaffected regions* with the same stretches you have already circled or highlighted, but on the *unaffected side*, starting with the next consecutive number.

B. Evaluate all of the remaining stretches on **Worksheet 2A1** in order of stiffness and asymmetry, and continue ranking those stretches (left then right for the same stretch) until you have numbered all 26 stretches and sides. Do not circle the stretch numbers or left/right for these stretches.

4. List stretches in order on Log Form C: Stretch/Mobilization Cycles:

A. You now have ranked 26 stretches beginning with the affected side and regions (both the stretch number and affected side are circled or highlighted), followed by the same stretches on the unaffected side (stretch number circled or highlighted, but not the side), then the stretches for unaffected regions (no stretch numbers or sides circled or highlighted). This is the order in which you will do your stretches in Phase Two.

B. Enter these numbers in order (1 through 26) on your first **Log Form C**. Be sure to *circle or highlight the rank number on the affected side* for each stretch on your "affected" list. At the top of Log Form C, write in your affected side and *possible affected regions* in the appropriate boxes. *Do not fill in the boxes for days or dates at this time.*

Worksheet 2A1: Mobility Self-Assessment

Circle *Possible Affected Region* and Side →		1: Toe	2: Arch	3: Heel	4: Shin	5: Calf	6: Knee	7: Band	8: Hams	9: Hip	10:Butt
		Left	Left	Left	Left	Left	Left	Left	Left	Left	Left
		Right	Right	Right	Right	Right	Right	Right	Right	Right	Right
Stretch	**SIDE / Rank #**										
11-1	**Left:**										
	Right:										
Notes:											
11-2	**Left:**										
	Right:										
Notes:											
11-3	**Left:**										
	Right:										
Notes:											
11-4	**Left:**										
	Right:										
Notes:											
11-5	**Left:**										
	Right:										
Notes:											
11-6	**Left:**										
	Right:										
Notes:											
11-7	**Left:**										
	Right:										
Notes:											
11-8	**Left:**										
	Right:										
Notes:											
11-9	**Left:**										
	Right:										
Notes:											
11-10	**Left:**										
	Right:										
Notes:											
11-11	**Left:**										
	Right:										
Notes:											
11-12	**Left:**										
	Right:										
Notes:											
11-13	**Left:**										
	Right:										
Notes:											

(A.) Ranking Affected Regions: Complete **Worksheet 2A2** below:

Instructions for Worksheet 2A2: Ranking Affected Regions

1. On **Worksheet 2A2: Ranking Affected Regions**, write in your affected SIDE (left or right). In the left-hand column, circle or highlight your *possible affected regions*. If you have *possible affected regions* on both sides, use a separate **Worksheet 2A2** for each side.

2. Go to your **Worksheet 2A1: Mobility Self-Assessment**. For each region, look down the column and find the *maximum stiffness* on each side (left and right) and enter those numbers in the appropriate columns in **Worksheet 2A2: Ranking Affected Regions**. Circle or highlight any number higher than 0.

3. Go again to **Worksheet 2A1: Mobility Self-Assessment**. For each region, find the circled or highlighted pair with the *maximum asymmetry* (greatest difference between left and right), and enter those numbers in the appropriate column in **Worksheet 2A2: Ranking Affected Regions**. These numbers may or may not be the same as those you entered for maximum stiffness. *Circle or highlight all asymmetrical pairs.*

4. Go to your **Worksheet 1D4: Summary of Original Injury** and copy the information for your affected side (left or right) to the appropriate columns in **Worksheet 2A2: Ranking Affected Regions**. Circle or highlight the following entries: any pain greater than 0, any swelling, and any injury stage (1 to 5).

5. Use all the signs and symptoms you have circled or highlighted in **Worksheet 2A2: Ranking Affected Regions** to assess problems in both your *affected* and *unaffected* region(s):

A. For each *possible affected region*, write "*possible affected region*" in the column for "Assessment."

B. If you have any stiffness or asymmetry in *unaffected* regions, write the main problems you need to work on in the column for "Assessment."

C. Under "Rank," number all the regions that have symptoms in order from the most severe to the least severe. These are the regions you will evaluate in your *Stretch/Mobilization Cycles.*

D. Do not rank any regions for which you recorded no symptoms.

Worksheet 2A2: Ranking Affected Regions								
SIDE:		**From Worksheet 2A1**			**From Worksheet 1D4**			**Summary**
Possible Affected Regions	**Maximum Stiffness**		**Maximum Asymmetry (left/right)**	**Pain (0-10)**	**Swelling yes/no**	**Injury Stage (1-5)**	**Assessment**	**Rank #**
	Left	Right						
1 Toe								
2 Arch								
3 Heel								
4 Shin								
5 Calf								
6 Knee								
7 Band								
8 Hams								
9 Hip								
10 Butt								

(B.) Select Self-Mobilizations for **Log Form C: Stretch/Mobilization Cycles** (see sample **Log Forms C** in *Case Studies*):

1. Find the *possible affected region* that you ranked #1 in **Worksheet 2A2: Ranking Affected Regions**

2. On your **Log Form C: Stretch/Mobilization Cycles**, find the stretch that you ranked #1. Locate that stretch in *Table 2A2: Injury Regions and Stretches* below, and see if the *possible affected region* that you ranked #1 is checked. If it is, write that region on your **Log Form C**, on the line for *"Self-Mobs"* below that stretch. If your region #1 is not checked, find the highest-ranked region (from your **Worksheet 2A2: Ranking Affected Regions**) for that stretch, and write that region on the line for *"Self-Mobs."*

Table 2A2: Injury Regions and Stretches											
		REGIONS									
STRETCHES		1	2	3	4	5	6	7	8	9	10
		Toe	Arch	Heel	Shin	Calf	Knee	Band	Hams	Hip	Butt
11-1	Wall/ Toe Stretch with Rope	X									
11-2	Wall Calf Stretch with Rope			X	X	X					
11-3	Wall Hamstring Stretch								X		
11-4	Ankle-Knee Wall Stretch								X	X	X
11-5	Toes to Nose Stretch	X	X	X	X	X	X		X		
11-6	Toes to Nose, Belt Stretch			X	X	X			X		
11-7	Straight-Leg Raise, Belt Stretch			X	X	X		X	X		
11-8	Straight-Leg Raise, Belt Stretch to Side							X			X
11-9	Cross-Leg Side Bend							X			X
11-10	Side Quadriceps Stretch						X			X	
11-11	Ankle-Knee Diagonal Stretch									X	X
11-12	Pelvic Stretch									X	
11-13	Back Incline Stretch		X	X	X	X					

3. Continue matching each of the stretches on your **Log Form C: Stretch/Mobilization Cycles** with the regions you identified in **Worksheet 2A2: Ranking Affected Regions**. Each stretch for *affected regions* on **Log Form C** should be matched with one of your *possible affected regions* from **Worksheet 2A2.** For all other stretches, choose any other region that you ranked in **Worksheet 2A2**. Double-check *Table 2A2: Injury Regions and Stretches* to make sure each region you choose matches that stretch. If a stretch does not match *any* region on your list, do not enter anything on the line for *Self-Mobs*.

4. When you are finished entering regions on the lines for *Self-Mobs*, double-check to make sure you have included all of the regions you ranked in **Worksheet 2A2: Ranking Affected Regions**

5. Go to the *Self-Mobilization Exercises* in **Box 10-2.** For each region listed in **Log Form C: Stretch/Mobilization Cycles** on the lines for *Self-Mobs*, choose one self-mobilization exercise, and write the exercise number next to the region (*e.g.* Calf #1).

What to do now:
• Your **Log Form C: Stretch/Mobilization Cycles** now contains your individualized recovery program for Phase Two PT Time.
• Check lines 11.7, 11.8, and 11.9 on your Course Map, and continue to *Self-Assessment 2B* to determine your *Phase Two Treatment Group and Complexity Subgroup*.

Self-Assessment 2B:
Phase Two Treatment Group and Complexity Subgroup

Course Map reference: 11.10

Instructions: Follow the guidelines in Chapter 11 to determine which treatment group you are in for Phase Two, and whether your injury is *simple or complex* (your complexity subgroup).

Self-Assessment: Complete **Worksheet 2B1** below.

***

What to do now:

• Check line 11.10 on your Course Map.
• Begin your daily schedule of Phase Two PT Time, following the instructions for your treatment group and subgroup (**Appendix G** *Tables 11-1 and 11-2*).
• Fill out one **Log Form C: Stretch/Mobilization Cycles** for each day in Phase Two (see **Instructions for Log Form C**), and continue to *Self-Assessment 3C:* **Evaluation of Log Form C for Symmetry.**

Worksheet 2B1: Phase Two Treatment Group and Sub-Group
1. Did you begin Phase One in Group 2 (with *Red Flags* or swelling)? 　　A. No 　　B. Yes
2. Do you *now* have any *Red Flags* or visible swelling in the injured region? 　　A. No 　　B. Yes
3. Based on your answers to questions 1 and 2, find your Phase Two treatment group:

Question 1:	Question 2:	Treatment Group
A. No	*and* A. No	Group 1
A. No	*and* B. Yes	Group 2
B. Yes	*and* A. No	Group 2
B. Yes	*and* B. Yes	Group 2

4. Go to your completed **Worksheet 2A2: Ranking Affected Regions**. How many regions did you assess as *possibly affected regions*?

   A. If you have only one *possible affected region* on one side (no regions on the other side), then count your injury as **one region**.

   B. If you have two or three *possible affected regions* on one side (and no regions on the other side), AND your *possible affected regions* are in closely associated areas (such as 1, 2, 3 or 6, 7, 8), AND you have decided, based on the guidelines in this book, that your symptoms are due to one simple injury, then count your injury as **one region**.

   C. If you circled one or more *possible affected region* on the left side AND one or more *possible affected region* on the right side, count your injury as **two or more regions**.

   D. If you circled two or more *possible affected regions* on one side, and they are NOT all closely associated with each other (such as 2, 3 and 7), count your injury as **two or more regions**.

5. Go to your **Self-Assessment 1C: Medical History**.

   A. If you answered NO to *all* questions in **Self-Assessment 1C**, you have **NO pre-existing condition** that might affect your running.

   B. If you answered YES to *any* question in **Self-Assessment 1C**, you have a **pre-existing condition** that might affect your running.

6. Based on your answers to questions 4 and 5 above, find your complexity subgroup below:

Question 4:	Question 5:	Subgroup
A or B (One region)	*and* A. NO pre-existing condition	*Simple Injury*
A or B (One region)	*and* B. Pre-existing condition	*Complex Injury*
C or D (Two or more regions)	*and* A.NO pre-existing condition	*Complex Injury*
C or D (Two or more regions)	*and* B. Pre-existing condition	*Complex Injury*

7. Fill in your Phase Two Recovery Group and Complexity Subgroup here:

   Entering Phase Two, I am in recovery group (*1 or 2*) _____, and I will follow

   the guidelines for (*simple or complex*) _____ injuries.

Self-Assessment 2C: Phase Two Clearance
(Evaluation of Log Form C for Symmetry by Complexity Subgroup)

Course Map reference: 11.12

Instructions:

1. Before beginning this evaluation, complete **Log Form C**, following the instructions for your treatment group and subgroup **[*Tables 11-1 and 11-2*]**. (See sample **Log Forms C** in *Case Studies*.)

2. At the end of each day of Phase Two PT Time, evaluate your **Log Form C** for the degree of symmetry and mobility required for clearance in your complexity subgroup.

Self-Assessment:

1. Monitor your *tenderness* in self-mobilizations on **Log Form C** to make sure your pain level does not go over a level of 5 or 6.

2. Evaluate each **Log Form C** for clearance, follow the clearance guidelines in *Table 2C1* below for your complexity subgroup. Evaluate *only* the *stiffness* in stretches, not the tenderness in self-mobilizations.

Table 2C1: Clearance Goals for Phase Two		
Complexity Subgroup	**Mobility Goals**	**Symmetry (Log Form C)**
Simple Injuries	Achieve *symmetrical* range of motion with the unaffected leg.	Symmetry is checked YES for all stretches.
Complex Injuries	1. Achieve *full* range of motion on both sides of the body, in all regions. 2. Able to exactly match the positions for stretching exercises shown in all of the figures in **Box 11-3**.	All entries for stiffness are at level 0.

What to do now:
• When you have achieved the *Mobility Goals* and *Symmetry* required for your complexity subgroup in *Table 2C1*, you are *Cleared* to enter Phase Three Part One.
• Follow the guidelines in *Appendix G Table 13-1:* Guidelines for Phase Three Part One.
• Check line 11.12 on your *Course Map*.
• Continue immediately to *Self-Assessment 2D:* **Evaluation of Log Form C for Regional Tenderness.**

Self-Assessment 2D: Evaluate Log Form C for Regional Tenderness

Course Map reference: 11.13

Instructions:

1. Before beginning this Self-Assessment, complete *all* of your Phase Two PT Time, following the instructions for your treatment group and subgroup **(Appendix G *Tables 11-1 and 11-2*).**

2. Evaluate your **Log Forms C** for *tenderness in possible affected regions* (see sample **Log Forms C** in *Case Studies*).

Self-Assessment: **Complete Worksheet 2D1 below:**

Instructions for Worksheet 2D1: Regional Tenderness

1. List all of your *possible affected regions* from **Log Form C** on **Worksheet 2D1**.

2. Look at all your **Log Forms C: Stretch/Mobilization Cycles**, and choose the form that shows the greatest amount of tenderness in your *possible affected regions*.

3. On your selected **Log Form C**, find the self-mobilization(s) for your *possible affected regions* that caused the most tenderness as compared to the same region on the unaffected side. Record those numbers on **Worksheet 2D1**, and calculate the left/right difference (subtract the higher number from the lower number).

4. Use the difference in tenderness to assess each region for injury. If any *possible affected region* has no increase in tenderness on the more affected side during any self-mobilization, you may eliminate that region from your list of *possible affected regions*.

Worksheet 2D1: Regional Tenderness				
List *possible affected regions* from **Log Form C**	Max tenderness on *more affected* side:	Max tenderness on *less affected* side:	Left/Right Difference	Assessment (affected or not)

What to do now:

• Narrow down your list of *possible affected regions* to include only those regions with greater tenderness on the affected side in **Worksheet 2D1**.

• Check line 11.13 on your Course Map and continue.

Instructions for Log Form C: Stretch/Mobilization Cycles

1. On your first day of Phase Two PT Time, begin with the **Log Form C** that you prepared in *Self-Assessment 2A*, which contains your individualized program of stretches and self-mobilizations for affected and unaffected regions.

2. At the top of the form, fill in today's day and date, the number of days that have passed since the *last day you ran* (from Worksheet 1B1: Running History, line 1). On the second line, enter "Phase Two" and "Day 1."

3. Perform your Stretch/Mobilization Cycles in order, beginning with the stretch ranked #1 for your affected side and region. Carefully follow the instructions for stretching exercises [**BOX 11-3**], and the instructions for self-mobilizations [**BOX 10-2**]. Refer to the figure accompanying each stretching exercise for correct form and degree of mobility. Remember to follow the appropriate instructions for stretch/mobilization cycles for affected or unaffected regions [**BOX 11-2**].

4. As you complete each stretch/mobilization cycle, record your results in the boxes located to the right of the Rank number on **Log Form C**. The upper line is for stiffness in the stretch (0 to 5), using the Mobility Scale in *Table C1* below. The lower line is for tenderness in the self-mobilization (0 to 5).

Table C1: Mobility Scale for Stretches		
Scale	**Flexibility**	**Guidelines**
0	No stiffness	Able to reach exact position shown in book, with no pain.
1	Almost no stiffness	Able to reach exact position shown in book, with slight pain.
2	Slight stiffness	Can almost reach exact position shown in book, with slight pain.
3	Moderate stiffness	Can't get very close to position shown in book, with moderate pain.
4	Very stiff	Can't get very close to position shown in book, with severe pain.
5	Extreme stiffness	Can't do the stretch at all, with severe pain.

5. When you have completed all stretch/mobilization cycles in order of Rank, evaluate your symmetry in each stretch. Compare the numbers you recorded for each stretch on left and right sides, and check the column for symmetry (No or Yes) on **Log Form C**. Evaluate only your symmetry in the stretches, not your tenderness.

6. Fill in one **Log Form C** for each day in Phase Two, until you have achieved the degree of symmetry required for your group and subgroup (*Self-Assessment 2C*).

Log Form C: Stretch/Mobilization Cycles

DAY/DATE:	Days since _last day you ran_:
PHASE #	Days in this Phase:
AFFECTED SIDE:	AFFECTED REGION(S):

Circle affected side →		Left		Right	Symmetry	
Enter your exercise list from _Worksheets 2A1_ and _2A2_	Rank #	**Stretches:** **Stiffness (0-5)** / **Self Mobs:** **Tenderness (0-5)**	Rank#	**Stretches:** **Stiffness (0-5)** / **Self Mobs:** **Tenderness (0-5)**	No	Yes
Stretch # 11-						
Self-Mob:						
Stretch # 11-						
Self-Mob:						
Stretch # 11-						
Self-Mob:						
Stretch # 11-						
Self-Mob:						
Stretch # 11-						
Self-Mob:						
Stretch # 11-						
Self-Mob:						
Stretch # 11-						
Self-Mob:						
Stretch # 11-						
Self-Mob:						
Stretch # 11-						
Self-Mob:						
Stretch # 11-						
Self-Mob:						
Stretch # 11-						
Self-Mob:						
Stretch # 11-						
Self-Mob:						
Stretch # 11-						
Self-Mob:						

PHASE THREE WORKBOOK

Phase Three Guidelines

The goal of Phase Three is to improve your strength and balance. All injuries involve dysfunctions that affect one side more than the other, resulting in an imbalance in strength and neuro-muscular control. Since running requires more stability than walking, we do balance and stabilization exercises to restore a proper balance before we can start to run in a functional manner.

Most of your injury-recovery work will be done is Phase Three, so this phase is divided into several smaller units and subgroups, each with their own clearance requirements. In Phase Three Part One, everyone is in the same treatment group. In this phase, you will use Basic Closed-Chain Exercises to evaluate and improve your strength and balance, based on four basic balance requirements. When you clear Phase Three Part One, you will be sorted into a new treatment group for post-injury training.

In Phase Three Part Two, there are separate *Guidelines* for Groups 1 and 2 (*Table 13-2* and *Table 13-3*), based on whether your injury is simple or complex, and how long it has been since you last ran in regular training.

Each group is further divided into subgroups A and B, based on whether or not you were able to clear Basic Closed-Chain Exercises in one week or less. Those who are sorted into Group 1B should note that there is a special *Group 1B Reassessment* in *Guidelines Table 13-2: Group 1 Guidelines for Phase Three Part Two*. In this reassessment, everyone in Group 1B will be reassigned to either Group 1A or Group 2A when they complete their Basic Closed-Chain Exercises. This is a special reassessment for Group 1B only, and does not appear in the general *Self-Assessments*.

Also note that, in Phase Three Part Two, the Course Map divides and Groups 1 and 2 take separate pathways. Along with the *Course Map*, there is also one set of *Self-Assessments* that is divided by treatment group. If you are following the *Course Map* for Group 1, you will be using the *Self-Assessment 3G1 for Self-Paced Plan*. If you are following the *Course Map* for Group 2, you will be using the *Self-Assessment 3G2 for Two-Week-Interval Plan*.

In P.T. Time, Groups 1A and 2A will clear Basic Closed-Chain Exercises (**Log Form B**) and change to Regional Closed-Chain Exercises (**Log Form R**) at the start of Phase Three Part Two. Groups 1B and 2B will continue with **Log Form B** when they start Phase Three Part Two, then change forms when they clear their Basic Closed-Chain Exercises.

Regional Closed-Chain Exercises are also divided into two stages (*see Instructions for Log Form R*). Stage 1 requires an *Initial Assessment* to determine your individualized *Symmetry Target* for each exercise, which you must meet for clearance in Phase Three Part Two. In Stage 2, you will continue your Regional Closed-Chain Exercises at a standard

Final Target level. This level will be used to maintain and monitor your condition through the end of Phase Four and does not require any further clearance.

In Phase Three Part Two, everyone will establish an individualized Base Schedule (**Log Form S: Base Schedule**) for post-injury training. Different groups will start at different levels, and follow different time schedules based on their *Worksheet T: Time Plan.* Your Base Schedule will always begin with a fitness walk to help you warm up and evaluate your progress. Group 1A will immediately start post-injury running with walk/glide

sets consisting of progressive amounts of fitness walking, controlled glides, and glide drills. Other groups will begin this phase by fitness walking their Base Schedule until they are cleared to progress to post-injury running.

Phase Three Part Two includes walk/glide sets and glide drills at Base Schedule Levels 1 though 5 (60-minute glides). Clearance to begin Phase Four requires Base Schedule Clearance at Level 5, and P.T. Time Clearance at the *Symmetry Target* level for all of the Regional Closed-Chain Exercises on your **Log Form R**.

Table 13-1

Guidelines: Phase Three Part One

PHASE THREE PART ONE	All Groups
P.T. Time	1. Basic Closed-Chain Exercises, 40 minutes per day, every day (**Log Form B**) 2. Continue with *Stretch/Mobilization Cycles* (flexibility training), 20 minutes per day, every day (**Log Form M**).
Phase Three Part One Clearance *(Self-Assessment 3A)*	1. Able to perform all 8 Basic Closed-Chain Exercises correctly and symmetrically, with no increase in symptoms. **OR** 2. Completed 1 week of Basic Closed-Chain Exercises, but still *unable* to perform all 8 Basic Closed-Chain exercises correctly, symmetrically, or with no increase in symptoms.

Table 13-2

Group 1 Guidelines: Phase Three Part Two

PHASE THREE PART TWO	GROUP 1	
Phase Three Part Two, Group 1 (*Self-Assessment 3D*)	1. Simple injury **AND** 2. Less than 6 weeks have passed since your last regular training run.	
	Subgroup 1A	**Subgroup 1B**
	Cleared all eight Basic Closed-Chain exercises in 1 week or less.	*Unable* to clear all 8 basic closed-chain exercises *after 1 week.*
Time Plan (*Worksheet T*)	Reduce P.T. Time to 2 days per week, and add your Base Schedule	Reduce P.T. Time to 2 days per week, and add your Base Schedule
Group 1 P.T. Time	1. Continue with *Stretch/Mobilization Cycles* (flexibility training), 2 days per week, 20 minutes per day (**Log Form M: Maintain Mobility**). 2. Begin Regional Closed-Chain Exercises for your one affected region, 2 days per week, 40 minutes per day (**Log Form R: Regional Closed-Chain**).	1. Continue with *Stretch/Mobilization Cycles* (flexibility training), 2 days per week, 20 minutes per day (**Log Form M: Maintain Mobility**). 2. Continue with Basic Closed-Chain Exercises, 2 days per week, 40 minutes per day, until you are able to perform all Basic Closed-Chain Exercises correctly and symmetrically, with no increase in symptoms (**Log Form B: Basic Closed-Chain**).
Group 1 Base Schedule (*Self-Assessment 3E*)	Walk/Glide your Base Schedule (**Log Form S**) starting at the appropriate level, following the **Self-Paced Plan**.	1. Fitness Walk your Base Schedule (**Log Form S: Level 0**), following the **Self-Paced Plan** until you have cleared all Basic Closed-Chain Exercises. 2. When you have cleared all Basic Closed-Chain Exercises, do the *Group 1B Reassessment* below.

(Table 13-2 cont)	Subgroup 1A	Subgroup 1B
Group 1B Reassessment	*(Subgroup 1 A: Skip this section)*	*Perform this self-assessment on the day that you clear all eight Basic Closed-Chain Exercises.* Look at the top section of today's **Log Form B: Basic Closed-Chain**, and find the box for "Days since last day you ran:" A. If today is 42 days (6 weeks) or less since your last regular training run, you can now move to **Group 1A** (Go to *Table 13-2, Group 1A PT Time* and *Base Schedule*). B. If today is 43 days or more (more than 6 weeks) since your last training run, you must move to **Group 2A** (Go to *Table 13-3, Group 2A PT Time* and *Base Schedule*).
Group 1: Phase Three Part Two Clearance *(Self-Assessment 3H)*	1. P.T. Time: Able to perform all regional closed-chain exercises for your one identified region, with symmetry and no increase in symptoms *(Self-Assessment 3F)*. 2. Base Schedule: Able to complete your Base Schedule with a 50-minute glide and glide drills for one week with no increase in symptoms *(Self-Assessment 3G1)*.	

Table 13-3

Group 2 Guidelines: Phase Three Part Two

PHASE THREE PART TWO	GROUP 2	
Phase Three Part Two, Group 2 *(Self-Assessment 3D)*	1. Complex injury **AND/OR** 2. More than 6 weeks have passed since your last regular training run.	
	Subgroup 2A *Cleared* all eight Basic Closed-Chain exercises in 1 week or less.	**Subgroup 2B** *Unable* to clear all eight Basic Closed-Chain Exercises *after 1 week*.
Time Plan *(Worksheet T)*	Reduce P.T. Time to 2 days per week, and add your Base Schedule.	Reduce P.T. Time to 2 days per week, and add your Base Schedule.
Group 2 P.T. Time	1. Continue with *Stretch/Mobilization Cycles* (flexibility training), 2 days per week, 20 minutes per day (**Log Form M: Maintain Mobility**). 2. Begin Regional Closed-Chain Exercises for all affected regions, 2 days per week, 40 minutes per day (**Log Form R: Regional Closed-Chain**).	1. Continue with *Stretch/Mobilization Cycles* (flexibility training), 2 days per week, 20 minutes per day (**Log Form M: Maintain Mobility**). 2. Continue with Basic Closed-Chain Exercises, 40 minutes per day, until you are able to perform all Basic Closed-Chain Exercises correctly and symmetrically, with no increase in symptoms (**Log Form B: Basic Closed-Chain**). 3. When you have cleared all Basic Closed-Chain Exercises, then begin Regional Closed-Chain Exercises for all affected regions, 2 days per week, 40 minutes per day (**Log Form R: Regional Closed-Chain**).

(Table 13-3 cont.)	Subgroup 2A	Subgroup 2B
Group 2 **Base Schedule,** **Part 1:** **Fitness Walking** (*Self-Assessment 3E*)	Fitness Walk your Base Schedule, following the **Two-Week Interval Plan**, until you have completed a minimum of 2 weeks, *and* you can complete 60 minutes of fitness walking with no increase in symptoms (**Log Form S: Level 0**).	1. Fitness Walk your Base Schedule until you have cleared all eight Basic Closed-Chain Exercises. 2. If you clear Basic Closed-Chain in less than 2 weeks, continue to Fitness Walk your Base Schedule, following the **Two-Week Interval Plan**, until you have completed a minimum of 2 weeks, *and* you can complete 60 minutes of fitness walking with no increase in symptoms (**Log Form S: Level 0**).
Group 2 **Base Schedule, Part 2: Walk/Glide**	Walk/Glide your Base Schedule, following the **Two-Week Interval Plan** (**Log Form S: Levels 0 through 5**).	
Group2: **Phase Three Part Two Clearance** (*Self-Assessment 3H*)	1. P.T. Time: Able to perform all Regional Closed-Chain Exercises for each of your identified regions, with symmetry and no increase in symptoms (*Self-Assessment 3F*). 2. Base Schedule: Able to complete your Base Schedule with a 50-minute glide and glide drills for two weeks with no increase in symptoms (*Self-Assessment 3G2*).	

Self-Assessment 3A: Basic Closed-Chain Clearance

Course Map Reference: 14.7, 14.8, 14.9

Instructions:

1. Before starting this Self-Assessment, complete your Course Map through line 14.6.

2. Follow the **Guidelines for Basic Closed-Chain Exercises [Box 14-3]**.

3. Fill out one **Log Form B** for each day of Basic Closed-Chain Exercises (See **Instructions for Log Form B: Basic Closed-Chain).**

4. Each day, evaluate your **Log Form B** for difficulty and clearance in individual exercises, and use this information to determine your exercise rotation for the following day.

5. Evaluate your **Log Form B** for Phase Three Part One clearance.

6. Complete **Worksheet 3A1** *on the same day* that you clear all eight Basic Closed-Chain Exercises, *or on Day 7* of Basic Closed-Chain Exercises without clearance

Self-Assessment 3A, Part 1: **Evaluate Log Form B (Phase Three Part One)**

1. Your **Log Forms B** for Day 1 and Day 2 contain your initial times and pain levels for all eight Basic Closed-Chain Exercises. Remember that all times entered on this form must indicate the amount of time that the exercise was done with correct form and no increase in pain. Follow the **Instructions for Log Form B: Basic Closed-Chain** to calculate your *Average Set Times* and *Left-Right Difference* for each exercise, and compare them to their *Symmetry Goals.*

2. On Day 1 and Day 2, evaluate your **Log Forms B** for initial difficulty and clearance of individual exercises:

    A. First, find any exercises for which you have already reached the *Target Time* and have symmetry (*Left-Right Difference* less than or equal to *Symmetry Goal*). These exercises are *cleared* and you can remove them from your next rotation. *Note:* Since exercise #6 does not have a *Left-Right Difference*, use your judgment to evaluate your ability to maintain form in this exercise.

    B. Note any exercises that are *cleared* on one side, and reduce the number of repetitions on the side that is cleared in your next rotation.

    C. Next, note which exercises show the most asymmetry (greatest *Left-Right Difference*). These are the exercises you will have to work on more often on the weaker side.

    D. Rank your eight Basic Closed-Chain Exercises in order of difficulty, based on how hard it was for you to maintain correct form (higher *Left-Right Difference*) and maximum pain levels (see **Worksheet 3A1**).

3. Determine which four Basic Closed-Chain Exercises you will do on the following day:

 A. On Day 3, start with the four exercises that had the greatest asymmetry on Days 1 and 2.

 B. On Day 4, do any exercises you didn't do on Day 3. If you have less than four exercises, add any of the other exercise(s) that you have *not* cleared to maintain a total of four exercises.

 C. Eliminate exercises as you reach clearance (symmetry). When you have less than four exercises remaining, add back exercises that you have already cleared to maintain a total of four exercises per day.

4. Monitor your pain levels from day to day. Note any change in pain levels during exercise for the same exercise and side. Pain levels should decrease over time, and should not exceed a level of 5 or 6 on any day. Also monitor your injury stage, to make sure you do not go above Stage 2 at any time [**Box 3-1**].

Self-Assessment 3A, Part 2: **Progress to Phase Three Part Two**

 Complete **Worksheet 3A1: Evaluation of Basic Closed-Chain Exercises** *on the same day* that you clear all eight Basic Closed-Chain exercises, *or on Day 7* of Basic Closed-Chain Exercises without clearance.

***

What to do now:
• Begin Phase Three Part Two.
• Follow the guidelines in Appendix G for *able* or *unable* to clear Basic Closed-Chain in treatment Group 1 (*Table 13-2*) or treatment Group 2 (*Table 13-3*).
• Check Course Map lines 14.7, 14.8, and 14.9.
• Continue immediately to *Self-Assessment 3B*: Injury Regions through *Self-Assessment 3E*: Base Schedule.

Worksheet 3A1: Evaluation of Basic Closed-Chain Exercises

1. Based on your daily assessments, list all eight Basic Closed-Chain Exercises **in order of difficulty**:

    1. CC#_____

    2. CC#_____

    3. CC#_____

    4. CC#_____

    5. CC#_____

    6. CC#_____

    7. CC#_____

    8. CC#_____

2. Count the number of days since you started your Basic Closed-Chain exercises, and **circle** the statement below that applies to you:

I was *able* to clear all Basic Closed-Chain Exercises in 7 days or less, and I am progressing to Regional Closed-Chain Exercises.	I was *unable* to clear all Basic Closed-Chain Exercises in 7 days or less, and I am continuing with Basic Closed-Chain Exercises.

Self-Assessment 3B: Injury Regions

Course Map Reference: 14.10

Instructions:

1. Complete this Self-Assessment *on the same day* that you clear all eight Basic Closed-Chain exercises, *or on Day 7* of Basic Closed-Chain Exercises without clearance (after you complete *Self-Assessment 3A, Part 2*).

2. Complete **Worksheet 3B1**: **Regional Self-Assessment Tables.**

3. Identify your Injury Region(s) using all available information to date, and list your Injury Regions in order from most severe to least severe (**Worksheet 3B2: Injury Regions in Order of Severity**).

4. Locate your **Regional Plans** in *Appendix R*.

Self-Assessment 3B, Part 1: Complete **Worksheet 3B1** below:

Instructions for Worksheet 3B1: Regional Self-Assessment Tables

1. Refer to the following sections in your Workbook to determine your *maximum symptoms* for this running injury:
   • Worksheet 1D4: Summary of Original Injury
   • Worksheet 2A2: Ranking Affected Regions
   • Worksheet 2D1: Regional Tenderness
   • Log Forms B: Basic Closed Chain
   • Worksheet 3A1: Evaluation of Basic Closed-Chain

2. In **Worksheet 3B1**, fill out the **Regional Self-Assessment Table** for each of your *possible affected regions*, and for each region where you found asymmetry in your mobility (in **Worksheet 2A2: Ranking Affected Regions**) or tenderness (in **Worksheet 2D1: Regional Tenderness**).

3. Check your *maximum symptoms* related to Self-Mobilizations, Stretches, and Basic Closed-Chain Exercises in the boxes for *left side* or *right side*. If you have no symptoms in a particular side or region, leave those boxes blank.

4. In the section for *Pre-Injury Stride Tendency*, use your best judgment to evaluate your running stride *at the time you were injured*. If you aren't sure, leave those boxes blank for now.

5. Fill out the **Regional Self-Assessment Table** for **Region 11: Regional Injury with Stress Fracture** to include or exclude stress fracture management

Worksheet 3B1: Regional Self-Assessment Tables

Region 1: Big Toe (1st Ray)
(Secondary Region: Outer Toes)

Activity	Self-Assessment		Left	Right
Self - mobilization	I have **tenderness** and/or bruising on the ball of the foot.			
Stretches	I have reduced range of motion **(stiffness)** in the toe region, *resulting in* difficulty flexing the toes up or down.			
Closed-Chain Exercises	I have **weakness** in the toe region, *resulting in*:	A. Difficulty flexing the toes during push off.		
		B. Difficulty flexing the toes during step-up.		
Pre-Injury Stride Tendency	While running, I have a tendency to:	A. Rotate the leg outward.		
		B. Push off from the inner or outer side of the big toe.		

Region 2: Arch

Activity	Self-Assessment		Left	Right
Self - mobilization	I have **tenderness** in or around the bottom of my foot; or under and/or to the outside of the heel and arch.			
Stretches	I have reduced range of motion **(stiffness)** in the ankle region, *resulting in* difficulty flexing the foot upward.			
Closed-Chain Exercises	I have **weakness** in the toe-flexing muscles, *resulting in* rolling the foot to the inside or outside when standing on one leg.			
Pre-Injury Stride Tendency	While running, I have a tendency to:	A. Turn the leg excessively out or in.		
		B. Overstrike and foot-slap into an overpronated foot.		

Region 3: Heel

Activity	Self-Assessment		Left	Right
Self - mobilization	I have **tenderness** at the Achilles tendon, and/or the outer side of the Achilles tendon.			
Stretches	I have reduced range of motion **(stiffness)** in the heel region, *resulting in* tightness in the heel area when standing on an uphill incline.			
Closed-Chain Exercises	I have **weakness** in the heel region, *resulting in*:	A. Difficulty keeping the foot flexed and straight.		
		B. Difficulty pushing off.		
Pre-Injury Stride Tendency	While running, I have a tendency to:	A. Overstrike, with the lower leg rotated outward.		
		B. Slap the foot, with the foot sticking out.		
		C. Overstrike on the outer edge of the heel and slap the foot.		
		D. Land too hard on the heel.		
		E. Overpronate and push off from the inner side of the big toe.		
		F. Roll the foot excessively inward.		

Region 4: Shin
(Secondary Region: Ankle)

Activity	Self-Assessment		Left	Right
Self - mobilization	I have **tenderness** on either side of the shin, extending down to the tendons near the foot.			
Stretches	I have reduced range of motion **(stiffness)** in the leg, *resulting in* reduced range of motion in the ankle.			
Closed-Chain Exercises	I have **weakness** in the shin region, *resulting in* twisting and leaning that causes excessive exertion in my shin.			
Pre-Injury Stride Tendency	While running, I have a tendency to:	A. A running stride that puts excessive stress on the shin.		
		B. Over-lean in any plane.		
		C. Overstrike on the heel.		
		D. Twist the knee and turn the foot outward.		
		E. Wobble at the hip.		

Region 5: Calf

Activity	Self-Assessment		Left	Right
Self - mobilization	I have **tenderness** in the thick part of the calf muscle			
Stretches	I have reduced range of motion **(stiffness)** in the calf region, *resulting in* difficulty flexing the foot upward.			
Closed-Chain Exercises	I have **weakness** in the calf region, *resulting in* difficulty flexing the foot downward.			
Pre-Injury Stride Tendency	While running, I have a tendency to:	A. Not be able to kick back straight and/or fully after pushoff.		
		B. Rotate the leg outward.		
		C. Have a circular movement of the lower leg.		
		D. Push off from the inner side of the big toe.		

Region 6: Knee
(Secondary Region: Thigh)

Activity	Self-Assessment		Left	Right
Self - mobilization	I have **tenderness** anywhere around the whole knee cap (usually to the outside of the knee cap), with or without generalized knee swelling.			
Stretches	I have reduced range of motion **(stiffness)** in the knee region, *resulting in* tightness and inability to bend the knee, and generalized stiffness.			
Closed-Chain Exercises	I have **weakness** in the knee region, *resulting in*:	A. Leg twisting inward during exercise.		
		B. difficulty bearing weight while stepping down.		
		C. Difficulty kicking back straight.		
		D. Difficulty balancing on one leg.		
		E. Inability to maintain knee control when stepping down stairs.		
Pre-Injury Stride Tendency	While running, I have a tendency to:	A. Twist at the knee.		
		B. Run with the foot pointed outward.		

Region 7: Band

Activity	Self-Assessment		Left	Right
Self - mobilization	I have **tenderness** on the outside of the knee, with or without visible swelling.			
Stretches	I have reduced range of motion **(stiffness)** from the hip and buttock down to the upper leg.			
Closed-Chain Exercises	I have **weakness** in the band region, *resulting in*:	A. Difficulty staying balanced on one leg.		
		B. Difficulty kicking out to the side.		
Pre-Injury Stride Tendency	While running, I have a tendency to:	A. Wobble side-to-side at the hip.		
		B. Lean to the outside with my foot sticking out, causing my knee to go to the inside.		

Region 8: Hamstring

Activity	Self-Assessment		Left	Right
Self - mobilization	I have **tenderness** in the back of the leg between the knee and buttock.			
Stretches	I have reduced range of motion **(stiffness)** in the Straight Leg Raise.			
Closed-Chain Exercises	I have **weakness** in the hamstring region, *resulting in* asymmetrical weakness and inflexibility in the hamstring area during kickback.			
Pre-Injury Stride Tendency	While running, I have a tendency to:	A. Push off from the inner side of the big toe.		
		B. Have a kickback that is short, asymmetrical, or twists.		

Region 9: Hip

Activity	Self-Assessment	Left	Right
Self - mobilization	I have **tenderness** and/or swelling in the front of the hip.		
Stretches	I have reduced range of motion **(stiffness)** in the hip region, *resulting in* inability to bring the ankle and/or knee all the way up, down, or back on the injured side when doing stretches.		
Closed-Chain Exercises	I have **weakness** in the hip region, *resulting in* difficulty kicking up to "high knees" position.		
Pre-Injury Stride Tendency	While running, I have a tendency to lean too far forward and toward the side of the injured hip.		

Region 10: Buttock
(Secondary Region: Lateral hip)

Activity	Self-Assessment		Left	Right
Self - mobilization	I have **tenderness** and swelling to the rear and side of the hip.			
Stretches	I have reduced range of motion **(stiffness)** in any hip stretching exercise.			
Closed-Chain Exercises:	I have **weakness** in the hip and buttock region that affects symmetrical kickback and overall balance.			
Pre-Injury Stride Tendency	While running, I have a tendency to:	A. Wobble side-to-side at the hip.		
		B. Be unable to kick back straight and/or fully.		
		C. Have asymmetrical rotation of the pelvis.		

Region 11: Regional Injury with Stress Fracture

Activity	Self-Assessment	Left	Right
Self - mobilization	I have **tenderness** in any weight-bearing bone in my injury region (anywhere from the foot to the pelvis), with or without pain in the associated soft tissues.		
Stretches	I have reduced range of motion **(stiffness)** in the region where I have bone tenderness.		
Closed-Chain Exercises:	After icing *and* not running for at least 3 weeks, I can *still* **reproduce my injury pain** when I hop on the injured leg (unable to clear CC#1 Square Hop Exercise).		
Pre-Injury Stride Tendency	While running, I feel pain in the region where I have bone tenderness.		

Self-Assessment 3B, Part 2: **Identify Injury Regions**

1. Use all the information you have gathered in your workbook, and compare it to the descriptions in **Worksheet 3B1: Regional Self-Assessment Tables** to select your Injury Region(s) for Regional Closed-Chain Exercises (Phase Three Part Two). This is a qualitative decision, so use your best judgment based on everything you have learned so far. It's okay if you are not 100% certain, as long as you are close.

2. If your injury is complex (see **Worksheet 2B1: Phase Two Treatment Group and Sub-Group**), you may choose more than one injury region. *Do not choose more than 2 regions on one side* – not including stress fracture. If you have affected regions on both sides, *do not choose more than 3 injury regions all together* (two on one side, one on the other side) – not including stress fracture.
      • Worksheet 2A2: Ranking Affected Regions
      • Worksheet 2D1: Regional Tenderness
      • Worksheet 3A1: Evaluation of Basic Closed-Chain

3. If you have selected two or three regions, use your **Worksheet 1D4: Summary of Original Injury**; **Worksheet 2A2: Ranking Affected Regions**; and **Worksheet 2D1: Regional Tenderness** to rank these regions in order of severity, from most severe to least severe. List your injury region(s) and side(s) in order, from most severe to least severe, on **Worksheet 3B2** below:

Worksheet 3B2: Injury Regions in Order of Severity		
Rank #	**Side (left/right)**	**Injury Region**
1.		Region #
2.		Region #
3.		Region #
4.		Region #

4. If you were *unable* to clear CC#1 Square Hops after icing *and* not running for at least 3 weeks, OR if you checked *any two* boxes in **Worksheet 3B1, Table 11: Regional Injury with Stress Fracture**, then add Region 11: Stress Fracture to **Worksheet 3B2**. Follow your Regional Plan(s) and add Recovery Plan 11 for Stress Fracture (*Appendix R*) to your Regional Closed-Chain Exercises.

What to do now:
• Go to *Appendix R: Regional Plans*, and familiarize yourself with the recovery plan(s) for each of your Injury Region(s).
• Check line 14.10 on your Course Map.
• Continue immediately to *Self-Assessment 3C* through *Self-Assessment 3F*.

Self-Assessment 3C:
Regional Closed-Chain Exercises (Prepare Log Form R)

Course Map Reference: 14.11

Instructions:

1. Complete this Self-Assessment *on the same day* that you clear all eight Basic Closed-Chain exercises, *or on Day 7* of Basic Closed-Chain Exercises without clearance (after you complete *Self-Assessment 3B*).

2. Fill out **Worksheet 3C1: Regional Closed-Chain Exercises in Order of Severity.**

3. Use **Worksheet 3C1:** to prepare your first **Log Form R**.

***Self-Assessment 3C, Part 1,* Regional Closed-Chain Exercises:** Complete **Worksheet 3C1:** below (see *Sample* **Worksheets 3C1** in *Case Studies*).

Instructions for Worksheet 3C1:
Regional Closed-Chain Exercises in Order of Severity

1. Copy your Injury Regions from **Worksheet 3B2: Injury Regions in Order of Severity** to **Worksheet 3C1**. Your list should contain one to three Injury Regions, plus Stress Fracture if applicable. Write your 1st Injury Region and side at the top of Box 1; your 2nd Injury Region and side at the top of the Box 2, and so on. Leave any unused boxes blank.

2. Refer to ***Table 3C1: Closed-Chain Exercises by Region*** below. Find your 1st Injury Region, and copy the list of six exercises to **Worksheet 3C1, Box 1**.

3. If you have a 2nd Injury Region, copy that list to the second box. *Then cross out any exercises in Box 2 that you already entered in Box 1, so there are no duplicate exercises.*

4. If you have a 3rd Injury Region, enter that information in Box 3, and cross out any exercises in Box 3 that duplicate an exercise in Box 1 or Box 2.

5. If you have added Stress Fracture to your list of regions, copy the information for Region 11: Stress Fracture to Box 4. Again, cross out any duplicated exercises.

6. **Worksheet 3C1** now contains your list of Regional Closed-Chain Exercises in order of severity.

Table 3C1: Closed-Chain Exercises by Region

Region 1: Big Toe (Outer Toes)

CC# 3	One-Leg Armswings, Barefoot
CC# 5	Barefoot Push-Up
CC# 11	Straight-Leg Raise with Theraband
CC# 16	Barefoot Push-Through
CC# 18	Shod Push-Through with Ankle Weights
CC# 19	Box Step-Up

Region 2: Arch

CC# 2	Side Step-Down
CC# 3	One-Leg Armswings, Barefoot
CC# 8	Box Step Up and Over
CC# 11	Straight-Leg Raise with Theraband
CC# 12	One-Leg Armswings, Double Pillows
CC# 16	Barefoot Push-Through

Region 3: Heel

CC# 5	Barefoot Push-Up
CC# 6	Quick Steps
CC# 8	Box Step Up and Over
CC# 11	Straight-Leg Raise with Theraband
CC# 12	One-Leg Armswings, Double Pillows
CC# 18	Shod Push-Through with Ankle Weights

Region 4: Shin (Ankle)

CC# 1	Square Hops
CC# 2	Side Step-Down
CC# 11	Straight-Leg Raise with Theraband
CC# 12	One-Leg Armswings, Double Pillows
CC# 13	One-Leg Armswings, Side Incline
CC# 17	Shod Push-Up with Ankle Weights

Region 5: Calf

CC# 2	Side Step-Down
CC# 6	Quick Steps
CC# 12	One-Leg Armswings, Double Pillows
CC# 17	Shod Push-Up with Ankle Weights
CC# 18	Shod Push-Through with Ankle Weights
CC# 19	Box Step-Up

Region 6: Knee (Thigh)	
CC# 2	Side Step-Down
CC# 7	Weighted Kickback
CC# 8	Box Step Up and Over
CC# 11	Straight-Leg Raise with Theraband
CC# 12	One-Leg Armswings, Double Pillows
CC# 18	Shod Push-Through with Ankle Weights

Region 7: Band	
CC# 2	Side Step-Down
CC# 8	Box Step Up and Over
CC# 9	Hip Abduction with Theraband
CC# 12	One-Leg Armswings, Double Pillows
CC# 13	One-Leg Armswings, Side Incline
CC# 20	Theraband Kickback

Region 8: Hamstring	
CC# 2	Side Step-Down
CC# 7	Weighted Kickback
CC# 8	Box Step Up and Over
CC# 12	One-Leg Armswings, Double Pillows
CC# 14	One-Leg Armswings, Double Weights
CC# 20	Theraband Kickback

Region 9: Hip (Groin or Inner Thigh)	
CC# 2	Side Step-Down
CC# 8	Box Step Up and Over
CC# 10	Lateral Straight-Leg Raise with Theraband
CC# 11	Straight-Leg Raise with Theraband
CC# 12	One-Leg Armswings, Double Pillows
CC# 15	High Knees with Theraband

Region 10: Buttock (Lateral Hip)	
CC# 6	Quick Steps
CC# 7	Weighted Kickback
CC# 8	Box Step Up and Over
CC# 9	Hip Abduction with Theraband
CC# 13	One-Leg Armswings, Side Incline
CC# 14	One-Leg Armswings, Double Weights

Region 11: Stress Fracture (Add to Regional Exercises)	
CC# 1	Square Hops
CC# 2	Side Step-Down
CC# 8	Box Step Up and Over

Worksheet 3C1: Regional Closed-Chain Exercises in Order of Severity

1st Injury Region and Side:

	Box1: Regional Closed-Chain Exercises
CC#	
CC#	
CC#	
CC#	
CC#	
CC#	

2nd Injury Region and Side:

	Box 2: Regional Closed-Chain Exercises
CC#	
CC#	
CC#	
CC#	
CC#	
CC#	

3rd Injury Region and Side:

	Box 3: Regional Closed-Chain Exercises
CC#	
CC#	
CC#	
CC#	
CC#	
CC#	

Stress Fracture, Side:

	Box 4: Regional Closed-Chain Exercises
CC# 1	
CC# 2	
CC# 8	

Self Assessment 3C, Part 2: **Prepare Your First Log Form R** (see *Sample* **Log Forms R** in *Case Studies*)

1. Read the **Instructions for Log Form R: Regional Closed Chain**, and review **Box 14-4: Guidelines for Regional Closed-Chain.**

2. Determine whether you are a Fitness Runner or Racer (see **Worksheet 1B1**) .

3. At the top of **Log Form R**, write "Phase Three Part Two, Stage 1" on the line for *Phase*. List your *Injury Region(s) and Side* on the appropriate line. Do not enter any information for days or dates at this time.

4. Copy the numbers and names of all your Regional Closed-Chain Exercises, in order, from **Worksheet 3C1: Regional Closed-Chain Exercises in Order of Severity** to **Log Form R**. If you have more than 8 exercises on your list, use additional **Log Forms R**, and number the pages in order on the title line.

5. Go to *Appendix Z: Regional Closed-Chain Tables for Fitness Runners and Racers*, and find the examples for each of your Regional Closed-Chain Exercises. Copy the information for *Rest Between Sets*, *Final Target*, and *Build Pace*, to each exercise in your **Log Form R**. Copy *only* the *Final Target* and *Rest* times for your group (Fitness Runner or Racer).

6. As you copy the information for each exercise from *Appendix Z* to **Log Form R**, be sure to copy any references to footnotes (any letters in parentheses) to the line for *"Notes."*

7. **Special Instructions for CC#6 (Quick Steps), CC#16 (Barefoot Push-Through), and CC#18 (Shod Push-Through):** For exercises that use both legs at the same time, you will record only one set time for both legs. For these exercises, modify your **Log Form R** to look like the examples in *Appendix Z*. Cross out *Left* and *Right* on the line for *Set Times*, and write in "Both." Cross out *one* of each pair of boxes numbered 1 through 5. Also cross out the boxes for *Left/Right Difference* and *Symmetry Goal* (see sample in *Case Studies*).

8. Your **Log Form R** now contains your schedule for Regional Closed-Chain Exercises in Phase Three Part Two, Stage 1. You will fill in your *Symmetry Target* and *Symmetry Goal* for each exercise when you start your exercises and do your *Initial Assessment* (see **Instructions for Log Form R**).

*** * ***

What to do now:
• Check line 14.11 on your Course Map.
• Use **Log Form B** until you have cleared all Basic Closed-Chain Exercises, then progress to **Log Form R: Regional Closed-Chain** (see **Instructions for Log Form R**).
• Continue immediately to *Self-Assessment 3D* through *Self-Assessment 3F*.

Self-Assessment 3D: Treatment Groups for Phase Three Part Two

Course Map References: 14.12 and 14.13

Instructions:

1. Complete this Self-Assessment *on the same day* that you clear all eight Basic Closed-Chain exercises, *or on Day 7* of Basic Closed-Chain Exercises without clearance (after you complete *Self-Assessment 3C*).

2. In *Self-Assessment 3D Part 1*, prepare *Impairment Statements* that correlate your Injury Region(s) to specific balance problems to address in your recovery program.

3. In *Self-Assessment 3D Part 2*, determine which treatment group and subgroup you will enter in Phase Three Part Two.

4. Use this information to start filling out **Worksheet T: Training Plan for Phase Three Part Two.**

Self-Assessment 3D Part 1, Impairment Statements:

1. Each Regional Closed-Chain Exercise is associated with one of the four basic requirements for balance (***Table 14-1***). Use the results of your Basic Closed-Chain Exercises to identify which of these four basic requirements you will focus on during your recovery.

2. Refer to your list of Basic Closed-Chain Exercises in order of difficulty (**Worksheet 3A1: Evaluation of Basic Closed-Chain Exercises**) and **Worksheet 3B2: Injury Regions in Order of Severity**.

3. Use *Table 3D1* below to identify your two main balance problems:

   A. Find the CC# of the first Basic Closed-Chain Exercise on your **Worksheet 3A1**, and circle the Basic Balance Problem for that exercise in *Table 3D1*.

   B. Find the CC# of the second Basic Closed-Chain Exercise on your **Worksheet 3A1**, and circle the Basic Balance Problem for that exercise in *Table 3D1*.

   C. You must circle two Basic Balance Problems. If your first two exercises have the same balance problem, go to the third exercise on your **Worksheet 3A1**, and circle the Basic Balance Problem for that exercise in *Table 3D1*.

Table 3D1: Basic Closed-Chain Balance Problems	
Basic Closed-Chain Exercise	**Basic Balance Problem**
CC# 1 or 2	Difficulty maintaining balance over a straight foot.
CC# 3 or 4	Difficulty using armswings to maintain balance while standing on one leg.
CC# 5 or 6	Difficulty maintaining balance while pushing off straight through the big toe.
CC# 7 or 8	Difficulty maintaining balance while kicking straight back.

4. Write an Impairment Statement for your first Basic Balance Problem. It should include three parts: (1) the *Side* of your injury; (2) all of the *Injury Regions* on that side; and (3) your first *Basic Balance Problem*. For example, if you have two Injury Regions in the left hip and left knee, and you had the most trouble with CC# 4, you might write this Impairment Statement: "I have trouble with my left hip and knee when using my arms to balance my body."

Impairment Statement 1:

5. Write a second Impairment Statement for your second Basic Balance Problem. For example, if your second problem exercise was CC#2, you might write this Impairment Statement: "My left knee and hip wobble when I try to balance on a straight foot."

Impairment Statement 2:

6. If you have a complex injury with separate injuries in your left and right legs, write one additional Impairment Statement for the second leg.

Impairment Statement 3 (for injuries in the second leg only):

Self-Assessment 3D, Part 2, **Treatment Groups:** Complete **Worksheet 3D1** below:

Worksheet 3D1: Treatment Groups for Phase Three Part Two

1. Which of the following statements applies to you?
   A. I have cleared all eight Basic Closed-Chain Exercises in 7 Days or less.
   B. I have completed Day 7 of Basic Closed-Chain Exercises, and I still have *not* cleared one or more of the eight Basic Closed-Chain Exercises.

2. Based on your **Self-Assessment 2B**, which complexity subgroup are you in?
   A. *Simple Injuries.*
   B. *Complex Injuries.*

3. How many Injury Regions did you list in **Worksheet 3B2: Injury Regions in Order of Severity**?
   A. One
   B. More than one

4. Look at the top section of today's **Log Form B: Basic Closed-Chain**, and find the box for "Days since *last day you ran.*" Which of the following statements applies to you?
   A. Today is 42 days or less (6 weeks or less) since the last day I ran.
   B. Today is 43 days or more (more than 6 weeks) since the last day I ran.

---

5. Based on questions 1 through 4, find your Treatment Group for Phase Three Part Two:

You are in:	If your answers to questions 1 though 4 are:
GROUP 1A	"A" to ALL FOUR questions
GROUP 1B	"B" to question 1 AND "A" to ALL of questions 2, 3 and 4
GROUP 2A	"A" to question 1 AND "B" to ONE OR MORE of questions 2, 3, and 4
GROUP 2B	"B" to question 1 AND "B" to ONE OR MORE of questions 2, 3, and 4

What to do now:
• Copy your *Impairment Statements* to **Worksheet T: Training Plan for Phase Three Part Two**, and work to correct these weaknesses throughout your recovery program.
• Write your treatment group for Phase Three Part Two on your **Worksheet T**.
• Follow the guidelines for Group 1 (**Table 13-2**) or Group 2 (**Table 13-3**).
• Check lines 14.12 and 14.13 on your Course Map and continue to the next line.

Self-Assessment 3E: Base Schedule and Training Plan

Course map references: 15.11 and 15.12

Instructions:

1. Complete this Self-Assessment *on the same day* that you clear all eight Basic Closed-Chain exercises, *or on Day 7* of Basic Closed-Chain Exercises without clearance (after you complete *Self-Assessment 3E*).

2. Establish your Base Schedule.

3. Plan your PT Time and Base Schedule for Phase Three Part Two.

4. Use this information to continue filling out **Worksheet T: Training Plan for Phase Three Part Two.**

Self-Assessment:

1. Review your *Self-Assessment 1B:* Running History.

2. Find the scheduling information that applies to you in *Tables 3E1, 3E2, and 3E3* below, and enter it on **Worksheet T: Training Plan for Phase Three Part Two.**

Table 3E1: Base Schedules for Fitness Runners and Racers

Fitness Runners

Schedule	Pre-Injury Training [1]	Base Schedule
Days Per Week	A. 2 days or less	Increase to 3 days per week
	B. 3 to 5 days	Same as pre-injury training
	C. More than 5 days	Decrease to 5 days per week
Miles Per Week	A. Less than 10 miles	Increase to 10 miles per week
	B. 10 to 25 miles	Same as pre-injury training
	C. More than 25 miles	Lower to 25 miles per week

[1] From *Self-Assessment 1B: Running History*

Racers

Schedule	Pre-Injury Training [1]	Base Schedule
Days Per Week	A. 2 days or less	Increase to 4 days per week
	B. 3 to 5 days	Same as pre-injury training
	C. More than 5 days	Decrease to 5 days per week
Miles Per Week	A. Less than 10 miles	Increase to 10 miles per week
	B. 10 to 25 miles	Same as pre-injury training
	C. More than 25 miles	Lower to 25 miles per week

[1] From *Self-Assessment 1B: Running History*

Table 3E2: Starting Your Self-Paced Plan or Two Week-Interval Plan			
Phase Three Part Two Base Schedule	**Group Number**	**Starting Level for Base Schedule (Log Form S)**	**Special Instructions** [1]
Self-Paced Plan	1A	*See Table 3E3:* Group 1 Self-Paced Plan	Start at appropriate level
	1B	Level 0: Fitness Walking	Reassess Group after clearing Basic Closed-Chain Exercises
Two-Week-Interval Plan	2A	Level 0: Fitness Walking	Begin walk/glides after 2 weeks.
	2B	Level 0: Fitness Walking	Begin walk/glides after clearing Basic Closed-Chain AND 2 weeks of fitness walking.

[1] See guidelines in Appendix G *Tables 13-2 and 13-3.*

Table 3E3: Group 1 Self-Paced Plan: Where to Begin Your Base Schedule		
With your original injury, if you had pain after running:	**Start your Walk/Glide Program with 10 minutes fitness walking followed by:**	**Base Schedule: Log Form S**
Less than 10 minutes or 1 mile	50 minutes of fitness walking	Level 0
10 to 20 minutes, or 1 to 2 miles	(1 minute glides + 4 minutes fitness walking) x 10 sets	Level 1
20 to 30 minutes, or 2 to 3 miles	(2 minutes glides + 3 minutes fitness walking) x 10 sets	Level 2
30 to 40 minutes, or 3 to 4 miles	(3 minutes glides + 2 minutes fitness walking) x 10 sets	Level 3
40 to 50 minutes, or 4 to 5 miles	(4 minutes glides + 1 minute fitness walking) x 10 sets	Level 4
More than 50 minutes or 5 miles	50 minutes of glides	Level 5

Worksheet T: Training Plan for Phase Three Part Two

1. I am a (Fitness Runner or Racer): _____.

2. I plan to do my P.T. Time (**Log Form M** and **Log Form B** or **Log Form R**) 60 minutes per day, two days per week, on these days: _____ and _____.
(*Note:* P.T. Time may be done on the same days as your Base Schedule, or on different days).

3. I plan to do my Base Schedule (**Log Form S**) 60 minutes per day, _____ days per week, on these days:

_____.

4. I am in Treatment Group Number (1A, 1B, 2A, or 2B) _____.

5. I am following the (*Self-Paced Plan* or *Two-Week-Interval Plan*):
_____.

6. I will start my Base Schedule at Level _____.

7. My weekly mileage *goal* is _____ miles per week.

8. My daily mileage *maximum* is _____ miles per day (divide line 7 by line 3).

Write your personalized *Impairment Statements* from *Self-Assessment 3D* here:

What to do now:

Group 1 ONLY:

• Follow the guidelines for Group 1 in Appendix G *Table 13-2* based on the individualized plan you prepared in **Worksheet T: Training Plan for Phase Three Part Two**.

• Use *Self-Assessment 3G1 for Self-Paced Plan* to evaluate your Base Schedule (**Log Form S**) for Phase Three clearance.

• Follow the Course Map for Group 1, beginning with line 15.13A.

• Check lines 15.11 and 15.12 on your Course Map and continue.

Group 2 ONLY:

• Follow the guidelines for Group 2 in Appendix G *Table 13-3* based on the individualized plan you prepared in **Worksheet T: Training Plan for Phase Three Part Two**.

• Use *Self-Assessment 3G2 for Two-Week-Interval Plan* to evaluate your Base Schedule (**Log Form S**) for Phase Three clearance.

• Follow the Course Map for Group 2, beginning with line 15.13B.

• Check lines 15.11 and 15.12 on your Course Map, and continue.

Self-Assessment 3F: Regional Closed-Chain Clearance

Group 1A Course Map reference: line 14.16A and 15.24A
Group 2A Course Map reference: line 15.15B and 15.32B
Group 2B Course Map reference: line 15.21B and 15.32B

Instructions:

1. Begin this Self-Assessment on your first day of P.T. Time for Regional Closed-Chain Exercises.

2. Read the **Instructions for Log Form R: Regional Closed-Chain, Stage 1** and perform an *Initial Assessment* (**Log Form R, Line 8**) on your first day for *each* new Regional Closed-Chain Exercise, to determine your *Symmetry Target* and *Symmetry Goal* for Stage 1.

3. For each day in Stage 1, perform a *Self-Assessment* to evaluate those exercises for symmetry and clearance.

4. Focus on clearing all of your Regional Closed-Chain Exercises as quickly as possible. You must clear all Regional Closed-Chain Exercises (including stress fracture if applicable) before you enter Phase Four.

Self-Assessment (see *Sample* **Log Forms R** in *Case Studies*):

1. Complete four Regional Closed-Chain Exercises on your daily **Log Form R**, and do the calculations (see **Instructions for Log Form R, Part 1**).

2. For each exercise, compare your *Left/Right Difference* to the *Symmetry Goal* on the line beneath it to see if you have met your symmetry requirements for that exercise. You have *Cleared* that exercise when the *Left/Right Difference* is equal to or less than your *Symmetry Goal*; and you have completed 10 minutes of that exercise, for equal amounts of time on each leg, with correct form and no increase in pain.

3. *Special instructions for Quick Steps and Push-Throughs:* For exercises that use both legs at the same time (CC#6: Quick Steps; CC#16: Barefoot Push-Throughs; and CC#18: Shod Push-Throughs), evaluate your symmetry and clearance based on correct form and pain levels rather than *Left/Right Difference* (see **Box 14-4**).

4. When you have cleared an exercise in Stage 1, write *Cleared* on that exercise in your **Log Form R**, and skip that exercise in your next rotation. When you have cleared all Regional Closed-Chain Exercises in Stage 1, progress to Stage 2 (see **Instructions for Log Form R, Part 2**).

What to do now:

• Follow the **Instructions for Log Form R** and **Log Form M** for P.T. Time.

• Check the appropriate line on your Course Map (see Course Map references above for Groups 1A, 2A, and 2B), and continue.

• When you have cleared all Regional Closed-Chain Exercises in Stage 1, follow the **Instructions for Log Form R: Regional Closed-Chain, Stage 2** to revise your **Log Form R** for Stage 2, and to monitor your symmetry while building toward your *Final Target*.

Self-Assessment 3G1 for Self-Paced Plan:
Base Schedule Clearance (Levels 0 through 5)

Course Map references: 15.13A through 15.23A

Instructions:

1. Do this Self-Assessment if you are in Group 1A or 1B.

2. Read the **Instructions for Log Form S**, and start with the form for your correct level (see your **Worksheet T: Training Plan for Phase Three Part Two**).

3. Complete one square of **Log Form S** for each day of your Base Schedule, and evaluate it for clearance to the next higher level.

4. At Level 5, you must clear a consecutive number of Base Schedule Days equal to your number of _Target Days per Week._

Self-Assessment: Complete **Worksheet 3G1** each day for clearance to the next level of **Log Form S** (see _Sample_ **Log Forms S** in _Case Studies_).

***

What to do now:

• If you answered _"Yes"_ to ANY question in **Worksheet 3G1**, continue with your Base Schedule at the same level.

• If you answered _"No"_ to ALL questions in **Worksheet 3G1**, write _"Cleared"_ on your **Log Form R** for that level (Levels 0 through 4), and progress to the next level in your Base Schedule.

• When you reach Level 5, continue until you have cleared your number of _target days per week_ (3, 4 or 5 days) consecutively. (_Note:_ the 3, 4 or 5 consecutive days do not have to be in the same calendar week.)

• When you have written _"Cleared"_ on the required number of consecutive Base Schedule days in Level 5, go to _Self-Assessment 3H_ for clearance to enter Phase Four.

Worksheet 3G1: Evaluate Log Form S for Self-Paced Plan (Level 0)

1. Evaluate your ability to fitness-walk your *Base Schedule* according to the instructions in Chapter 15 of *The Running Injury Recovery Program*:	Did you have any increase in pain or break in form during your 60-minute fitness walk?	Yes	No
2. Evaluate your notes:	A. Did you note any weakness, asymmetry, or problem with your stride?	Yes	No
	B. Are you aware of any other problem that you need to work on before progressing to Walk/Glide sets?	Yes	No

Worksheet 3G1: Evaluate Log Form S for Self-Paced Plan (Levels 1 through 5)

1. Evaluate your ability to perform each part of your *Base Schedule* according to the instructions in Chapter 15 of *The Running Injury Recovery Program*:	A. *Warmup:* Did you have any increase in pain or break in form during your 10-minute fitness walk?	Yes	No
	B. *Walk/glide sets:* Did you have any increase in pain or break in form during walk/glide sets?	Yes	No
	C. *Glide drills:* Did you have any difficulty performing any of the drills with correct form (as described in the instructions for that drill)?	Yes	No
	D. *Cooldown:* Did you have any increase in pain or break in form during your 5-minute fitness walk?	Yes	No
2. Evaluate completion of all drills:	A. Were you *unable* to complete the required time (*duration*) for any drill?	Yes	No
	B. Were you *unable* to complete the required number of sets (*repetitions*) for any drill?	Yes	No
3. Evaluate your notes:	A. Did you note any weakness, asymmetry, or problem with your stride?	Yes	No
	B. Do you have any other problem that you need to work on before progressing to the next level?	Yes	No
4. Level 5 only: Continue until the two numbers on the right match:	Write your number of *Target Days per Week* (3, 4, or 5).		
	Write the number of consecutive days you have cleared your Base Schedule at Level 5 with no break in form and no increase in symptoms.		

Self-Assessment 3G2 for Two-Week-Interval Plan: Base Schedule Clearance (Levels 0 through 5)

Course Map references: 15.13B through 15.31B

Instructions:

1. Do this Self-Assessment if you are in Group 2A or 2B.

2. Read the **Instructions for Log Form S**, and start with the form for **Level 0**.

3. Complete one square of **Log Form S** for each day of your Base Schedule, and evaluate it for clearance to the next higher level.

4. At each level, clear a consecutive number of Base Schedule Days equal to two times your number of *Target Days per Week.*

Self-Assessment: Complete one **Worksheet 3G2** for each Level of **Log Form S** (see *Samples* in *Case Studies*).

***

What to do now:

• If you answered *"No"* to ALL questions in **Worksheet 3G2**, write *"Cleared"* on your **Log Form R** for that day, and continue at the same level until you have *cleared* the number of consecutive Base Schedule days that equals two times your number of *target days per week.*

• If you answered *"Yes"* to ANY question in **Worksheet 3G2**, continue with your Base Schedule at the same level, and start over counting toward the number of consecutive days required for clearance at that level.

• When you have *cleared* the number of consecutive Base Schedule days that equals two times your number of *target days per week* (6 to 10 consecutive Base Schedule days) you may progress to the next level of **Log Form S** (Levels 0 through 5).

• When you have written *"Cleared"* on the required number of consecutive Base Schedule days in Level 5, go to *Self-Assessment 3H* for clearance to enter Phase Four.

Worksheet 3G2: Evaluate Log Form S for Two-Week-Interval Plan (Level 0)

1. Evaluate your ability to fitness-walk your Base Schedule according to the instructions in Chapter 15 of *The Running Injury Recovery Program*:	Did you have any increase in pain or break in form during your 60-minute fitness walk?	Yes	No
2. Evaluate your notes:	A. Did you note any weakness, asymmetry, or problem with your stride?	Yes	No
	B. Are you aware of any other problem that you need to work on before progressing to Walk/Glide sets?	Yes	No
3. Level 0: Continue until the two numbers on the right match:	Multiply your number of *Target Days per Week* (3, 4, or 5) times two.		
	Write the number of consecutive days you have cleared your Base Schedule at Level 0 with no break in form and no increase in symptoms.		

Worksheet 3G2: Evaluate Log Form S for Two-Week-Interval Plan (Levels 1 through 5)

1. Evaluate your ability to perform each part of your Base Schedule according to the instructions in Chapter 15 of *The Running Injury Recovery Program*:	A. *Warmup:* Did you have any increase in pain or break in form during your 10-minute fitness walk?	Yes	No
	B. *Walk/glide sets:* Did you have any increase in pain or break in form during walk/glide sets?	Yes	No
	C. *Glide drills:* Did you have any difficulty performing any of the drills with correct form (as described in the instructions for that drill)?	Yes	No
	D. *Cooldown:* Did you have any increase in pain or break in form during your 5-minute fitness walk?	Yes	No
2. Evaluate completion of all drills:	A. Were you *unable* to complete the required time (*duration*) for any drill?	Yes	No
	B. Were you *unable* to complete the required number of sets (*repetitions*) for any drill?	Yes	No
3. Evaluate your notes:	A. Did you note any weakness, asymmetry, or problem with your stride?	Yes	No
	B. Do you have any other problem that you need to work on before progressing to the next level?	Yes	No
4. Levels 1 through 5: Continue until the two numbers on the right match.	Multiply your number of *Target Days per Week* (3, 4, or 5) times two.		
	Write the number of consecutive days you have cleared your Base Schedule at this level with no break in form and no increase in symptoms?		

Self Assessment 3H:
Phase Three Clearance and Preparation for Phase Four

Group 1 Course map references: 15.24A, 15.25A, 15.26A
Group 1 Course map references: 15.32B, 15.33B, 15.34B

Instructions:

1. Follow the instructions in *Self-Assessment Part 1* for clearance to enter Phase Four.

2. Follow the instructions in *Self-Assessment Part 2* to write your *Specific Mental Focus Statement* and prepare your log forms for Phase Four.

Self-Assessment 3H Part 1: **Phase Three Clearance**

Complete **Worksheet 3H1** below:

Worksheet 3H1: Phase Three Clearance		
1. Have you cleared all of your Regional Closed-Chain Exercises through Stage 1 (*Self-Assessment 3F*)?	No	Yes
2. Have you cleared your Base Schedule through Level 5 (*Self-Assessment 3G1 or 3G2*)?	No	Yes

A. If you answered YES to both questions, you are cleared to enter Phase Four.

B. If you have cleared your Base Schedule through Level 5, but have *not* cleared Regional Closed-Chain Exercises through Stage 1, continue with your Base Schedule at Level 5 until all Regional Closed-Chain Exercises are cleared.

C. If you have cleared all of your Regional Closed-Chain Exercises through Stage 1, but have *not* cleared your Base Schedule through Level 5, continue with your Regional Closed-Chain Exercises in Stage 2 until you have cleared your Base Schedule at Level 5.

**Self-Assessment 3H Part 2:** **Prepare your Log Forms for Phase Four** (see _Sample_ **Log Forms R** and **S** in _Case Studies_).

1. Add Hill Closed-Chain Exercises to your P.T. Time (**Log Form R**):

   A. Go to _Appendix Z: Regional Closed-Chain Tables for Fitness Runners and Racers,_ and find the examples for Hill Closed-Chain Exercises.

   B. Copy the information for Hill CC#1 and Hill CC#2 to your **Log Form R**, after your Regional Closed-Chain Exercises.

   C. Copy only the _Final Target_ for your group (Fitness or Racing).

   D. Copy _Footnote A_ to Log Form R _Notes_.

2. Write your _Specific Mental Focus Statement_ for Phase Four:

   A. Review your _Impairment Statements_ (**Worksheet T: Training Plan for Phase Three Part Two**).

   B. Go to _Appendix R: Regional Plans_ and locate the plans for your injury regions. For each injury region, find the line for _Specific Mental Focus Statement_ in the section for _Goals._

   C. Write your own _Specific Mental Focus Statement_ for Phase Four. It must be a positive statement that helps you focus on what you need to do to improve your stride, as it relates to your specific injury. Write your statement in any words that make sense to you.
   • If you have a _simple injury_, you may use the _Specific Mental Focus Statement_ in _Appendix R_ for your one region, or you may modify this statement based on your _Impairment Statement._
   • If you have a _complex injury_ involving two or more regions, write a personalized statement that includes all of your regions and impairments.

Specific Mental Focus Statement:

---

3. Prepare **Log Form S** for Phase Four:

A. In the box at the top of each **Log Form S** (Level 6, Level 7, and Level 8), find the time goals for your group (Fitness Runners or Racers). Circle the goals for your group and cross out the goals for the other group.

B. Copy your *Specific Mental Focus Statement* for Phase Four to the line for Mental Focus Statement.

C. Fill in your number of Target Days per Week (3, 4, or 5). If you have less than 5 target days per week, cross out the extra squares for each week.

What to do now:

1. As you enter Phase Four:
• Continue with your PT Time (**Log Form M** and **Log Form R, Stage 2**) two days per week.
• Continue with your Base Schedule, starting with **Log Form S, Level 6** (accelerations).

2. Check the lines on your Course Map that are appropriate for your group and continue.

***

Instructions for Log Form M: Maintain Mobility

1. Do not use this form until you have cleared Phase Two, and met the mobility requirements for your treatment group (*Table 11-1 or 11-2*).

2. When you begin Phase Three, you can start using this short form to record your Stretch/Mobilization Cycles, in place of *Log Form C*: **Stretch/Mobilization Cycles.** Continue using this form throughout Phases Three and Four. There is no clearance requirement for this form.

3. In Phases Three and Four, 20 minutes of P.T. time are allocated to stretches and self/mobilizations. During this time you should do all 13 stretches, in any order you prefer, following the instructions for *Stretch/Mobilization Cycles for Unaffected Regions* [**Box 11-2B**].

4. Monitor your pain level, stiffness in stretches, and tenderness in self-mobilizations, and record the maximum levels for each stretch, on each side.

5. Check the boxes for symmetry based on stiffness – not pain or tenderness in the self-mobilizations. Your goal is to maintain the flexibility and symmetry you achieved in Phase Two, with no increase in pain.

Log Form M: Maintain Mobility

DAY/DATE	Days since *last day you ran*:
PHASE #	Days in this Phase:

	Stretch/Mobilization Cycles	Left		Right		Symmetry	
Enter your exercise list from *Self-Assessment*		**Pain** (0-10)	**Stiffness / Tenderness** (0-5)	**Pain** (0-10)	**Stiffness / Tenderness** (0-5)	**No**	**Yes**
Set 1	Stretch #						
	Self-Mob s						
Set 2	Stretch #						
	Self-Mobs						
Set 3	Stretch #						
	Self-Mobs						
Set 4	Stretch #						
	Self-Mobs						
Set 5	Stretch #						
	Self-Mobs						
Set 6	Stretch #						
	Self-Mobs						
Set 7	Stretch #						
	Self-Mobs						
Set 8	Stretch #						
	Self-Mobs						
Set 9	Stretch #						
	Self-Mobs						
Set 10	Stretch #						
	Self-Mobs						
Set 11	Stretch #						
	Self-Mobs						
Set 12	Stretch #						
	Self-Mobs						
Set 13	Stretch #						
	Self-Mobs						

Instructions for Log Form B: Basic Closed-Chain

1. At the top of **Log Form B**, enter the day and date, and the number of days that have passed since the *last day you ran* (**Worksheet 1B1: Running History**, line 1).

2. Fill in the boxes for Phase Three Part One or Part Two, and the number of consecutive days since you began Phase Three.

3. Fill in the box for your affected side (right or left) and list your affected regions on that side. If you have affected regions on both sides, list each injury separately (*example:* left knee, right knee).

4. Choose four of the eight Basic Closed-Chain Exercises to do on the first day. Perform each exercise for 10 minutes, carefully following the guidelines in **BOX 14-3** and the instructions for exercises CC# 14-1 through CC#14-8 in **BOX 14-2.**

5. In the boxes marked *Set Times* (1 through 5) on your **Log Form B**, record the times for 5 sets of each exercise on each leg (preferably the first two sets and the last three sets). Your goal is to match your set times with the *Target Time* for each exercise.

6. For each exercise, record your maximum level of *Pain* (0 to 10) on each side.

7. When you have completed your daily P.T. Time, calculate your average time per set. [Add the set times in each column. Enter the total number of seconds for each side under *Total*. Divide the Total by the number of sets.] Write the result (rounded off to the nearest whole second) in the box marked *Average Set Time*.

8. Calculate the difference in average set time between left and right sides [subtract the lower number from the higher number], and enter that number in the box marked *Left-Right Difference*. For each exercise, compare your *Left-Right Difference* to the *Symmetry Goal* (on the line below) to see whether or not you have achieved symmetry of time for that exercise.

9. *Special instructions for exercise CC#6 (Quick Steps):* Enter the average time per set, and evaluate your symmetry based on correct form and pain levels rather than time (see **Box 14-3 line 11**: Special Instructions for Quick Steps).

Log Form B: Basic Closed-Chain

DAY/DATE		Days since *last day you ran:*
PHASE 3, Part#		Days in this Phase
AFFECTED SIDE and REGION(S)		

Basic Closed-Chain Exercise	CC#1 Square Hops		CC#2 Side Step-Down		CC#3 One-Leg Armswings, Barefoot		CC#4 One-Leg Armswings, 1 Pillow	
Target Time	20 sec		20 sec		15 sec		30 sec	
Rest Between Sets	10 sec		0		0		0	
Set Times	Left	Right	Left	Right	Left	Right	Left	Right
1								
2								
3								
4								
5								
Total								
Avg Set Time								
L/R Difference								
Symmetry Goal	1 sec		1 sec		1 sec		2 sec	
Max Pain (0-10)	L:	R:	L:	R:	L:	R:	L:	R:
NOTES:								

DAY/DATE		Days since *last day you ran:*	Days in this Phase

Basic Closed-Chain Exercise	CC#5 Barefoot Push-Up		CC#6 Quick Steps	CC#7 Weighted Kickback		CC#8 Box Step Up and Over	
Target Time	15 sec		20 sec	60 sec		60 sec	
Rest Between Sets	0		10 sec	0		0	
Set Times	Left	Right	Both Legs [A]	Left	Right	Left	Right
1							
2							
3							
4							
5							
Total							
Avg Set Time							
L/R Difference							
Symmetry Goal	1 sec			3 sec		3 sec	
Max Pain (0-10)	L:	R:	L: R:	L:	R:	L:	R:
NOTES:							

[A] See instructions line 9: *Special Instructions for Quick Steps*

Instructions for Log Form R: Regional Closed-Chain

Note: See examples of **Log Forms R** in *Section 3: Case Studies*. Review the guidelines in **Box 14-4** for *Regional Closed-Chain, Stage 1* (Symmetry and Clearance); and *Regional Closed-Chain, Stage 2* (Building to Final Target).

Part 1: Regional Closed-Chain, Stage 1 (Symmetry and Clearance)

1. On your first day of Regional Closed-Chain Exercises, use the **Log Form(s) R** that you prepared in *Self-Assessment 3C*.

2. Note that one **Log Form R** contains sections for two days of PT Time. Fill in one section of Log **Form R** (and one **Log Form M**) for each day of PT Time.

3. Enter your tracking information at the top of **Log Form R**: the day and date, the number of days that have passed since the *last day you ran* (**Worksheet 1B1: Running History**, line 1), the phase you are in, and the number of days you have been using this form.

4. On each day of PT Time, perform 4 exercises from your **Log Form R**. Carefully follow the instructions in **Box 14-2** for each exercise. Note that exercises 1 through 8 have instructions for both Regional Closed-Chain and Basic Closed-Chain. If your Regional Plan includes any of these exercises, skip the instructions for *Basic Closed-Chain Clearance*.

5. Before you begin each exercise, note whether that exercise is to be performed continuously, or with rest between sets (*Log Form R, line 2*). Spend a total of 10 minutes on each exercise. Perform each exercise first on your stronger leg, and continue until you start to become fatigued or break form. Record this time as *Set Time 1* for that leg. Repeat on the other leg. Record the times for 5 sets on each leg (preferably the first two sets and the last three sets). If an exercise has less than 5 sets in 10 minutes, record all completed sets. Count only sets that are completed with correct form and no increase in pain.

6. For each exercise, record your maximum level of *Pain* (0 to 10) on each side.

7. When you have completed your PT Time, calculate your *Average Set Times*. [Add the set times in each column, and enter the total for each side under *Total*. Divide the *Total* by the number of sets.] Write the result (rounded off to the nearest whole second) in the box marked *Average Set Time*. Calculate the difference in average set time between left and right sides [subtract the lower number from the higher number], and enter that number in the box marked *Left-Right Difference*.

8. Initial Assessment, Stage 1: Fill In Symmetry Target and Symmetry Goal

A. Perform this assessment *only* on the first day for each Regional Closed-Chain Exercise. After the first day for each exercise, skip to line 9.

B. After you complete **Log Form R**, look at the *Average Set Times* for left and right sides, and circle or highlight the higher number in each pair, even if it is on the injury side.

C. Copy the highlighted number to the line for *Symmetry Target* for that exercise.

D. Compare the *Symmetry Target* time to the *Final Target* time. For Stage 1, cross out the *higher* number and use the remaining number as your *Symmetry Target* time per leg for that exercise.

E. Go to *Table R1*: **Symmetry Goals for Closed-Chain** below. Find the *Symmetry Goal* that corresponds to your *Symmetry Target* for each exercise, and enter it on the appropriate line on **Log Form R.**

F. Use this *Symmetry Target* and *Symmetry Goal* on all of your **Log Forms R**, until you have cleared all Regional Closed-Chain Exercises in Stage 1.

9. At the end of each P.T. Time, evaluate your **Log Form R** for symmetry and pain level (*Self-Assessment 3F*).

10. As you achieve clearance for each exercise, write "*Cleared*" on your log form and skip that exercise during your next P.T. Time (to clear Stage 1 more quickly). When you have less than 4 exercises to clear in Stage 1, add back exercises you have already cleared, so you always have 4 closed-chain exercises during P.T. Time.

11. Proceed to *Part 2* when you have cleared all Regional Closed-Chain Exercises in Stage 1.

Part 2: Regional Closed-Chain, Stage 2 (Build to Final Target)

1. Revise **Log Form R** for Stage 2 (Build to Final Target):

A. Start over with a clean copy of the **Log Form R** that you prepared in *Self-Assessment 3C*.

B. Cross out the line for *Symmetry Target* on your **Log Form R**.

C. Make sure the lines for *Rest Between Sets*, *Final Target*, and *Build pace as* are filled in with the correct information for your group from *Appendix Z: Regional Closed-Chain Tables for Fitness Runners and Racers*.

D. The line for *Symmetry Goal* is blank. Go to *Table R1*: **Symmetry Goals for Closed-Chain**, and enter the appropriate symmetry goals for your *Final Target* for each exercise.

E. During your P.T. Time, rotate though all of the Regional Closed-Chain Exercises on **Log Form R**, in order, four at a time, and record your time per set as in

Stage 1. Do not skip any exercises. Follow this schedule until you complete Phase Four in your recovery program. There is no further clearance for these exercises.

2. Evaluate **Log Form R** for symmetry (not clearance):

A. In Stage 2, restart all Regional Closed-Chain Exercises on **Log Form R** at symmetry level (Stage 1 clearance level) and build your time and pace toward your *Final Target*. Follow the guidelines in the line for *Build pace as* (glide pace or acceleration).

B. Build your time and pace slowly to maintain symmetry and prevent any increase in pain level. After each day of PT Time, compare your *Left/Right Difference* with your *Symmetry Goal* for Stage 2. (For exercises that use both legs, monitor your symmetry in form and pain levels only.)

Part 3: Hill Closed-Chain

1. When you begin Phase Four (Base Schedule Level 6), add Hill Closed-Chain Exercises [**Box 16-2**] to your **Log Form R**, and follow the guidelines for *Clearance* to begin Hill Training.

2. Continue using this form in Phase Four to monitor symmetry and pain levels for all your Regional Closed-Chain Exercises, and build your time and pace toward your *Final Target*.

Table R1: Symmetry Goals for Closed-Chain (Left/Right time within 5%)			
For Symmetry Target		**For Final Target**	
Average time on better leg:	**L/R Difference no more than:**	**Final Target:**	**L/R Difference no more than:**
05 *to* 20 sec	1 sec	30 sec	2 sec
21 *to* 40 sec	2 sec	50 to 60 sec	3 sec
41 *to* 60 sec	3 sec	90 sec	5 sec
61 *to* 80 sec	4 sec	2.5 min	8 sec
81 *to* 90 sec	5 sec	5 min	15 sec

Log Form R: Regional Closed-Chain

DAY/DATE:		Days since *last day you ran:*	
PHASE (3 or 4):		Days in this Phase:	
Injury Region(s) and Side:			

Regional Closed-Chain Exercise (number and name)	CC#		CC#		CC#		CC#	
Symmetry Target								
Rest Between Sets								
Final Target								
Build pace as:								
Set Times	Left	Right	Left	Right	Left	Right	Left	Right
1								
2								
3								
4								
5								
Total								
Avg Set Time								
L/R Difference								
Symmetry Goal		sec		sec		sec		sec
Max Pain (0-10)	L:	R:	L:	R:	L:	R:	L:	R:
NOTES:								
FOOTNOTES:								

DAY/DATE:		Days since *last day you ran:*	Days in this Phase:

Regional Closed-Chain Exercise (number and name)	CC#		CC#		CC#		CC#	
Symmetry Target								
Rest Between Sets								
Final Target								
Build pace as:								
Set Times	Left	Right	Left	Right	Left	Right	Left	Right
1								
2								
3								
4								
5								
Total								
Avg Set Time								
L/R Difference								
Symmetry Goal		sec		sec		sec		sec
Max Pain (0-10)	L:	R:	L:	R:	L:	R:	L:	R:
NOTES:								
FOOTNOTES:								

Instructions for Log Form S:
Base Schedule Levels 0 through 5

1. Start using **Log Form S: Base Schedule**, when you begin Phase Three Part Two. Groups 1B, 2A, and 2B will start with **Log Form S, Level 0** and progress through each level in order to Level 5. Group 1A will begin at the level determined in *Self-Assessment 3E* and progress through each level in order to Level 5.

2. Use the correct **Log Form S** for each Level (0 through 5).

3. Follow the guidelines for the *Self-Paced Plan* or the *Two-Week Interval Plan* in **BOX 15-1:** *HOW TO* **Build Your Walk/Glide Program.**

4. In Phase Three Part Two (Levels 0 through 5), carefully follow the instructions for fitness walking [**Box 15-2**], glides [**Box 15-3**], and glide drills [**Box 15-4**]. Follow the guidelines in *Table 15-4 A through E* for inserting glide drills into your glide time. (Guidelines for each level are also summarized at the top of each **Log Form S**.)

5. On your *first day* at each Level, fill in the following tracking information at the top of the form: *Starting Day/Date, Days since the last day you ran (on starting day)* and *Target Days per week* (from your **Worksheet T**). **Log Form S** has squares for five Target Days per week on each line. If your target is 3 or 4 days per week, *cross out* the extra squares and leave either 3 or 4 empty squares on each line.

6. On each day of Base Schedule time, fill in *one square* on your **Log Form S**. Enter the *Day* and *Date* on the top line. Enter your maximum level of *Pain (0-10)* during exercise on the second line. On the line for *Drills/Form*, enter the number of sets of drills (*i.e.* glide drills, acceleration drills, hills, or plyometrics) you completed that day with correct form, symmetry, and no increase in pain. Use the line for *Notes* to list any areas of difficulty (*e.g.* symmetry, balance, stability on landing or pushoff) or write "*Cleared.*" Feel free to use a separate journal if you need more room for your notes.

7. Evaluate each **Log Form S** for clearance before moving to the next higher level.

8. On your *last day* in each Level, fill in the *Clearance date* at the top of the form, and start your next level of **Log Form S**.

9. Clear your Base Schedule through Level 5 (*Self-Assessment 3G1 or 3G2*), and Regional Closed-Chain Exercises (*Self Assessment 3F: Regional Closed-Chain, Stage 1*), before progressing to Phase Four /Base Schedule Level 6.

Log Form S: Base Schedule
Level 0 (Groups 1B, 2A and 2B Only)

	Activity	Type	Repetitions	Duration	Total Time
Starting Day/Date:			Days since *last day you ran* (on starting day):		
Target Days per week (3, 4, 5)			Clearance date:		
Warmup	Fitness walk				10 min
Base Schedule	Fitness walk				50 min
Cooldown	Fitness walk				5 min

	Day/Date	Day/Date	Day/Date	Day/Date	Day/Date
Week 1	/	/	/	/	/
Pain (0-10)					
Notes:					
Week 2	/	/	/	/	/
Pain (0-10)					
Notes:					
Week 3	/	/	/	/	/
Pain (0-10)					
Notes:					
Week 4	/	/	/	/	/
Pain (0-10)					
Notes:					

Log Form S: Base Schedule
Level 1

Starting Day/Date:			**Days since *last day you ran*** (on starting day):	
Target Days per week (3, 4, 5)			**Clearance date:**	

	Activity	**Type**	**Repetitions**	**Duration**	**Total Time**
Warmup	Fitness Walk				10 min
Base Schedule (*Table 15-4A*)	Walk/glide sets	Glide 1min/walk 4 min	10		50 min
	10 Glide Drills:	Drill #1	2	15 sec	
		Drill #2	2	15 sec	
		Drill #3	2	15 sec	
		Drill #4	2	15 sec	
		Drill #5	2	15 sec	
Cooldown	Fitness Walk				5 min

	Day/Date	Day/Date	Day/Date	Day/Date	Day/Date
Week 1	/	/	/	/	/
Pain (0-10)					
Drills/Form					
Notes:					
Week 2	/	/	/	/	/
Pain (0-10)					
Drills/Form					
Notes:					
Week 3	/	/	/	/	/
Pain (0-10)					
Drills/Form					
Notes:					
Week 4	/	/	/	/	/
Pain (0-10)					
Drills/Form					
Notes:					

Log Form S: Base Schedule
Level 2

Starting Day/Date:			**Days since *last day you ran* (on starting day):**		
Target Days per week (3, 4, 5)			**Clearance date:**		
	Activity	Type	Repetitions	Duration	Total Time
Warmup	Fitness Walk				10 min
Base Schedule (*Table 15-4B*)	Walk/glide sets	Glide 2 min/walk 3 min	10		
	15 Glide Drills:	Drill #1	3	15 sec	50 min
		Drill #2	3	15 sec	
		Drill #3	3	15 sec	
		Drill #4	3	15 sec	
		Drill #5	3	15 sec	
Cooldown	Fitness Walk				5 min

	Day/Date	Day/Date	Day/Date	Day/Date	Day/Date
Week 1	/	/	/	/	/
Pain (0-10)					
Drills/Form					
Notes:					
Week 2	/	/	/	/	/
Pain (0-10)					
Drills/Form					
Notes:					
Week 3	/	/	/	/	/
Pain (0-10)					
Drills/Form					
Notes:					
Week 4	/	/	/	/	/
Pain (0-10)					
Drills/Form					
Notes:					

Log Form S: Base Schedule
Level 3

Starting Day/Date:			Days since *last day you ran* (on starting day):		
Target Days per week (3, 4, 5)			Clearance date:		
	Activity	Type	Repetitions	Duration	Total Time
Warmup	Fitness Walk				10 min
Base Schedule (*Table 15-4C*)	Walk/glide sets	Glide 3 min/walk 2 min	10		50 min
	15 Glide Drills:	Drill #1	3	15 sec	
		Drill #2	3	15 sec	
		Drill #3	3	15 sec	
		Drill #4	3	15 sec	
		Drill #5	3	15 sec	
Cooldown	Fitness Walk				5 min

	Day/Date	Day/Date	Day/Date	Day/Date	Day/Date
Week 1	/	/	/	/	/
Pain (0-10)					
Drills/Form					
Notes:					
Week 2	/	/	/	/	/
Pain (0-10)					
Drills/Form					
Notes:					
Week 3	/	/	/	/	/
Pain (0-10)					
Drills/Form					
Notes:					
Week 4	/	/	/	/	/
Pain (0-10)					
Drills/Form					
Notes:					

Log Form S: Base Schedule
Level 4

	Starting Day/Date:			Days since *last day you ran* (on starting day):		
	Target Days per week (3, 4, 5)			Clearance date:		
	Activity	**Type**	**Repetitions**	**Duration**	**Total Time**	
Warmup	Fitness Walk				10 min	
Base Schedule (*Table 15-4D*)	Walk/glide sets	Glide 4 min/walk 1 min	10		50 min	
	15 Glide Drills:	Drill #1	3	15 sec		
		Drill #2	3	15 sec		
		Drill #3	3	15 sec		
		Drill #4	3	15 sec		
		Drill #5	3	15 sec		
Cooldown	Fitness Walk				5 min	

	Day/Date	Day/Date	Day/Date	Day/Date	Day/Date
Week 1	/	/	/	/	/
Pain (0-10)					
Drills/Form					
Notes:					
Week 2	/	/	/	/	/
Pain (0-10)					
Drills/Form					
Notes:					
Week 3	/	/	/	/	/
Pain (0-10)					
Drills/Form					
Notes:					
Week 4	/	/	/	/	/
Pain (0-10)					
Drills/Form					
Notes:					

Log Form S: Base Schedule
Level 5

Starting Day/Date:			Days since *last day you ran* (on starting day):		
Target Days per week (3, 4, 5)			**Clearance date:**		
	Activity	**Type**	**Repetitions**	**Duration**	**Total Time**
Warmup	Fitness Walk				10 min
Base Schedule	Glides	50-minute glides			
(*Table 15-4E*)	15 Glide Drills:	Drill #1	3	15 sec ea	
		Drill #2	3	15 sec ea	
		Drill #3	3	15 sec ea	50 min
		Drill #4	3	15 sec ea	
		Drill #5	3	15 sec ea	
Cooldown	Fitness Walk				5 min

	Day/Date	Day/Date	Day/Date	Day/Date	Day/Date
Week 1	/	/	/	/	/
Pain (0-10)					
Drills/Form					
Notes:					
Week 2	/	/	/	/	/
Pain (0-10)					
Drills/Form					
Notes:					
Week 3	/	/	/	/	/
Pain (0-10)					
Drills/Form					
Notes:					
Week 4	/	/	/	/	/
Pain (0-10)					
Drills/Form					
Notes:					

PHASE FOUR WORKBOOK

When you reach Phase Four, all signs and symptoms of your injury should be gone, and you will start doing running drills that are harder than gliding so that you can increase the load on your injured region and strengthen your body for post-recovery running. In Phase Four, everyone is in the same treatment group (*Table 16-1*), but the intensity of your training will depend upon your goals as a *Fitness Runner* or a *Racer*.

During P.T. Time, you'll continue your Stretch/Mobilization Cycles to maintain mobility **(Log Form M)**, and you'll continue your Regional Closed-Chain Exercises at the *Final Target* level **(Log Form R, Stage 2)**. Your specific *Final Target* level will depend upon whether you are a *Ftiness Runner* or *Racer* (see *Appendix Z: Closed-Chain Exercises for Fitness Runners and Racers*). Remember that *Final Target* levels are long-term goals, not clearance requirements, so always build up your time and effort slowly.

When you start Phase Four, you'll also add two Hill Closed-Chain Exercises to your Log Form R (CC#16-1 and 16-2) which you must clear at the *Symmetry Target* level before you can progress to Hill Training in your Base Schedule.

Your Base Schedule will continue through three new levels: Accelerations (**Log Form S level 6**), Hill Training (**Log Form S Level 7**) and Plyometrics (**Log Form S Level 8**). Everyone will do the same drills, but the length of the drills and the amount of rest between drills are different for *Fitness Runners* and *Racers* (see *Tables 16-2, 16-3,* and *17-1*). Once again, remember that you can't start Level 7 Hill Training until you have cleared the Hill Closed-Chain Exercises in P.T. Time.

When you have cleared Base Schedule Level 8, you are physically prepared to return to your normal running routine, but don't forget to complete your final clearance (*Self-Assessment 4D: Clearance for Post-Recovery Running*). Fill in Worksheeet 4D1, Habits For Post-Recovery Running, and take few moments to consider everything you have learned during your Recovery Program about running habits and mental focus. These are the skills that will prepare you mentally for functional running, and will actually help you avoid reinjuring yourself.

Finally, when you return to running, remember to always monitor your Injury Stages. If you address any running dysfunctions right away, and take steps to correct any factors that might contribute to an injury, you will always be a smarter and safer runner.

Table 16-1

Guidelines: Phase Four

	All Groups
P.T. Time	Continue with Stretch/Mobilization Cycles, 2 days per week, 20 minutes per day **(Log Form M).**
	1. Continue with your Regional Closed-Chain Exercises, 2 days per week, 40 minutes per day **(Log Form R).**
	2. Add Hill Closed-Chain Exercises and clear the *Symmetry Target* before progressing to Hill Drills in your Base Schedule.
Base Schedule	Continue your Base Schedule.
Acceleration Drills *(Self-Assessment 4A)*	Add Acceleration Drills (3 drills, 3 times each) into your Base Schedule **(Log Form S: Level 6).**
Hill Drills *(Self-Assessment 4B)*	Add Hill Drills (2 drills, 3 times each) into your Base Schedule **(Log Form S: Level 7).**
Plyometric Exercises *(Self-Assessment 4C)*	Add Plyometric Drills (4 drills, 3 times each) into your Base Schedule. **(Log Form S: Level 8).**
Clearance to Start Regular Training *(Self-Assessment 4D)*	Able to perform all Phase Four exercises correctly for the specified amount of time with no increase in symptoms.

Phase Four Self-Assessments

Self-Assessment 4A: Base Schedule Level 6 Clearance

Course Map reference: 16.5 through 16.12

Instructions:
1. **Log Form S Level 6**:
• Use the **Log Form S: Base Schedule Level 6** that you prepared in *Self Assessment 3H*.
• Following the **Instructions for Log Form S**, and the guidelines for acceleration drills in Chapter 16, fill in one square on **Log Form S Level 6** for each day of your Base Schedule.
• At the end of each day, evaluate your **Log Form S** for clearance.

2. Log Form R (Stage 2):
• Use the **Log Form R** that you prepared in *Self Assessment 3H*.
• At the end of each day, evaluate your **Log Form R** for clearance in Hill Closed-Chain Exercises.

Self-Assessment: Complete **Worksheet 4A1** below:

Worksheet 4A1: Level 6 Clearance			
Log Form S Level 6:	1. Are you able to perform all nine of your acceleration drills for the time required for your group (Fitness Runner or Racer), with no break in form and no increase in pain?	No	Yes
	2. Are you able to complete your Base Schedule (glides and acceleration drills) continuously for 50 minutes, with no break in form or significant increase in pain?	No	Yes
Log Form R (Stage 2)	3. Are you maintaining symmetry in all of your Regional Closed-Chain Exercises, with no significant increase in pain?	No	Yes
	4. Have you reached your *Symmetry Target* for Hill Closed-Chain Exercises 1 and 2?	No	Yes

What to do now:
• When you can answer "Yes" to all questions in **Worksheet 4A1**, you are cleared to progress to Hill Drills in your Base Schedule (**Log Form S Level 7**).
• On your next **Log Form R**, cross out the *Symmetry Target* for Hill Closed-Chain Exercises 1 and 2, and use the *Final Target* time.
• Check lines 16.5 through 16.12 on your Course Map and continue.

Self-Assessment 4B: Base Schedule Level 7 Clearance

Course Map references: 16.14 through 16.18

Instructions:
• Use the **Log Form S: Base Schedule Level 7** that you prepared in *Self Assessment 3H*.
• Following the **Instructions for Log Form S**, and the guidelines for Hill Training drills in Chapter 16, fill in one square on **Log Form S Level 7** for each day of your Base Schedule.
• At the end of each day, evaluate your **Log Form S** for clearance.

Self-Assessment: Complete **Worksheet 4B1** below:

Worksheet 4B1: Level 7 Clearance			
Log Form S Level 7:	1. Are you able to perform all six of your Hill Training drills for the time required for your group (Fitness Runner or Racer), with no break in form and no increase in pain?	No	Yes
	2. Are you able to complete your Base Schedule (glides and Hill-Training drills) continuously for 50 minutes, with no break in form or significant increase in pain?	No	Yes

What to do now:
• When you can answer "Yes" to all questions in Worksheet 4B1, you are cleared to progress to Plyometric Drills in your Base Schedule (**Log Form S Level 8**).
• Continue with **Log Form R** and **Log Form M** during your PT Time.
• Check lines 16.4 through 16.18 on your Course Map and continue.

Self-Assessment 4C:
Base Schedule Level 8 Clearance (Return to Running)

Course Map reference: 17.5 through 17.10

Instructions:
• Use the **Log Form S: Base Schedule Level 8** that you prepared in *Self Assessment 3H.*
• Read the instructions for Plyometric Drills, and carefully practice any movements that you are not familiar with before you try to insert them into your glide program.
• Following the **Instructions for Log Form S**, the guidelines for Plyometric Drills in chapter 17, and the guidelines for Glide Drills, fill in one square on **Log Form S Level 8** for each day of your Base Schedule.
• At the end of each day, evaluate your **Log Form S** for clearance.

Self-Assessment: Complete **Worksheet 4C1** below:

Worksheet 4C1: Level 8 Clearance			
Log Form S Level 8:	1. Are you able to perform all twelve of your Plyometric Drills for the time required for your group (Fitness Runner or Racer), with no break in form and no increase in pain?	No	Yes
	2. Are you able to complete your Base Schedule (glides and Plyometric Drills and Glide Drills) continuously for 50 minutes, with no break in form or significant increase in pain?	No	Yes

What to do now:
• When you can answer "Yes" to all questions in **Worksheet 4C1**, you have completed your *Running Injury Management Program.*
• Check line 17.10 on your Course Map, and continue to *Self-Assessment 4D*: Clearance for Post-Recovery Running.

Self-Assessment 4D: Clearance for Post-Recovery Running

Course map references: 18.1 through 18.8

Instructions: Prepare yourself for post-recovery running.

Self-Assessment: Complete **Worksheet 4D1** below:

Worksheet 4D1: Habits for Post-Recovery Running		
Post-Recovery Running Habits Checklist:	1. I will make a plan, and train consistently.	
	2. I will set realistic running goals.	
	3. I will start each run with a proper warmup.	
	4. I will pay close attention to my equipment, particularly my footwear.	
	5. I will focus on functional running.	
	6. I will manage my running injuries early, before they become severe.	

The most important lessons I have learned from my *Running Injury Recovery Program* that I will use when I return to regular training are:

What to do now:

• Check lines 18.1 through 18.8 on your Course Map and continue to the **Checkpoint to Return to Running.**

• Return to your regular training program, and use what you have learned to become a smarter and safer runner.

Phase Four Log Forms

Instructions for Log Form S:
Base Schedule Levels 6, 7, and 8

Lines 1 through 9: See *Instructions for Log Form S, Base Schedule Levels 0-5*. Clear your Base Schedule through Level 5 (*Self-Assessment 3G1 or 3G2: Base Schedule Clearance*), and Regional Closed-Chain Exercises (*Self Assessment 3F: Regional Closed-Chain Clearance*), before progressing to Base Schedule Level 6.

10. In Phase Four, build your drill times toward the goals for Fitness Runners or for Racers at the top of each log form.

11. At Level 6, carefully follow the instructions for acceleration drills in **Box 16-1**. Follow the guidelines in *Table 16.2* for inserting acceleration drills into your glide time (also summarized at the top of **Log Form S, Level 6**).

12. Clear Hill Closed-Chain Exercises and acceleration drills (*Self-Assessment 4A*) before progressing to Level 7.

13. At Level 7, carefully follow the guidelines for Hill Training in *Chapter16, Techniques for Hill Training*. Follow the guidelines in *Table 16.3* for inserting hill-training drills into your glide time (also summarized at the top of **Log Form S, Level 7**). Clear hill-training drills (*Self-Assessment 4B*) before progressing to Level 8.

14. At Level 8, carefully follow the instructions for plyometric drills in **Box 17-1.** Follow the guidelines in *Table 17.1* for inserting plyometric drills and glide drills into your glide time (also summarized at the top of **Log Form S, Level 8**).

15. Base Schedule Level 8 is the final clearance level in your Running Injury Recovery Program (see *Self-Assessment 4C*).

Log Form S: Base Schedule
Level 6

Starting Day/Date:				Days since *last day you ran* (on starting day):		
Target Days per week (3, 4, 5)				Clearance date:		
	Activity	Type	Reps	A. Fitness Runners	B. Racers	Total Time
Warmup	Fitness Walk					10 min
Base Schedule (*Table 16-2*)	Glides	50-min. glides				
	9 Acceleration Drills:	Drill #1	3	30 sec each	Build to 90 sec each	
		Drill #2	3			
		Drill #3	3			50 min
Cooldown	Fitness Walk					5 min
Mental Focus Statement:						

	Day/Date	Day/Date	Day/Date	Day/Date	Day/Date
Week 1	/	/	/	/	/
Pain (0-10)					
Drills/Form					
Notes:					
Week 2	/	/	/	/	/
Pain (0-10)					
Drills/Form					
Notes:					
Week 3	/	/	/	/	/
Pain (0-10)					
Drills/Form					
Notes:					
Week 4	/	/	/	/	/
Pain (0-10)					
Drills/Form					
Notes:					

Log Form S: Base Schedule
Level 7

Starting Day/Date:			**Days since _last day you ran_ (on starting day):**			
Target Days per week (3, 4, 5)			**Clearance date:**			
	Activity	**Type**	**Reps**	**A. Fitness Runners**	**B. Racers**	**Total Time**
Warmup	Fitness Walk					10 min
Base Schedule (_Table 16-3_)	Glides	50-min. glides				50 min
	6 Hill Drills:	Uphill Drill	3	90 sec each	Build to 4.5 min each	
		Downhill Drill	3	90 sec each	Build to 4.5 min each	
Cooldown	Fitness Walk					5 min
Mental Focus Statement:						

	Day/Date	Day/Date	Day/Date	Day/Date	Day/Date
Week 1	/	/	/	/	/
Pain (0-10)					
Drills/Form					
Notes:					
Week 2	/	/	/	/	/
Pain (0-10)					
Drills/Form					
Notes:					
Week 3	/	/	/	/	/
Pain (0-10)					
Drills/Form					
Notes:					
Week 4	/	/	/	/	/
Pain (0-10)					
Drills/Form					
Notes:					

Log Form S: Base Schedule
Level 8

Starting Day/Date:			Days since *last day you ran* (on starting day):			
Target Days per week (3, 4, 5)			Clearance date:			
	Activity	**Type**	**Reps**	**A. Fitness Runners**	**B. Racers**	**Total Time**
Warmup	Fitness Walk					10 min
Base Schedule (*Table 17-1*)	Glides	50-min. glides				
	12 Plyometric Drills:	Drill #1	3	15 sec each	Build to 45 sec each	50 min
		Drill #2	3			
		Drill #3	3			
		Drill #4	3			
	10 Glide Drills	5 glide drills	2 each	15 sec each	15 sec each	
Cooldown	Fitness Walk					5 min
Mental Focus Statement:						

	Day/Date	Day/Date	Day/Date	Day/Date	Day/Date
Week 1	/	/	/	/	/
Pain (0-10)					
Drills/Form					
Notes:					
Week 2	/	/	/	/	/
Pain (0-10)					
Drills/Form					
Notes:					
Week 3	/	/	/	/	/
Pain (0-10)					
Drills/Form					
Notes:					
Week 4	/	/	/	/	/
Pain (0-10)					
Drills/Form					
Notes:					

Section 3: Case Studies

Example #1: Simple Injury
"Sarah"

Example #2: Complex Injury
"Karl"

Example #3 Simple Injury with Other Running Dysfunctions
"Erica"

This section contains three examples of runners who completed *The Running Injury Recovery Workbook*. These examples will show you how runners with different histories and different types of injuries have filled out their forms, done the calculations for their Self-Assessments, and worked through the phases of recovery. No matter what your injury is like, you should find these examples helpful when you start filling out your own forms.

Note that in *Example #1*, "Sarah" has filled out all of her Worksheets and Log Forms. However, in Example #2 "Karl" and *Example #3* "Erica" only certain Worksheets and Log Forms are shown. Some of the forms they filled out were omitted because there were many copies of the same form that were very similar. Other forms are not shown simply because they chose not to fill them out.

These examples show that it is possible to benefit from doing the exercises and Self-Assessments even if you are not able to fill in your Log Forms completely, or if you just don't want to do the math. These forms are intended to help you, not to frustrate you. When you fill out your forms, do the best you can, but don't let the forms get in the way of completing your Recovery Program.

Example #1:
Simple Injury ("Sarah")

"Sarah" is a healthy young college student who is concerned because, every time she runs, she feels a pain (about 3 fingers wide) on the outside of her right knee, and a little bit behind her knee (about 2 fingers wide). The pain grabs her while she is running, and makes her stop running. When she stops running, the pain ceases and does not bother her while she is at rest (not moving). However, if she continues running after the pain starts, she feels some pain later that day when she stands up, or when she tries to climb stairs. The pain soon goes away as long as she doesn't run, and she does not take any pain medication for it. She does not notice any swelling.

Sarah reads *The Running Injury Recovery Program* textbook and decides to start the *Workbook*. She follows the Course Map, and on lines 1.1, 1.2, and 1.3 she completes Self-Assessments 1A, 1B, and 1C in her Phase One Self-Assessment.

Self-Assessment 1A:
Identifying a Running Injury

Sarah first has to find out if she has a running injury. Sarah answers "yes" to all three questions in **Worksheet 1A1: Identifying a Running Injury**, which indicates that she may indeed have a running injury.

Self-Assessment 1B:
Running History

Sarah is a Fitness Runner who has been running for about six months. Before her injury, she was trying to run about 3 days per week, about 5 miles per day (15 miles per week) – but when other things came up, she often skipped her workouts. She doesn't stretch, and she is wearing old shoes that she bought online because she liked the color. Her last training run was on Monday 3/5. At that time, she could only run about 15 minutes before her pain started. Sarah documents her Running History in **Worksheet 1B1: Running History**, and copies her answer to question 1 (*last day you ran*) at the top of **Worksheet 1D: Document Your Injury.**

Sarah reads the examples in Chapter 1 of *The Running Injury Recovery Program* and considers what risk factors may have contributed to her running injury. She lists the fact that she has been running less than one year, her lack of mobility, and her inconsistent workouts as *intrinsic* factors that she needs to work on. She lists her old shoes as an *extrinsic* factor that she can change right away.

Worksheet 1A1: Identifying a Running Injury		
1. Do you think you might have a running injury?	No	**(Yes)**
2. Do you have pain that only appears or gets worse *while* you are running OR that only appears in a regular pattern some time *after* you run?	No	**(Yes)**
3. Do your symptoms always lessen when you *stop* running (either immediately or after not running for up to two weeks)?	No	**(Yes)**

Worksheet 1B1: Running History

1. Write the exact day and date of the **last day you ran** (your last regular training session):

   _____ *Monday 3/5* _____.

2. How many years have you been running on a regular basis?
   - **(a)** Less than 1 year
   - b. 1 to 3 years
   - c. More than 3 years

3. Which type of runner are you?
   - **(a)** My primary goal is to improve my fitness (**Fitness Runner**).
   - b. My primary goal is to run faster in competitions (**Racer**).

4. Before your injury, how many *days* per week were you running on a regular basis?
   - a. 2 days or less per week
   - **(b)** 3 to 5 days per week
   - c. More than 5 days per week

5. Before your injury, how many *miles* per week were you running on a regular basis?
   - a. Less than 10 miles per week
   - **(b)** 10 to 25 miles per week
   - c. More than 25 miles per week

6. With this injury, how long could you run before the pain started?
   - a. Less than 10 minutes or 1 mile
   - **(b)** 10 to 20 minutes, or 1 to 2 miles
   - c. 20 to 30 minutes, or 2 to 3 miles
   - d. 30 to 40 minutes, or 3 to 4 miles
   - e. 40 to 50 minutes, or 4 to 5 miles
   - f. More than 50 minutes or 5 miles

7. Based on the examples in Chapter 1 of *The Running Injury Recovery Program*, list any *intrinsic* or *extrinsic* factors that you need to work on:

Intrinsic factors: Running less than 1 year, mobility, skipping workouts

Extrinsic factors: Get new shoes

Self-Assessment 1C:
Medical History

Sarah has no previous injuries, surgeries, or illnesses that might affect her running; and she takes no medication of any kind. Sarah answers "No" to all questions in **Worksheet 1C1: Medical History**, indicating that her recovery should not be complicated by medical factors.

When Sarah has completed *Self-Assessment 1C*, she checks off lines 1.1, 1.2, and 1.3 on her Course Map, and continues to the next line.

Worksheet 1C1: Medical History		
1. Have you had any previous running injuries that are not completely resolved and may still affect your running?	Yes	(No)
2. Have you had any traumatic injuries such as a fall, twist, sprain, or other accident within the past 12 months that affect your running?	Yes	(No)
3. Have you ever had surgery on any body part that might affect your running?	Yes	(No)
4. Do you have any pre-existing medical condition that affects your ability to run, such as osteoarthritis?	Yes	(No)
5. Do you take any medication for a medical condition which affects your ability to feel pain, such as a steroid or anti-inflammatory medication?	Yes	(No)

If you answered "Yes" to any question, list your conditions and/or medications here:

None

Self-Assessment 1D:
Document Your Injury and Phase One Treatment Group

Sarah has reached line 3.2 on her Course Map and is ready to document her injury in *Self-Assessment 1D*.

When Sarah runs for 15 minutes, she feels a lot of pain on the outside and back of her right knee, which she describes as a pain level of 5 or 6 (on a scale of 0 to 10). The pain goes away when she stops running but, for a day or so after she runs, she occasionally feels some pain in that area (when she stands up or climbs stairs) but not enough to make her limp or to prevent her from going about her daily routine (her "activities of daily living" or "ADLs"). She doesn't notice any swelling in her leg.

On **Worksheet 1D1: Pain Pattern**, Sarah shades in the areas where she feels pain. She now turns to *Appendix A: Index of Affected Regions* and compares her pain pattern with the regions diagrams. She finds that the areas she has shaded on **Worksheet 1D1** are included in both Region 7 (Band) and Region 8 (Hamstring). She lists both of these regions as *possible affected regions* in the box on **Worksheet 1D1.**

On **Worksheet 1D2: Swelling Within Past 2 Weeks**, she writes "no swelling."

At the top of **Worksheet 1D3: Injury Stage**, Sarah copies her two *possible affected regions* from **Worksheet 1D1**. In **Table A: Maximum Symptoms *within the past 2 weeks***, Sarah circles her maximum symptoms: She has Stage 1 symptoms (pain while running) and Stage 3 symptoms (pain when standing up and climbing stairs). She has no Red Flag symptoms. Since her injury is less than two weeks old, she leaves **Table B: Maximum Symptoms *from more than 2 weeks ago*** blank.

Sarah now fills out **Worksheet 1D4: Summary of Original Injury** (for the right side only). She circles both Region 7 (Band) and Region 8 (Hamstring) as *possible affected regions*. She has only one pain, but she has not yet identified which of these two regions is causing it. Since she doesn't know which of the two *possible affected regions* is causing her pain, she fills out the same information for both regions.

She decides that her *maximum* pain in the affected region, while running, was at level 6. She records no swelling from **Worksheet 1D2**. Her *maximum* Injury Stage (from **Worksheet 1D3**) was Stage 3, and she has no Red Flags.

When Sarah has filled in **Worksheet 1D4**, she returns to *Self-Assessment 1D* to complete her evaluation and determine her Phase One Treatment Group. Sarah finds that, since **Worksheet 1D4** shows no swelling and no Red Flags, she does not have to ICE. She circles the statement for Group 1 in **Worksheet 1D5: Phase One Treatment Group**, and begins Phase One in Group 1. She will follow the guidelines for Group 1 in *Table 5-1*: Guidelines for Phase One Treatment Groups.

Sarah checks off lines 3.2 through 3.5 on her Course Map and continues to the next line.

Worksheet 1D:
Document Your Injury and Phase One Treatment Group

Last day you ran: _Monday 3/5_   **Today's date:** _Saturday 3/10_

Worksheet 1D1: Pain Pattern

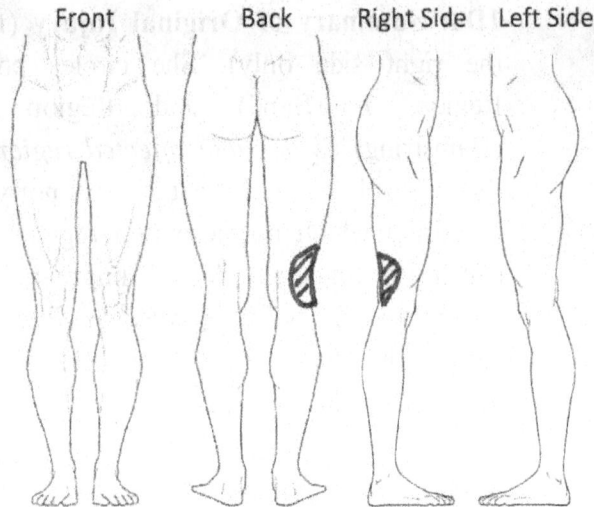

Front   Back   Right Side   Left Side

Compare to *Appendix A* and list your *possible affected regions* and side here:

_____

_____ 7. Right Band _____

_____ 8. Right Hamstring _____

_____

_____

_____

Worksheet 1D2: Swelling Within Past 2 Weeks

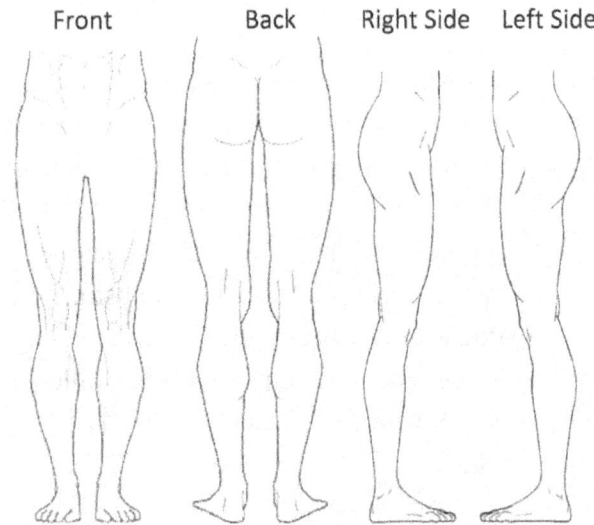

Front   Back   Right Side   Left Side

Compare to *Appendix A* and list your *possible affected regions* and side here:

_____

_____

_____ No Swelling _____

_____

_____

_____

Worksheet 1D3: Injury Stage

Injury Side and *possible affected region(s)*: ___Right Band, Right Hamstring___

Table A: Maximum Symptoms *within the past 2 weeks*

Injury Stages	Emerging Symptoms	Red Flags	Which region(s)?
Stage 1	(Pain while running)	Pain that alters your stride	Band Hamstring
Stage 2	Pain at rest (after running)	Pain that disturbs your rest	
(Stage 3)	(Pain during your normal daily activities)	Pain that interferes with or makes you avoid ADLs	Band Hamstring
Stage 4	Running injury pain that you take medication for	Being in Stage 4	
Stage 5	Pain that cripples you	Being in Stage 5	

Table B: Maximum Symptoms *from more than 2 weeks ago*   NO

Injury Stages	Emerging Symptoms	Red Flags	Which region(s)?
Stage 1	Pain while running	Pain that alters your stride	
Stage 2	Pain at rest (after running)	Pain that disturbs your rest	
Stage 3	Pain during your normal daily activities	Pain that interferes with or makes you avoid ADLs	
Stage 4	Running injury pain that you take medication for	Being in Stage 4	
Stage 5	Pain that cripples you	Being in Stage 5	

Worksheet 1D4: Summary of Original Injury

Refer to →	Worksheet 1D1: Pain Pattern	Worksheet 1D2: Swelling	Worksheet 1D3: Table A Injury Stage in Past 2 Weeks	
Left Leg Circle *Possible Affected Regions*	Pain Severity (1-10)	Swelling in past 2 weeks (yes/no)	Injury Stage Scale (1-5)	Red Flag (yes/no)
1 Toe				
2 Arch				
3 Heel				
4 Shin				
5 Calf				
6 Knee				
7 Band				
8 Hamstring				
9 Hip				
10 Buttock				

Refer to →	Worksheet 1D1: Pain Pattern	Worksheet 1D2: Swelling	Worksheet 1D3: Table A Injury Stage in Past 2 Weeks	
Right Leg Circle *Possible Affected Regions*	Pain Severity (1-10)	Swelling in past 2 weeks (yes/no)	Injury Stage Scale (1-5)	Red Flag (yes/no)
1 Toe				
2 Arch				
3 Heel				
4 Shin				
5 Calf				
6 Knee				
(7) Band	6	No	Stage 3	No
(8) Hamstring	6	No	Stage 3	No
9 Hip				
10 Buttock				

Worksheet 1D5: Phase One Treatment Group

Circle ONE of the two statements below:

I will enter Phase One injury management in treatment Group 1, and I do not have to ICE.	I will enter Phase One injury management in treatment Group 2, and I will now begin to ICE (**Log Form I**).

Self-Assessment 1E:
Document Your Injury and Phase One Treatment Group

When Sarah reaches line 9.4 on her Course Map, she has finished her Phase One education and she is ready to complete **Worksheet 1E1: Phase One Clearance**. She has protected and rested her injury, and her symptoms have improved, so she circles "yes" on all questions (skipping the last question because she is in Group 1) and continues to the next line on her Course Map.

Worksheet 1E1: Phase One Clearance

I have *no* Red Flag symptoms or visible swelling.	No	Yes
All of the emerging symptoms I recorded in Worksheets 1D1 through 1D4 have improved.	No	Yes
My sleep is not disturbed by pain due to this injury.	No	Yes
I can perform my activities of daily living (ADLs) normally, with less pain.	No	Yes
I do not need to take medication for pain and inflammation due to my running injury.	No	Yes
I have checked lines 5.1 through 9.4 on my Course Map.	No	Yes
I have followed all of the instructions in chapters 5 through 9 to implement protection and recovery for my running injury.	No	Yes
Group 2 ONLY: I have Iced 3 times a day, and the symptoms I have recorded on **Log Form I** have improved.	No	Yes

Sarah has now reached line 11.7 on her Course Map. She understands the goals of Phase Two, and she has followed the instructions for Protection and Recovery, including a new pair of well-fitted training shoes. She has assembled the equipment she needs for self-mobilizations and stretches, she has studied the instructions for Stretch/ Mobilization Cycles, and she is ready to begin *Self-Assessment 2A*.

Sarah follows the **Instructions for Worksheet 2A1: Mobility Self-Assessment** and fills in her mobility numbers for all 37 pairs of stretches. She is pleased to find out that she can match the positions shown in the book, or nearly match those positions, for most of the stretches – so her overall mobility isn't as bad as she was afraid it might be when she listed her *intrinsic* risk factors in **Worksheet 1B1: Running History.**

When Sarah has completed **Worksheet 2A1**, she returns to *Self-Assessment 2A* to evaluate her worksheet and prepare for Phase Two.

***

1. Evaluate Symmetry

After filling out her **Worksheet 2A1**, Sarah circles 15 left/right pairs with *two different numbers* (lack of symmetry).

She finds that *all* of the left/right pairs in regions 1, 2, 3, 4, and 6 have matching numbers, so these regions have symmetry. Pairs in regions 5, 7, 8, 9 and 10 do not match (have asymmetry), but she notices that region 7 (hamstring) has a greater amount of asymmetry than the other regions (a greater difference between the higher and lower numbers).

2. Order Stretches for Affected Regions

On her **Worksheet 2A1**, Sarah has circled regions 7 and 8 on the *right* side as *possible affected regions*. In these columns, she sees that exercises 11-3 and 11-6 have the greatest differences in mobility and the greatest stiffnesses on the right side, so she circles the *right* side for exercises 11-3 and 11-6 and numbers them #1 and #2.

There are 7 stretches (11-3 through 11-9) associated with regions 7 and 8. Sarah continues to circle and number these stretches, *on the right side only*, in order of asymmetry and stiffness. She checks to make sure she has circled all of the stretch numbers and "right" for each of these stretches.

3. Order Stretches for Unaffected Regions

Sarah has ranked stretches 11-3 through 11-9 on the *affected* (right) side with numbers 1 through 7, so she numbers the same stretches on the *unaffected* (left) side with numbers 8 through 14. (She does not circle the word "left.")

Sarah now numbers all of the remaining stretches on **Worksheet 2A1** in pairs (left and right), in order of asymmetry and stiffness. Stretches 11-11, 11-2, and 11-13 show some asymmetry, so she numbers them 15/16, 17/18, and 19/20, respectively.

Worksheet 2A1: Mobility Self-Assessment

Circle *Possible Affected Region* and Side →

Stretch	SIDE / Rank #	1: Toe	2: Arch	3: Heel	4: Shin	5: Calf	6: Knee	(7: Band)	(8: Hams)	9: Hip	10:Butt
		Left	Left	Left	Left	Left	Left	Left	Left	Left	Left
		Right	Right	Right	Right	Right	Right	(Right)	(Right)	Right	Right
11-1	Left: #25	0									
	Right: #26	0									
Notes:											
11-2	Left: #17			0	1	(0)					
	Right: #18			0	1	(1)					
Notes:											
(**11-3**)	Left: #8								1		
	(Right: #1)								4		
Notes:											
(**11-4**)	Left: #10								2	1	0
	(Right: #3)								4	2	0
Notes:											
(**11-5**)	Left: #11	0	0	0	1	(0)	0		2		
	(Right: #4)	0	0	0	1	(2)	0		4		
Notes:											
(**11-6**)	Left: #9			0	1	(0)			1		
	(Right: #2)			0	1	(2)			4		
Notes:											
(**11-7**)	Left: #12			0	1	(0)		2	2		
	(Right: #5)			0	1	(2)		3	4		
Notes:											
(**11-8**)	Left: #13							2			0
	(Right: #6)							3			0
Notes:											
(**11-9**)	Left: #14							2			0
	(Right: #7)							3			0
Notes:											
11-10	Left: #21					0				1	
	Right: #22					0				1	
Notes:											
11-11	Left: #15									1	0
	Right: #16									2	0
Notes:											
11-12	Left: #23									1	
	Right: #24									1	
Notes:											
11-13	Left: #19		0	0	1	(0)					
	Right: #20		0	0	1	(2)					
Notes:											

Stretches 11-10 and 11-12 show some stiffness but not asymmetry, so they are next on the list at numbers 21/22 and 23/24. Finally, stretch number 11-1 shows neither asymmetry nor stiffness, and is at the end of the list with numbers 25/26. She does not circle the stretch numbers or left/right for any of these stretches.

Sarah's **Worksheet 2A1** now has a list of 26 stretches in the order in which she will do her exercises in Phase Two.

4. List stretches in order on Log Form C: Stretch/Mobilization Cycles

Sarah enters the stretch numbers from her **Worksheet 2A1** in order (1 through 26) on her first **Log Form C** [*see Sample 1A Log Form C*]. She circles the rank number on the *affected* (right) *side only* for stretches 11-3 through 11-9.

At the top of her **Log Form C**, Sarah writes in her affected side (right) and *possible affected regions* (hamstring and band).

5. Complete Worksheet 2A2: Ranking Affected Regions

Before Sarah can finish her **Log Form C**, she must complete **Worksheet 2A2: Ranking Affected Regions.** At the top, she writes in her affected side (right). In the left-hand column, she circles her two *possible affected regions* (hamstring and band).

She looks at her **Worksheet 2A1: Mobility Self-Assessment** and finds the *maximum stiffness* on each side (left and right) in each region, and enters those numbers in the appropriate columns in

Worksheet 2A2: Ranking Affected Regions. She circles all of the entries that are greater than zero (for shin, calf, band, hamstring, and hip).

Sarah looks again at her **Worksheet 2A1: Mobility Self-Assessment** and finds the highlighted pair in each region that has the *maximum asymmetry* (greatest difference between left and right), and enters those numbers in the appropriate column in **Worksheet 2B: Ranking Affected Regions.** She circles all of the entries that have asymmetry (calf, band, hamstring, and hip).

Sarah then goes to her **Worksheet 1D4: Summary of Original Injury** and copies her information to the appropriate columns in **Worksheet 2A2: Ranking Affected Regions**. She circles all of the outstanding entries for calf, band, hamstring, and hip.

Looking at all of her entries in **Worksheet 2A2: Ranking Affected Regions**, Sarah writes an *assessment* of each region that has any highlighted signs or symptoms. For band and hamstring, she writes "*possible affected region.*" For the unaffected regions (shin, calf, and hip) she writes the main problems she needs to work on in each region.

Sarah now ranks all the regions she needs to work on in order of severity, starting with her *possible affected regions*. The right hamstring is #1, followed by the right band (#2). She ranks the right calf next highest (#3) based on asymmetry, followed by the right hip (#4) and right shin (#5).

Sample 1A <u>Log Form C: Stretch/Mobilization Cycles</u>

DAY/DATE:	Days since *last day you ran*:
PHASE #	Days in this Phase:
AFFECTED SIDE: Right	AFFECTED REGION(S): Hamstring, Band?

Circle affected side →		Left		(Right)	Symmetry	
Enter your exercise list from *Worksheets 2A1* and *2A2*	Rank #	Stretches: Stiffness (0-5) / Self Mobs: Tenderness (0-5)	Rank#	Stretches: Stiffness (0-5) / Self Mobs: Tenderness (0-5)	No	Yes
Stretch # 11- 3 / Self-Mob:	8		①			
Stretch # 11- 6 / Self-Mob:	9		②			
Stretch # 11- 4 / Self-Mob:	10		③			
Stretch # 11- 5 / Self-Mob:	11		④			
Stretch # 11- 7 / Self-Mob:	12		⑤			
Stretch # 11- 8 / Self-Mob:	13		⑥			
Stretch # 11- 9 / Self-Mob:	14		⑦			
Stretch # 11- 11 / Self-Mob:	15		16			
Stretch # 11- 2 / Self-Mob:	17		18			
Stretch # 11- 13 / Self-Mob:	19		20			
Stretch # 11- 10 / Self-Mob:	21		22			
Stretch # 11- 12 / Self-Mob:	23		24			
Stretch # 11- 1 / Self-Mob:	25		26			

Worksheet 2A2: Ranking Affected Regions								
SIDE: *Right*	From Worksheet 2A1			From Worksheet 1D4			Summary	
Possible Affected Regions	Maximum Stiffness		Maximum Asymmetry (left/right)	Pain (0-10)	Swelling yes/no	Injury Stage (1-5)	Assessment	Rank #
	Left	Right						
1 Toe	0	0		0	no			
2 Arch	0	0		0	no			
3 Heel	0	0		0	no			
4 Shin	1	1		0	no		Work on stiffness	#5
5 Calf	0	2	0/2	1	no		Work on symmetry	#3
6 Knee	0	0		0	no			
7 Band	2	3	2/3	3	no	4	Possible affected region	#2
8 Hams	1	4	1/4	6	yes	4	Possible affected region	#1
9 Hip	1	2	1/2	1	no		Stiff + asymmetry	#4
10 Butt	0	0		0	no			

6. Select Self-Mobilizations

Sarah must now choose a self-mobilization for each stretch on her **Log Form C**. For each stretch associated with a *possible affected region* she must choose either a hamstring self-mobilization or a band self-mobilization.

She checks *Table 2A2:* **Injury Regions and Stretches** and finds that, for her first four stretches (11-3, 11-6, 11-4, and 11-5) the hamstring region is checked, but not the band. She writes "hams" on the line for "Self-Mob" below each of these stretches on her **Log Form C**.

For stretch 11-7, Sarah sees that both "hams" and "band" are checked, and she chooses "hams." For stretches 11-8 and 11-9, Sarah sees that "band" is checked, but not "hams" so she writes "band" below each of these stretches.

The remaining 6 stretches are for *unaffected* regions. Based on her **Worksheet 2A2**, the unaffected regions Sarah needs to work on are her calf, hip, and shin. She checks *Table 2A2* and finds that only two of her remaining stretches (11-2 and 11-13) are associated with the calf and shin, so she chooses "calf" for 11-13, and "shin" for 11-2. She now has four stretches left (11-1, 11-10, 11-11, and 11-12) and one more region, the hip, which needs mobilization. Stretches 11-10, 11-11, and 11-12 are associated with the hip, so she writes "hip" below those stretch numbers. Since exercise 11-1 is not associated with any area of concern from **Worksheet 2B**, Sarah lists no region for that stretch. She has now listed each region of concern at least once on her **Log Form C** [*See Sample 1B Log Form C*].

Sarah then goes to **Box 10-2** and chooses a self-mobilization number for each region she listed on the "self-mob" lines of **Log Form C**. Her **Log Form C** is now ready for her first day of Phase Two P.T. Time. Sarah check lines 11.7, 11.8, and 11.9 on her Course Map, and continues to the next line.

Sample 1B Log Form C: Stretch/Mobilization Cycles

DAY/DATE:	Days since *last day you ran*:
PHASE #	Days in this Phase:
AFFECTED SIDE: Right	AFFECTED REGION(S): Hamstring, Band?

Circle affected side →		Left		Right	Symmetry	
Enter your exercise list from *Worksheets 2A1 and 2A2*	Rank #	Stretches: Stiffness (0-5) / Self Mobs: Tenderness (0-5)	Rank#	Stretches: Stiffness (0-5) / Self Mobs: Tenderness (0-5)	No	Yes
Stretch # 11- 3 / *Self-Mob:* Hams 1	8		(1)			
Stretch # 11- 6 / *Self-Mob: :* Hams 2	9		(2)			
Stretch # 11- 4 / *Self-Mob:* Hams 1	10		(3)			
Stretch # 11- 5 / *Self-Mob:* Hams 2	11		(4)			
Stretch # 11- 7 / *Self-Mob:* Hams 1	12		(5)			
Stretch # 11- 8 / *Self-Mob:* Band 1	13		(6)			
Stretch # 11- 9 / *Self-Mob:* Band 2	14		(7)			
Stretch # 11- 11 / *Self-Mob:* Hip 1	15		16			
Stretch # 11- 2 / *Self-Mob:* Shin 1	17		18			
Stretch # 11- 13 / *Self-Mob:* Calf 1	19		20			
Stretch # 11- 10 / *Self-Mob:* Hip 1	21		22			
Stretch # 11- 12 / *Self-Mob:* Hip 2	23		24			
Stretch # 11- 1 / *Self-Mob:* none	25		26			

Self-Assessment 2B:
Phase Two Treatment Group and Complexity Subgroup

Sarah is now on line 11.10 of her Course Map, and she fills in **Worksheet 2B1: Phase Two Treatment Group and Subgroup.**

Since she started Phase One in Group 1 (with no Red Flags or swelling), and she does not now have any Red Flags or visible swelling, Sarah will enter Phase Two in Group 1.

Now Sarah will determine whether her injury is simple or complex. In **Worksheet 2A2: Ranking Affected Regions**, Sarah listed two *possible affected regions* on the right side and no regions on the left side, AND the regions she circled are in closely associated areas (regions 7 and 8), AND she has decided,

based on the guidelines in *The Running Injury Recovery Program*, that her symptoms are due to one simple injury. Therefore, she will count her injury as **one region**.

In **Self-Assessment 1C: Medical History**, Sarah lists **no pre-existing condition** that might affect her running.

Based on her answers in **Worksheet 2B1: Phase Two Treatment Group and Sub-Group**, Sarah will follow the instructions for *Simple Injuries* in Phase Two.

Sarah begins her daily Phase Two P.T. Time, following the Guidelines for Group 1 (*Table 11-1*) and simple injuries (*Table 11-2*).

Sarah checks line 11.10 on her Course Map, and continues to the next line.

Worksheet 2B1: Phase Two Treatment Group and Subgroup

1. Did you begin Phase One in Group 2 (with *Red Flags* or swelling)?
   (A. No)
   B. Yes

2. Do you *now* have any *Red Flags* or visible swelling in the injured region?
   (A. No)
   B. Yes

3. Based on your answers to questions 1 and 2, find your Phase Two treatment group:

Question 1:	Question 2:	Treatment Group
(A. No)	*and* (A. No)	(Group 1)
A. No	*and* B. Yes	Group 2
B. Yes	*and* A. No	Group 2
B. Yes	*and* B. Yes	Group 2

4. Go to your completed **Worksheet 2A2: Ranking Affected Regions**. How many regions did you assess as *possibly affected regions*?

A. If you have only one *possible affected region* on one side (no regions on the other side), then count your injury as **one region**.

B. If you have two or three *possible affected regions* on one side (and no regions on the other side), AND your *possible affected regions* are in closely associated areas (such as 1, 2, 3 or 6, 7, 8), AND you have decided, based on the guidelines in this book, that your symptoms are due to one simple injury, then count your injury as **one region**.

C. If you circled one or more *possible affected region* on the left side AND one or more *possible affected region* on the right side, count your injury as **two or more regions**.

D. If you circled two or more *possible affected regions* on one side, and they are NOT all closely associated with each other (such as 2, 3 and 7), count your injury as **two or more regions**.

5. Go to your **Self-Assessment 1C: Medical History**.

A. If you answered NO to *all* questions in **Self-Assessment 1C**, you have **NO pre-existing condition** that might affect your running.

B. If you answered YES to *any* question in **Self-Assessment 1C**, you have a **pre-existing condition** that might affect your running.

6. Based on your answers to questions 4 and 5 above, find your complexity subgroup below:

Question 4:	Question 5:	Subgroup
A or B (One region)	*and* A. NO pre-existing condition	Simple Injury
A or B (One region)	*and* B. Pre-existing condition	Complex Injury
C or D (Two or more regions)	*and* A. NO pre-existing condition	Complex Injury
C or D (Two or more regions)	*and* B. Pre-existing condition	Complex Injury

7. Fill in your Phase Two Recovery Group and Complexity Subgroup here:

Entering Phase Two, I am in recovery group (*1 or 2*) ___Group 1___, and I will follow the guidelines for (*simple or complex*) ___Simple___ injuries.

Self-Assessment 2C:
Phase Two Clearance (Evaluation of Log Form C for Symmetry by Complexity Subgroup)

Sarah has reached lines 11.11 and 11.12 on her Course Map. She is in treatment Group 1, following the guidelines for a *simple injury* (although she has not yet identified whether her injury is in the right hamstring or right band). On her first day of Phase Two P.T. Time, Sarah uses the **Log Form C** she prepared in *Self-Assessment 2A*, and fills in the tracking information at the top of the form.

Sarah performs her Stretch/ Mobilization Cycles in order, following the **Instructions for Log Form C**. She first performs the circled stretches ranked 1 through 7 on her *affected (right) side only*, following the instructions in **BOX 11-2** for Stretch/Mobilization Cycles for *affected regions*. On the line for each stretch and side, Sarah records her *stiffness* in that stretch. On the line below, she records her *tenderness* in the self-mobilization for that stretch. She regulates the pressure she exerts during self-mobilizations so that her tenderness level does not go above a 5 or 6.

Once she has completed the circled exercises numbered 1 through 7 on her *affected* side, Sarah does the exercises numbered 8 through 26, following the instructions in **BOX 11-2** for Stretch/ Mobilization Cycles for *unaffected regions*, and records her stiffness and tenderness for those exercises.

When she has completed her first day of P.T. Time, Sarah evaluates her left/right symmetry for stiffness (not tenderness) in each stretch. In **Sample 2 Log Form C**, she has recorded different left/right numbers for stiffness in the first nine stretches on her list. For these stretches she checks "No" in the column for *Symmetry*. Her last 4 stretches have matching left/right numbers for stiffness, so she checks "Yes" for *Symmetry*.

***

Sarah continues with one hour of P.T. Time each day, filling in a new **Log Form C** each day and evaluating it for symmetry. On Day 7 [*see Sample 3 Log Form C*] Sarah achieves symmetry in all stretches. The numbers for stiffness match in each left/right pair, although there is still some general, level-1 stiffness. This meets the mobility requirements in *Table 11-2* for Phase Two Clearance for a person with *simple injuries* (but not for those with complex injuries).

Now that Sarah has achieved symmetry in her mobility, she is finished with **Log Form C: Stretch/Mobilization Cycles.** When she enters Phase Three, she will follow the guidelines for P.T. Time in *Table 13-1:* Guidelines for Phase Three Part One, and she will maintain her flexibility using **Log Form M: Maintain Mobility**.

Sarah checks off lines 11.11 and 11.12 on her Course Map, and continues to the next line.

Sample 2 **Log Form C: Stretch/Mobilization Cycles** (Day 1)

DAY/DATE: Mon. 3/12	Days since *last day you ran*: (7)
PHASE # Two	Days in this Phase: (1)
AFFECTED SIDE: Right	AFFECTED REGION(S): Hamstring, Band?

Circle affected side →		Left		Right	Symmetry	
Enter your exercise list from *Worksheets 2A1 and 2A2*	Rank #	Stretches: Stiffness (0-5) / Self Mobs: Tenderness (0-5)	Rank#	Stretches: Stiffness (0-5) / Self Mobs: Tenderness (0-5)	No	Yes
Stretch # 11- 3	8	(2)	(1)	(5)	(X)	
Self-Mob: Hams 1		1		5		
Stretch # 11- 6	9	(2)	(2)	(4)	(X)	
Self-Mob: : Hams 2		2		5		
Stretch # 11- 4	10	(1)	(3)	(4)	(X)	
Self-Mob: Hams 1		2		4		
Stretch # 11- 5	11	(1)	(4)	(4)	(X)	
Self-Mob: Hams 2		2		4		
Stretch # 11- 7	12	(1)	(5)	(3)	(X)	
Self-Mob: Hams 1		1		1		
Stretch # 11- 8	13	(0)	(6)	(1)	(X)	
Self-Mob: Band 1		1		1		
Stretch # 11- 9	14	(1)	(7)	(2)	(X)	
Self-Mob: Band 2		1		1		
Stretch # 11- 11	15	(0)	16	(1)	(X)	
Self-Mob: Hip 1		1		1		
Stretch # 11- 2	17	(0)	18	(1)	(X)	
Self-Mob: Shin 1		0		0		
Stretch # 11- 13	19	1	20	1		X
Self-Mob: Calf 1		0		1		
Stretch # 11- 10	21	1	22	1		X
Self-Mob: Hip 1		0		1		
Stretch # 11- 12	23	0	24	0		X
Self-Mob: Hip 2		0		1		
Stretch # 11- 1	25	0	26	0		X
Self-Mob: none		-		-		

Sample 3 **Log Form C: Stretch/Mobilization Cycles** (Clearance)

DAY/DATE:	Mon. 3/19	Days since *last day you ran*:	14
PHASE #	Two	Days in this Phase:	7
AFFECTED SIDE:	Right	AFFECTED REGION(S):	Hamstring, Band?

Circle affected side →		Left		Right		Symmetry	
Enter your exercise list from *Worksheets 2A1 and 2A2*	Rank #	Stretches: Stiffness (0-5) / Self Mobs: Tenderness (0-5)	Rank#	Stretches: Stiffness (0-5) / Self Mobs: Tenderness (0-5)		No	Yes
Stretch # 11- 3	8	1 ✓	1	1 ✓			(X)
Self-Mob: Hams 1		1		2			
Stretch # 11- 6	9	1 ✓	2	1 ✓			(X)
Self-Mob: : Hams 2		1		2			
Stretch # 11- 4	10	1 ✓	3	1 ✓			(X)
Self-Mob: Hams 1		1		2			
Stretch # 11- 5	11	1 ✓	4	1 ✓			(X)
Self-Mob: Hams 2		1		2			
Stretch # 11- 7	12	1 ✓	5	1 ✓			(X)
Self-Mob: Hams 1		1		2			
Stretch # 11- 8	13	0 ✓	6	0 ✓			(X)
Self-Mob: Band 1		1		1			
Stretch # 11- 9	14	1 ✓	7	1 ✓			(X)
Self-Mob: Band 2		1		1			
Stretch # 11- 11	15	1 ✓	16	1 ✓			(X)
Self-Mob: Hip 1		0		1			
Stretch # 11- 2	17	1 ✓	18	1 ✓			(X)
Self-Mob: Shin 1		0		0			
Stretch # 11- 13	19	0 ✓	20	0 ✓			(X)
Self-Mob: Calf 1		1		1			
Stretch # 11- 10	21	1 ✓	22	1 ✓			(X)
Self-Mob: Hip 1		-		-			
Stretch # 11- 12	23	0 ✓	24	0 ✓			(X)
Self-Mob: Hip 2		-		-			
Stretch # 11- 1	25	0 ✓	26	0 ✓			(X)
Self-Mob: none		-		-			

Self-Assessment 2D:
Evaluation of Log Form C
for Regional Tenderness

Sarah has reached line 11.13 on her Course Map. She must now evaluate her **Log Form C** for *tenderness*, which will help identify her specific injury region.

Looking at all of her **Log Forms C**, Sarah finds that she had maximum tenderness on Phase Two, Day 1 [*see Sample 4 Log Form C*], so she will use this form for her self-assessment.

Sample 4 Log Form C shows that Sarah has two *possible affected regions*: the right hamstring and the right band. On this form, Sarah rated her self-mobilizations for the *affected* right hamstring at a tenderness level of 4 to 5 (extremely tender), compared to the unaffected left hamstring, which she rated at tenderness level 1 to 2. However, she rated her self-mobilizations for the right band region at a tenderness level of only 1 on both sides. None of her other self-mobilizations resulted in tenderness levels above 1.

Sarah enters the maximum tenderness for each side in each *possible affected region* on her **Worksheet 2D1**, and fills in the left/right differences. Since her self-mobilizations for the band region did not result in greater tenderness in the affected leg, Sarah eliminates the band as a *possible affected region*. In this case, high levels of tenderness in hamstring self-mobilizations identify the hamstring as her only remaining *possible affected region*.

Sarah checks line 11.13 on her Course Map and continues to the next line.

Worksheet 2D1: Regional Tenderness				
List *possible affected regions* from **Log Form C**	Max tenderness on *more affected* side:	Max tenderness on *less affected* side:	Left/Right Difference	Assessment (affected or not)
Hamstring	5	2	3	Yes
Band	1	1	0	No

Sample 4 **Log Form C: Stretch/Mobilization Cycles** (Day 1)

DAY/DATE:	Mon. 3/12	Days since *last day you ran*:	(7)
PHASE #	Two	Days in this Phase:	(1)
AFFECTED SIDE:	Right	AFFECTED REGION(S):	Hamstring, Band?

Circle affected side →		Left		(Right)		Symmetry	
Enter your exercise list from *Worksheets 2A1 and 2A2*	Rank #	Stretches: Stiffness (0-5) / Self Mobs: Tenderness (0-5)	Rank#	Stretches: Stiffness (0-5) / Self Mobs: Tenderness (0-5)		No	Yes
Stretch # 11- 3	8	2	(1)	5		X	
Self-Mob: (Hams 1)		(1)		(5)			
Stretch # 11- 6	9	2	(2)	4		X	
Self-Mob: : (Hams 2)		(2)		(5)			
Stretch # 11- 4	10	1	(3)	4		X	
Self-Mob: (Hams 1)		(2)		(4)			
Stretch # 11- 5	11	1	(4)	4		X	
Self-Mob: (Hams 2)		(2)		(4)			
Stretch # 11- 7	12	1	(5)	3		X	
Self-Mob: (Hams 1)		1 ✓		1 ✓			
Stretch # 11- 8	13	0	(6)	1		X	
Self-Mob: (Band 1)		1 ✓		1 ✓			
Stretch # 11-9	14	1	(7)	2		X	
Self-Mob: (Band 2)		1 ✓		1 ✓			
Stretch # 11- 11	15	0	16	1		X	
Self-Mob: Hip 1		1		1			
Stretch # 11- 2	17	0	18	1		X	
Self-Mob: Shin 1		0		0			
Stretch # 11- 13	19	1	20	1			X
Self-Mob: Calf 1		0		1			
Stretch # 11- 10	21	1	22	1			X
Self-Mob: Hip 1		0		1			
Stretch # 11- 12	23	0	24	0			X
Self-Mob: Hip 2		0		1			
Stretch # 11- 1	25	0	26	0			X
Self-Mob: none		-		-			

Self-Assessment 3A:
Basic Closed-Chain Clearance

Following her Course Map, Sarah has learned how to use Basic Closed-Chain Exercises to evaluate her injury in Phase Three Part One. She has studied the guidelines and instructions for Basic Closed-Chain Exercises [**Boxes 14-2 and 14-3**], and she has collected the equipment she will need (*Table 14-2:* Equipment for Closed-Chain Exercises).

Sara has now reached lines 14.7 through 14.9 on her Course Map, and she is following the **Instructions for Log Form B: Basic Closed-Chain**.

On Day 1 of Phase Three Part One, Sarah chooses to do Basic Closed-Chain Exercises 2, 3, 4, and 5. Starting out, she wants to get accurate set times, so she asks a friend to time her with a stopwatch that has a memory function, while she concentrates on doing her exercises correctly. Following the instructions for each exercise, she alternates between the left leg and the right leg with no *Rest Between Sets*, and she is careful not to exceed the *Target Time* for each set. She spends 10 minutes on each exercise, then stops briefly to record the times for her two longest sets and her three shortest sets on each side. She also records her *Maximum Pain* level on each side. When she completes her P.T. Time, Sarah calculates her *Average Set Times* and *Left/Right Differences*. On Day 2, she does the same for exercises 1, 6, 7, and 8, then evaluates her log forms.

In *Sample 1 Log Form B*, Sarah sees that she has reached the *Target Times*

and is symmetrical for two exercises: her CC#3 (One-leg armswings, barefoot) has a left-right difference of 0, and her CC#4 (One-leg armswings, 1 pillow) has a right-left difference of 1 second, which meet the *Symmetry Goals* for these exercises. She writes *"Cleared"* on both of these exercises, and she does not have to do them again. Also in *Sample 1 Log Form B*, Sarah sees that she has cleared CC#2 on the left side only. She can now work this exercise mostly on the right side, and reduce the number of sets on the left side.

In *Sample 1* and *Sample 2 Log Forms B*, Sarah finds that she is most asymmetrical in CC#7 (Weighted kickback) and CC#8 (Step up and over). She is somewhat asymmetrical in CC#5 (Push-ups) and CC#6 (Quick Steps). CC#1(Square Hops) and CC#2 (Side Step-Down) show less asymmetry. For each of these exercises, Sarah will spend more time working on the weaker side.

Sarah chooses her exercises for Day 3 based on her evaluation of days 1 and 2. In *Sample 3*, she starts with the four exercises that had the greatest asymmetry, which are exercises 7, 8, 6, and 5.

On Day 4 (*Sample 4*) Sarah does the exercises she didn't do on the previous day (1 and 2), then repeats the exercises she had the most trouble with (7 and 8).

Sarah clears exercises 6, 1, and 2 on days 3 and 4, and eliminates these exercises from her schedule. On Day 5 (*Sample 5*), she has less than four exercises remaining on her list, so she adds back exercise 6 at the *Final Target* level, to keep a minimum four exercises in her P.T. Time.

DAY/DATE	Monday 3-20	Days since *last day you ran:*	15
PHASE 3, Part#	Part 1	Days in this Phase	1
AFFECTED SIDE and REGION(S)	Right Hamstring, right band		

Basic Closed-Chain Exercise	CC#1 Square Hops		CC#2 Side Step-Down		CC#3 One-Leg Armswings, Barefoot		CC#4 One-Leg Armswings, 1 Pillow	
Target Time	20 sec		20 sec		15 sec		30 sec	
Rest Between Sets	10 sec		0		0		0	
Set Times	Left	Right	Left	Right	Left	Right	Left	Right
1			20	20	15	15	30	30
2			20	18	15	15	30	30
3			20	15	15	15	30	29
4			20	15	15	15	30	28
5			20	15	15	15	30	28
Total			100	80	75	75	30	30
Avg Set Time			20	17	15	15	30	29
L/R Difference			3 sec		0 sec		1 sec	
Symmetry Goal	1 sec		1 sec		1 sec		2 sec	
Max Pain (0-10)	L:	R:	L: 0	R: 1	L: 0	R: 0	L: 0	R: 0
NOTES:			Cleared on left		(Cleared)		(Cleared)	

DAY/DATE		Days since *last day you ran:*	Days in this Phase

Basic Closed-Chain Exercise	CC#5 Barefoot Push-Up		CC#6 Quick Steps	CC#7 Weighted Kickback		CC#8 Box Step Up and Over	
Target Time	15 sec		20 sec	60 sec		60 sec	
Rest Between Sets	0		10 sec	0		0	
Set Times	Left	Right	Both Legs [A]	Left	Right	Left	Right
1	15	10					
2	15	10					
3	15	5					
4	13	5					
5	10	2					
Total	68	32					
Avg Set Time	14	6					
L/R Difference	8 sec						
Symmetry Goal	1 sec			3 sec		3 sec	
Max Pain (0-10)	L: 1	R: 1	L: R:	L:	R:	L:	R:
NOTES:							

[A] See Instructions line 9: *Special Instructions for Quick Steps*

Sample 2 **Log Form B: Basic Closed-Chain** (Day 2)

DAY/DATE	Tuesday 3-21	Days since *last day you ran:*	16
PHASE 3, Part#	Part 1	Days in this Phase	2
AFFECTED SIDE and REGION(S)	Right Hamstring, right band?		

Basic Closed-Chain Exercise	CC#1 Square Hops		CC#2 Side Step-Down		CC#3 One-Leg Armswings, Barefoot		CC#4 One-Leg Armswings, 1 Pillow	
Target Time	20 sec		20 sec		15 sec		30 sec	
Rest Between Sets	10 sec		0		0		0	
Set Times	Left	Right	Left	Right	Left	Right	Left	Right
1	20	20						
2	20	18						
3	15	13						
4	15	10						
5	13	10						
Total	75	75						
Avg Set Time	17	14						
L/R Difference	3 sec							
Symmetry Goal	1 sec		1 sec		1 sec		2 sec	
Max Pain (0-10)	L: 0	R: 1	L:	R:	L:	R:	L:	R:
NOTES:								

DAY/DATE		Days since *last day you ran:*		Days in this Phase

Basic Closed-Chain Exercise	CC#5 Barefoot Push-Up		CC#6 Quick Steps	CC#7 Weighted Kickback		CC#8 Box Step Up and Over	
Target Time	15 sec		20 sec	60 sec		60 sec	
Rest Between Sets	0		10 sec	0		0	
Set Times	Left	Right	Both Legs [A]	Left	Right	Left	Right
1			18	52	40	55	40
2			16	52	35	55	40
3			14	47	30	50	35
4			12	46	25	45	30
5			10	43	20	45	25
Total			70	240	150	250	170
Avg Set Time			14	48	30	50	34
L/R Difference				18 sec		16 sec	
Symmetry Goal	1 sec			3 sec		3 sec	
Max Pain (0-10)	L:	R:	L: 1 R: 3	L: 1	R: 4	L: 1	R: 3
NOTES:			Weak pushoff on right side				

[A] See Instructions line 9: *Special Instructions for Quick Steps*

Sample 3 **Log Form B: Basic Closed-Chain** (Day 3)

DAY/DATE	Wednesday 3-22	Days since *last day you ran:* 17
PHASE 3, Part#	Part 1	Days in this Phase 3
AFFECTED SIDE and REGION(S)	Right Hamstring, Right band?	

Basic Closed-Chain Exercise	CC#1 Square Hops		CC#2 Side Step-Down		CC#3 One-Leg Armswings, Barefoot		CC#4 One-Leg Armswings, 1 Pillow	
Target Time	20 sec		20 sec		15 sec		30 sec	
Rest Between Sets	10 sec		0		0		0	
Set Times	Left	Right	Left	Right	Left	Right	Left	Right
1								
2								
3								
4								
5								
Total								
Avg Set Time								
L/R Difference								
Symmetry Goal	1 sec		1 sec		1 sec		2 sec	
Max Pain (0-10)	L:	R:	L:	R:	L:	R:	L:	R:
NOTES:								

DAY/DATE		Days since *last day you ran:*		Days in this Phase

Basic Closed-Chain Exercise	CC#5 Barefoot Push-Up		CC#6 Quick Steps	CC#7 Weighted Kickback		CC#8 Box Step Up and Over	
Target Time	15 sec		20 sec	60 sec		60 sec	
Rest Between Sets	0		10 sec	0		0	
Set Times	Left	Right	Both Legs [A]	Left	Right	Left	Right
1	15	15	20	60	50	60	54
2	15	13	20	60	50	58	52
3	15	12	20	58	45	55	50
4	15	12	20	56	45	55	50
5	15	10	20	54	45	52	48
Total	75	62	100	288	235	280	254
Avg Set Time	15	12	20	58	47	56	51
L/R Difference	3 sec			11 sec		5 sec	
Symmetry Goal	1 sec			3 sec		3 sec	
Max Pain (0-10)	L: 0	R: 1	L: 0 R: 2	L: 0	R: 2	L: 0	R: 2
NOTES:	Cleared on left		Cleared				

[A] See Instructions line 9: *Special Instructions for Quick Steps*

Sample 4 **Log Form B: Basic Closed-Chain** (Day 4)

DAY/DATE Thursday 3-23		Days since *last day you ran:* 18
PHASE 3, Part# Part 1		Days in this Phase 4
AFFECTED SIDE and REGION(S) Right Hamstring, Right band?		

Basic Closed-Chain Exercise	CC#1 Square Hops		CC#2 Side Step-Down		CC#3 One-Leg Armswings, Barefoot		CC#4 One-Leg Armswings, 1 Pillow	
Target Time	20 sec		20 sec		15 sec		30 sec	
Rest Between Sets	10 sec		0		0		0	
Set Times	Left	Right	Left	Right	Left	Right	Left	Right
1	20	20	--	20				
2	20	20	--	20				
3	20	20	20	20				
4	20	20	20	20				
5	20	20	20	20				
Total	100	100	60	100				
Avg Set Time	20	20	20	20				
L/R Difference	0		0					
Symmetry Goal	1 sec		1 sec		1 sec		2 sec	
Max Pain (0-10)	L: 0	R: 0	L: 0	R: 0	L:	R:	L:	R:
NOTES:	Cleared		Cleared					

| DAY/DATE | | Days since *last day you ran:* | Days in this Phase |

Basic Closed-Chain Exercise	CC#5 Barefoot Push-Up		CC#6 Quick Steps	CC#7 Weighted Kickback		CC#8 Box Step Up and Over	
Target Time	15 sec		20 sec	60 sec		60 sec	
Rest Between Sets	0		10 sec	0		0	
Set Times	Left	Right	Both Legs [A]	Left	Right	Left	Right
1				60	60	60	58
2				60	60	60	56
3				60	55	60	54
4				60	55	60	52
5				60	50	60	52
Total				300 sec	280 sec	300 sec	272 sec
Avg Set Time				60	56	60	54
L/R Difference				4 sec		6 sec	
Symmetry Goal	1 sec			3 sec		3 sec	
Max Pain (0-10)	L:	R:	L: R:	L: 0	R: 1	L: 0	R: 1
NOTES:							

[A] See Instructions line 9: *Special Instructions for Quick Steps*

~ 143 ~

Sample 5 **Log Form B: Basic Closed-Chain** (Clearance)

DAY/DATE	Friday 3-24	Days since *last day you ran:* 19
PHASE 3, Part#	Part 1	Days in this Phase 5
AFFECTED SIDE and REGION(S)	Right Hamstring, Right band?	

Basic Closed-Chain Exercise	CC#1 Square Hops		CC#2 Side Step-Down		CC#3 One-Leg Armswings, Barefoot		CC#4 One-Leg Armswings, 1 Pillow	
Target Time	20 sec		20 sec		15 sec		30 sec	
Rest Between Sets	10 sec		0		0		0	
Set Times	Left	Right	Left	Right	Left	Right	Left	Right
1								
2								
3								
4								
5								
Total								
Avg Set Time								
L/R Difference								
Symmetry Goal	1 sec		1 sec		1 sec		2 sec	
Max Pain (0-10)	L:	R:	L:	R:	L:	R:	L:	R:
NOTES:								

DAY/DATE		Days since *last day you ran:*		Days in this Phase	

Basic Closed-Chain Exercise	CC#5 Barefoot Push-Up		CC#6 Quick Steps	CC#7 Weighted Kickback		CC#8 Box Step Up and Over	
Target Time	15 sec		20 sec *	60 sec		60 sec	
Rest Between Sets	0		10 sec	0		0	
Set Times	Left	Right	Both Legs [A]	Left	Right	Left	Right
1	--	15	40	60	60	60	60
2	--	15	35	60	58	60	58
3	15	14	30	60	58	60	56
4	15	14	25	60	56	60	56
5	15	14	20	60	56	60	56
Total	45 sec	72 sec	150 sec	300 sec	288 sec	300 sec	286 sec
Avg Set Time	15	14	30	60	58	60	57
L/R Difference	1 sec			2 sec		3 sec	
Symmetry Goal	1 sec			3 sec		3 sec	
Max Pain (0-10)	L: 0	R: 0	L: 0 R: 1	L: 0	R: 1	L: 0	R: 1
NOTES:	(Cleared)		Cleared* Final Target 50	(Cleared)		(Cleared)	

[A] See Instructions line 9: *Special Instructions for Quick Steps*

Sarah has been monitoring her pain levels and Injury Stage from day to day. In *Sample 2 Log Form B*, she found maximum pain levels of 3 to 4 on the right side for exercises 6, 7, and 8. On Day 5 (*Sample 5*), all pain levels were at 1 or less. Her Injury Stage does not go above Stage 2.

On Day 5, Sarah clears exercises 5, 7, and 8. She has now cleared all eight Basic Closed-Chain Exercises in less than 7 days. Sarah can now complete her **Worksheet 3A1: Evaluation of Basic Closed-Chain Exercises**. Based on difficulty (measured by left/right difference) and maximum pain levels, she ranks her Basic Closed-Chain Exercises in this order: 7, 8, 6, 5, 1, 2, 4, and 3.

Sarah is now cleared to progress to Regional Closed-Chain Exercises. She checks off lines 14.7 through 14.9 on her Course Map, and continues immediately to *Self-Assessments 3B, 3C, 3D, and 3E* to prepare for Phase Three Part Two.

Worksheet 3A1: Evaluation of Basic Closed-Chain Exercises

1. Based on your daily assessments, list all eight Basic Closed-Chain Exercises **in order of difficulty**:

1. CC# ___7___ Weighted Kickback

2. CC# ___8___ Box Step Up and Over

3. CC# ___6___ Quick Steps

4. CC# ___5___ Barefoot Push Up

5. CC# ___1___ Square Hops

6. CC# ___2___ Side Step-Down

7. CC# ___4___ One-Leg Armswings, 1 pillow

8. CC# ___3___ One-Leg Armswings, barefoot

2. Count the number of days since you started your Basic Closed-Chain exercises, and **circle** the statement below that applies to you:

I was *able* to clear all Basic Closed-Chain Exercises in 7 days or less, and I am progressing to Regional Closed-Chain Exercises.	I was *unable* to clear all Basic Closed-Chain Exercises in 7 days or less, and I am continuing with Basic Closed-Chain Exercises.

Self-Assessment 3B:
Injury Regions

Although Sarah is now fairly sure that she can eliminate the right band as a *possible affected region*, she still needs to do *Self-Assessment 3B* to finally determine her Injury Region(s) for Regional Closed-Chain Exercises. She completes the sections of **Worksheet 3B1: Regional Self-Assessment Tables** for *Region 7: Band* and *Region 8: Hamstring*, and for *Region 11: Stress Fracture*.

Sarah considers all the symptoms listed for each region. Although she checked two lines in the table for *Region 7: Band*, she doesn't think the entire table really describes her injury. On the other hand, she has checked every line in the table for *Region 8: Hamstring*, and she thinks this table describes her symptoms pretty well. She has none of the symptoms pointing to stress fracture in the table for *Region 11: Stress Fracture,* so she checks no boxes in that table.

Sarah now considers all of the information she has gathered so far to determine her Injury Region:

1. Her **Worksheet 1D4: Summary of Original Injury** highlights several regions in the right leg.
2. Her **Worksheet 2A2: Ranking Affected Regions** shows *possible affected regions* in both the right hamstring and right band.
3. Her **Worksheet 2D1: Regional Tenderness** identified maximum tenderness in the hamstring region, but not in the band region.
4. Her **Log Form B: Basic Closed Chain** shows no symptoms for Square Hops, and all Basic Closed-Chain Exercises were cleared in less than 7 days (**Worksheet 3A1**).
5. Her **Worksheet 3B1: Regional Self-Assessment Tables** suggests a running injury in the right hamstring region with no stress fracture.

Looking at all of this information together, Sarah decides that it is most likely that her symptoms in the right band region are actually due to a hamstring injury, and are not a separate injury. Therefore, Sarah's list of injury regions in order of severity (*Worksheet 3B2*) has only one region: the right hamstring.

Sarah will follow the Regional Plan for one region (*Region 8: Hamstring*), found in *Appendix R*. She checks line 14.10 on her Course Map and continues to *Self-Assessment 3C*.

Worksheet 3B2: Injury Regions in Order of Severity			
Rank #	Side (left/right)	Injury Region	
1.	Right	Region #	8 Hamstring
2.		Region #	
3.		Region #	
4.		Region #	

Worksheet 3B1: Regional Self-Assessment Tables

Region 7: Band

Activity	Self-Assessment		Left	Right
Self-mobilization	I have **tenderness** on the outside of the knee, with or without visible swelling.			
Stretches	I have reduced range of motion **(stiffness)** from the hip and buttock down to the upper leg.			X
Closed-Chain Exercises	I have **weakness** in the band region, *resulting in*:	A. Difficulty staying balanced on one leg.		X
		B. Difficulty kicking out to the side.		
Pre-Injury Stride Tendency	While running, I have a tendency to:	A. Wobble side-to-side at the hip.		
		B. Lean to the outside with my foot sticking out, causing my knee to go to the inside.		

Region 8: Hamstring

Activity	Self-Assessment		Left	Right
Self-mobilization	I have **tenderness** in the back of the leg between the knee and buttock.			X
Stretches	I have reduced range of motion **(stiffness)** in the Straight Leg Raise.			X
Closed-Chain Exercises	I have **weakness** in the hamstring region, *resulting in* asymmetrical weakness and inflexibility in the hamstring area during kickback.			X
Pre-Injury Stride Tendency	While running, I have a tendency to:	A. Push off from the inner side of the big toe.		X
		B. Have a kickback that is short, asymmetrical, or twists.		X

Region 11: Regional Injury with Stress Fracture

Activity	Self-Assessment	Left	Right
Self-mobilization	I have **tenderness** in any weight-bearing bone in my injury region (anywhere from the foot to the pelvis), with or without pain in the associated soft tissues.		
Stretches	I have reduced range of motion **(stiffness)** in the region where I have bone tenderness.	NO	
Closed-Chain Exercises:	After icing *and* not running for at least 3 weeks, I can *still* **reproduce my injury pain** when I hop on the injured leg (unable to clear CC#1 Square Hop Exercise).		
Pre-Injury Stride Tendency	While running, I feel pain in the region where I have bone tenderness.		

Self-Assessment 3C:
Regional Closed-Chain Exercises
(Prepare Log Form R)

Sarah is now on line 14.11 of her Course Map. Since she has a *simple injury* in one region (the right hamstring), she copies only the list of six Regional Closed-Chain Exercises for *Region 8: Hamstring* from *Table 3C1: Closed-Chain Exercises by Region* to **Worksheet 3C1, Regional Closed-Chain Exercises in Order of Severity**, and to her first **Log Form R**.

Sarah then goes to *Appendix Z*, and finds the examples for her six Regional Closed-Chain Exercises. For each exercise, she copies the information for *Rest Between Sets*, *Final Target* and *Build Pace*, to her first **Log Form R** [*see Sample 1 Log Form R*]. She copies *only* the *Final Target* and *Rest* times for Fitness Runners, not for Racers. She also copies footnote A for CC#2 and CC#8. This is her list of Regional Closed-Chain Exercises for Phase Three Part Two.

Sarah clears Basic Closed-Chain Exercises on Day 5 [*Sample 5 Log Form B*] and begins Regional Closed-Chain Exercises (**Log Form R**) on her next day of P.T. Time. She will fill in her *Symmetry Targets* and *Symmetry Goals* on **Log Form R** when she does her *Initial Assessment* for each exercise [*see Instructions for Log Form R*].

Sarah checks line 14.11 on her Course Map and continues immediately to *Self-Assessment 3D*.

Worksheet 3C1: Regional Closed-Chain Exercises in Order of Severity	
1st Injury Region and Side: Right hamstring	
Box1: Regional Closed-Chain Exercises	
CC# 2	Side Step-Down
CC# 7	weighted kickback
CC# 8	Box step up and over
CC# 12	1-leg armswing, 2 pillows
CC# 14	1-leg armswing, double weights
CC# 20	Theraband kickback

Sample 1 **Log Form R: Regional Closed-Chain**

DAY/DATE:	Days since *last day you ran:*	
PHASE (3 or 4): 3B, Stage 1	Days in this Phase:	
Injury Region(s) and Side: Right hamstring		

Regional Closed-Chain Exercise (number and name)	CC# 2 Side Step-Down		CC# 7 weighted kickback		CC# 8 Box step up and over		CC# 12 1-leg armswing, 2 pillows	
Symmetry Target								
Rest Between Sets	0		0		0		0	
Final Target	30 sec		2.5 min		2.5 min		30 sec	
Build pace as:	glide (A)		glide		glide (A)		acceleration	
Set Times	Left	Right	Left	Right	Left	Right	Left	Right
1								
2								
3								
4								
5								
Total								
Avg Set Time								
L/R Difference								
Symmetry Goal		sec		sec		sec		sec
Max Pain (0-10)	L:	R:	L:	R:	L:	R:	L:	R:
NOTES:								
FOOTNOTES: (A) See instructions to build box height (Box 14-2).								

DAY/DATE	Days since *last day you ran:*	Days in this Phase

Regional Closed-Chain Exercise (number and name)	CC# 14 1-leg armswing, double weights		CC# 20 Theraband kickback		CC#		CC#	
Symmetry Target								
Rest Between Sets	0		0					
Final Target	30 sec		60 sec					
Build pace as:	acceleration		acceleration					
Set Times	Left	Right	Left	Right	Left	Right	Left	Right
1								
2								
3								
4								
5								
Total								
Avg Set Time								
L/R Difference								
Symmetry Goal		sec		sec		sec		sec
Max Pain (0-10)	L:	R:	L:	R:	L:	R:	L:	R:
NOTES:								
FOOTNOTES:								

Self-Assessment 3D:
Treatment Groups for Phase Three Part Two

Sarah is now at Course Map lines 14.12 and 14.13.

First, she writes her *Impairment Statements* to correlate her balance problems with her injury region. In **Worksheet 3A1: Evaluation of Basic Closed-Chain Exercises**, Sarah ranked her Basic Closed-Chain Exercises in this order: 7, 8, 6, 5, 1, 2, 4, and 3. Her most difficult Basic Closed-Chain Exercise was CC#7. She checks *Table 3D1*: **Basic Closed-Chain Balance Problems**, and finds that the Balance Problem for CC#7 is "Difficulty maintaining balance while kicking straight back." Since she lists only one injury region in **Worksheet 3B2: Injury Regions in Order of Severity**, she writes this impairment statement: *"I am not able to control my right hamstring to kick back straight."*

Since her second most-difficult exercise is CC#8, which has the same Balance Problem as CC#7, she goes to the third exercise on her list, CC#6, to find a second Balance Problem, which is "Difficulty maintaining balance while pushing off straight through the big toe." She writes a second impairment statement for her second balance problem: *"I have difficulty using my right hamstring to push off straight through my right big toe."*

Sarah copies her two *Impairment Statements* to her **Worksheet T: Training Plan for Phase Three Part Two**, and continues to **Worksheet 3D1.**

***

In **Worksheet 3D1**, Sarah answers "A" to questions 1 through 4, and determines that she will enter Phase Three Part Two in Group 1A.

Sarah copies her group number to **Worksheet T.** She checks lines 14.12 and 14.13 on her Course Map, and continues to the next line.

Impairment Statement 1:

I am not able to control my right hamstring to kick back straight."

Impairment Statement 2:

I have difficulty using my right hamstring to push off straight through my right big toe."

Worksheet 3D1: Treatment Groups for Phase Three Part Two

1. Which of the following statements applies to you?

A. I have cleared all eight Basic Closed-Chain Exercises in 7 Days or less.

B. I have completed Day 7 of Basic Closed-Chain Exercises, and I still have *not* cleared one or more of the eight Basic Closed-Chain Exercises.

2. Based on your **Self-Assessment 2B**, which complexity subgroup are you in?

A. *Simple Injuries.*

B. *Complex Injuries.*

3. How many Injury Regions did you list in **Worksheet 3B2: Injury Regions in Order of Severity**?

A. One

B. More than one

4. Look at the top section of today's **Log Form B: Basic Closed-Chain**, and find the box for "Days since *last day you ran*." Which of the following statements applies to you?

A. Today is 42 days or less (6 weeks or less) since the last day I ran.

B. Today is 43 days or more (more than 6 weeks) since the last day I ran.

5. Based on questions 1 through 4, find your Treatment Group for Phase Three Part Two:

You are in:	If your answers to questions 1 though 4 are:
GROUP 1A	"A" to ALL FOUR questions
GROUP 1B	"B" to question 1 AND "A" to ALL of questions 2, 3 and 4
GROUP 2A	"A" to question 1 AND "B" to ONE OR MORE of questions 2, 3, and 4
GROUP 2B	"B" to question 1 AND "B" to ONE OR MORE of questions 2, 3, and 4

Self-Assessment 3E:
Base Schedule and Training Plan

Sarah is now on Course Map lines 15.11 and 15.12. She has studied the techniques for fitness walking and glides, and she understands the goals of a Base Schedule.

Based on her **Worksheet 1B1: Running History**, Sarah is a Fitness Runner who had been running 3 days per week, about 5 miles per day, for a total of 15 miles per week (although not very consistently). With this injury, she could run for about 15 minutes before the pain started. She consults *Table 3E1: Base Schedules for Fitness Runners and Racers* and finds that she should maintain the same number of miles and days per week as in her pre-injury training. She chooses two days for her P.T. Time and three days for her Base Schedule.

Sarah is in treatment Group 1A. Following the guidelines in *Tables 3E2 and 3E3*, she finds that she will start her Base Schedule on the *Self-Paced Plan* at *Level 1*. She enters all the information for her Base Schedule on her **Worksheet T.**

***

Sarah is now ready to begin her Base Schedule in Phase Three Part Two. She will follow the Guidelines for Group 1A in *Table 13-2*, based on her individualized plan in **Worksheet T.** She must now follow the Course Map for Group 1, and use *Self-Assessment 3G1 for Self-Paced Plan* to evaluate her Base Schedule for Phase Three clearance.

Sarah checks lines 15.11 and 15.12 on her Course Map, and continues to line 15.13A.

Self-Assessment 3F:
Regional Closed-Chain Clearance

Following the guidelines for Group 1A, Sarah has reached line 15.16A on her Course Map.

On her first day of Regional Closed-Chain Exercises, she uses the **Log Form R: Regional Closed-Chain** that she prepared in *Self-Assessment 3C: Regional Closed-Chain Exercises*, and enters her tracking information in the first section only. She does her first four exercises (CC 2, 7, 8, and 12) and performs an *Initial Assessment* [See **Instructions for Log Form R, Line 8**]. She records the set times for each exercise, calculates her *Average Set Time* for left and right legs, and enters that number as her *Symmetry Goal*. Since her first four *Symmetry Goals* are lower than her *Final Target*, she crosses out the *Final Target*. She goes to *Table R1: Symmetry Goals for Closed-Chain*, finds the *Symmetry Goals* that correspond to her *Symmetry Targets*, and enters those *Symmetry Goals* on **Log Form R** [*see Sample 2 Log Form R*].

When Sarah evaluates her **Log Form R** for Day 1, she compares her *Left/Right Difference* to her *Symmetry Goal*. Since her first three exercises duplicate Basic Closed-Chain Exercises, she is able to clear them with symmetry and no increase in pain during her *Initial Assessment*. She writes *"Cleared"* for these exercises, and she will skip these exercises in her next rotation.

Worksheet T: Training Plan for Phase Three Part Two

1. I am a (Fitness Runner or Racer): _____ Fitness Runner _____ .

2. I plan to do my P.T. Time (**Log Form M** and **Log Form B** or **Log Form R**) 60 minutes per day, two days per week, on these days: __Tuesday__ and __Thursday__ .
(*Note:* P.T. Time may be done on the same days as your Base Schedule, or on different days).

3. I plan to do my Base Schedule (**Log Form S**) 60 minutes per day, __3__ days per week, on these days:

_____ Monday, Wednesday, and Friday _____ .

4. I am in Treatment Group Number (1A, 1B, 2A, or 2B) __1A__ .

5. I am following the (*Self-Paced Plan* or *Two-Week-Interval Plan*):

_____ Self-Paced-Plan _____

6. I will start my Base Schedule at Level __1__ .

7. My weekly mileage *goal* is __15__ miles per week.

8. My daily mileage *maximum* is __5__ miles per day (divide line 7 by line 3).

Write your personalized *Impairment Statements* from *Self-Assessment 3D* here:

1. I am not able to control my right hamstring to kick back straight.

2. I have difficulty using my right hamstring to push off straight through my right big toe.

For her fourth exercise (CC#12), Sarah has determined a *Symmetry Target* of 22 seconds, and a *Symmetry Goal* of 2 seconds. Since her *Left/Right Difference* is greater than 2 seconds, and she also recorded a slight increase in pain level in the affected leg, this exercise is not cleared.

She will perform the *Initial Assessment* for her remaining exercises on Day 2. In the tracking information at the top of the second section of *Sample 2 Log Form R,* Sarah counts two more calendar days in *Days since last training run* (from 23 to 25), but she enters the next consecutive number for *Days in this Phase* (from 1 to 2).

Since Sarah has a simple injury with only six Regional Closed-Chain Exercises, she only has two new exercises (CC# 14 and CC# 20) remaining for *Initial Assessment* on Day 2. To keep four Closed-Chain Exercises during her P.T. Time, she adds two of the exercises from Day 1 to her schedule. The first exercise she adds is CC#12, which she did not clear on Day 1 – keeping the same *Symmetry Target* and *Symmetry Goal*. The second exercise she adds is CC#8, which she did clear on Day 1. For this exercise, she switches from her *Symmetry Target* to her *Final Target*, and finds her new *Symmetry Goal* in **Table R1**: **Symmetry Goals for Closed-Chain**. She also makes a note that she has raised her box height in CC#8 to the *Final Target* level.

When Sarah evaluates her **Log Form R** for Day 2, she finds that she has cleared CC#12 (her *Left/Right Difference* is equal to her *Symmetry Goal*, with no increase in pain level). She writes *"Cleared"* on this exercise, and she does not have to repeat it on her next day of P.T. Time.

On Day 3 [*Sample 3 Log Form R*], Sarah still has two Regional Closed-Chain Exercises to clear (CC#14 and CC#20), so she puts these first on her schedule. She can choose any of the other exercises for her last two exercises. For her third exercise, Sarah adds CC#7 at the *Final Target* level, and changes the *Symmetry Goal* for that exercise. For her fourth exercise, she continues with CC#8 at the *Final Target* level.

When Sarah evaluates her **Log Form R** for Day 3, she finds that she has met her symmetry goals for CC#14 and CC#20, and she writes *"Cleared"* on these exercises. On this date (4/5) Sarah has cleared all six of her Regional Closed-Chain exercises at the level required for clearance in Phase Three Part Two, Stage 1. She can now check line 15.24A on her Course Map and revise her **Log Form R** for Stage 2 (see *Self-Assessment 3H*).

However, Sarah cannot enter Phase Four until she completes her Base Schedule through Level 5. Until that time, Sarah will continue her P.T. Time with the same six Regional Closed-Chain Exercises, but working toward her *Final Target* level. When she has cleared **Log Form S: Base Schedule Level 5**, she can go to *Self-Assessment 3I* for clearance to enter Phase Four, and to prepare her log forms for Phase Four.

Sample 2 **Log Form R: Regional Closed-Chain** (Day 1)

DAY/DATE: Tuesday 3-28	Days since *last day you ran*: 23
PHASE (3 or 4): 3B, Stage 1	Days in this Phase: 1
Injury Region(s) and Side: Right hamstring	

Regional Closed-Chain Exercise (number and name)	CC# 2 Side Step-Down		CC# 7 weighted kickback		CC# 8 Box step up and over		CC# 12 1-leg armswing, 2 pillows	
Symmetry Target	(20 sec)		(60 sec)		(60 sec)		(22 sec)	
Rest Between Sets	0		0		0		0	
Final Target	(30 sec)		(2.5 min)		(2.5 min)		(30 sec)	
Build pace as:	glide (A)		glide		Glide (A)		acceleration	
Set Times	Left	Right	Left	Right	Left	Right	Left	Right
1	20	20	60	60	60	ue	27	20
2	20	20	60	58	60	58	25	18
3	20	20	60	58	60	56	22	16
4	20	20	60	56	60	56	20	12
5	20	20	60	56	60	56	15	12
Total	100	100	300 sec	288 sc	300 sec	286 sec	109	78
Avg Set Time	20	20	60	58	60	57	22	16
L/R Difference	1 sec		2 sec		3 sec		6 sec	
Symmetry Goal	1 sec		3 sec		3 sec		2 sec	
Max Pain (0-10)	L: 0	R: 1	L: 0	R: 1	L: 0	R: 1	L: 0	R: 2
NOTES:	CLEARED BASIC		CLEARED BASIC		CLEARED BASIC			

FOOTNOTES: (A) See instructions to build box height (Box 14-2).

DAY/DATE: Thursday 3-30	Days since *last day you ran*: 25	Days in this Phase: 2

Regional Closed-Chain Exercise (number and name)	CC# 14 1-leg armswing, double weights		CC# 20 Theraband kickback		CC# 12 1-leg armswing, 2 pillows		CC#8 Box step up and over	
Symmetry Target	(24)		(38)		(22 sec)		----	
Rest Between Sets	0		0		0		0	
Final Target	(30 sec)		(60 sec)		(30 sec)		2.5 min (150 sec)	
Build pace as:	acceleration		acceleration		acceleration		Glide (A)	
Set Times	Left	Right	Left	Right	Left	Right	Left	Right
1	30	25	45	40	27	25	90	60
2	25	20	45	40	25	25	90	58
3	25	20	35	30	22	20	90	56
4	20	20	35	25	20	20	60	56
5	20	15	30	20	15	10	60	56
Total	120	100	190	155	109	100	390 sec	286 sec
Avg Set Time	24	20	38	31	22	20	78 sec	57sec
L/R Difference	4 sec		7 sec		2 sec		21 sec	
Symmetry Goal	2 sec		2 sec		2 sec		8 sec	
Max Pain (0-10)	L: 0	R: 0	L: 0	R: 0	L: 0	R: 1	L: 0	R: 2
NOTES					CLEARED		Final Target Level	

FOOTNOTES: CC#8 Final Target: Raised box height to 90/90 position.

Sample 3 **Log Form R: Regional Closed-Chain** (Clearance)

DAY/DATE:	Tuesday 4-5		Days since *last day you ran:*	30
PHASE (3 or 4):	3B, Stage 1		Days in this Phase:	3
Injury Region(s) and Side:				

Regional Closed-Chain Exercise (number and name)	CC# 14 1-leg armswing, double weights		CC# 20 Theraband kickback		CC# 7 Weighted Kickbacks		CC#8 Box step up and over	
Symmetry Target	(24)		(38)		------		-----	
Rest Between Sets	0		0		0		0	
Final Target	(30 sec)		(60 sec)		(2.5 min)		(2.5 min)	
Build pace as:	acceleration		acceleration		glide		Glide (A)	
Set Times	Left	Right	Left	Right	Left	Right	Left	Right
1	25	25	40	40	60	60	60	60
2	25	25	40	40	60	58	60	58
3	25	25	40	38	60	58	60	56
4	25	20	35	35	60	56	60	56
5	25	20	35	30	60	56	60	56
Total	125	115	190	183	300 sec	288 sec	300 sec	286 sec
Avg Set Time	25	23	38	36	60	58	60	57
L/R Difference	(2 sec)		(2 sec)					
Symmetry Goal	(2)	sec	(2)	sec	8	sec	8	sec
Max Pain (0-10)	L: 0	R: 0	L: 0	R: 0	L: 0	R: 1	L: 0	R: 1
NOTES:	(CLEARED)		(CLEARED)		Final Target Level		Final Target Level	
FOOTNOTES: CC#8 Final Target: Raised box height to 90/90 position.								

Sarah is in Group 1A (Self-Paced Plan) and is now at lines 15.17A through 15.23A in her Course Map. Based on her **Worksheet T**, she starts her **Log Form S: Base Schedule** at Level 1, three days per week (Monday, Wednesday, and Friday), with a target mileage of 5 miles per day.

She enters the *Starting Day/Date*, the number of *Days since last training run* (on the day she begins this form), and her number of *Target Days per week* (3) in the tracking information at the top of the form. She does not enter the *Clearance date* at this time. She crosses out the squares for two days per week, leaving spaces for three days. The *Day/Date* on the first square in the Base Schedule Log is the same as the *Starting Day/Date*.

She fills in one square for each day of her Base Schedule [*see Group 1A Sample 1 Log Form S: Base Schedule*]. She evaluates her workout at the end of each day, following the guidelines in **Worksheet 3G1: Evaluate Log Form S for Self-Paced Plan (Levels 1 through 5)** [*see Sample 1 Worksheet 3G1*].

Monday 3/27: On the first day of her Base Schedule, Sarah notes her maximum *Pain* level during exercise is 4, which is slightly higher than before. After her 7th glide drill, she observes that, during her glides, she is not able to use equal force on both legs as she pushes off. She discontinues her walk/glide sets and

finishes her Base Schedule with fitness walking. She records the 7 *Drills* that she completed with correct form. In her *Notes*, she writes her area of difficulty (pushoff on the right leg), and how many minutes of her Base Schedule she completed with correct form (40 minutes).

Wednesday 3/29: Sarah fills in the second day of her Base Schedule in the second square of Week 1. On this day, she slows her pace to reduce her symptoms. Her maximum pain level has decreased from 4 to 3, and she is able to complete all of her walk/glide sets. However, she notes that she is having trouble keeping her balance in two glide drills with hands on head, and her pace is too slow.

Friday 3/31: Sarah fills in the third day of her Base Schedule in the third square of Week 1. On this day, her pain level has decreased from 3 to 2 and she has mastered all of her glide drills, but she notes that her pace is still too slow.

Monday 4/3: Sarah fills in her fourth day of Base Schedule in the first square for Week 2. On this day, her maximum pain level remains at 2. She increases her pace, and successfully completes all 10 of her glide drills at glide pace, with symmetrical form and no increase in pain. She writes "*Cleared*" in her notes for that day, and enters the *Clearance date* at the top of the form.

On her next Base Schedule day (Wednesday 4/5) Sarah will start on a new **Log Form S Level 2**. She continues in the same manner though Levels 2, 3, and 4.

Log Form S: Base Schedule
Level 1

Starting Day/Date: Monday 3/27				Days since *last day you ran* (on starting day):		22
Target Days per week (3, 4, 5) 3				Clearance date:	Monday 4/3	

	Activity	Type	Repetitions	Duration	Total Time
Warmup	Fitness Walk				10 min
Base Schedule (*Table 15-4A*)	Walk/glide sets	Glide 1min/walk 4 min	10		
	10 Glide Drills:	Drill #1	2	15 sec	50 min
		Drill #2	2	15 sec	
		Drill #3	2	15 sec	
		Drill #4	2	15 sec	
		Drill #5	2	15 sec	
Cooldown	Fitness Walk				5 min

	Day/Date	Day/Date	Day/Date	Day/Date	Day/Date
Week 1	Monday /3/27	Wednesday/3/29	Friday/3/31	/	/
Pain (0-10)	4	3	2		
Drills/Form	7	8	10		
Notes:	Difficulty pushing off on right leg, 40 minutes.	Difficulty with balance, hands on head. Slow pace.	All drills with good form. Slow pace.		
Week 2	Monday /4/3	/	/	/	/
Pain (0-10)	2				
Drills/Form	10				
Notes:	(CLEARED)				
Week 3	/	/	/	/	/
Pain (0-10)					
Drills/Form					
Notes:					
Week 4	/	/	/	/	/
Pain (0-10)					
Drills/Form					
Notes:					

Example 1 (Monday 3/27)

Worksheet 3G1: Evaluate Log Form S for Self-Paced Plan (Level 0)

1. Evaluate your ability to fitness-walk your *Base Schedule* according to the instructions in Chapter 15 of *The Running Injury Recovery Program*:	Did you have any increase in pain or break in form during your 60-minute fitness walk?	Yes	No
2. Evaluate your notes:	A. Did you note any weakness, asymmetry, or problem with your stride?	Yes	No
	B. Are you aware of any other problem that you need to work on before progressing to Walk/Glide sets?	Yes	No

Worksheet 3G1: Evaluate Log Form S for Self-Paced Plan (Levels 1 through 5)

1. Evaluate your ability to perform each part of your *Base Schedule* according to the instructions in Chapter 15 of *The Running Injury Recovery Program*:	A. *Warmup:* Did you have any increase in pain or break in form during your 10-minute fitness walk?	Yes	(No)
	B. *Walk/glide sets:* Did you have any increase in pain or break in form during walk/glide sets?	(Yes)	No
	C. *Glide drills:* Did you have any difficulty performing any of the drills with correct form (as described in the instructions for that drill)?	(Yes)	No
	D. *Cooldown:* Did you have any increase in pain or break in form during your 5-minute fitness walk?	Yes	(No)
2. Evaluate completion of all drills:	A. Were you *unable* to complete the required time (*duration*) for any drill?	(Yes)	No
	B. Were you *unable* to complete the required number of sets (*repetitions*) for any drill?	(Yes)	No
3. Evaluate your notes:	A. Did you note any weakness, asymmetry, or problem with your stride?	(Yes)	No
	B. Do you have any other problem that you need to work on before progressing to the next level?	Yes	(No)
4. Level 5 only: Continue until the two numbers on the right match:	Write your number of *Target Days per Week* (3, 4, or 5).		
	Write the number of consecutive days you have cleared your Base Schedule at Level 5 with no break in form and no increase in symptoms.		

It takes Sarah seven more Base Schedule days to clear Levels 2, 3, and 4, and she has now reached Level 5. She fills in her starting *Day/Date, Days since last training run*, and *Target Days* at the top of **Log Form S, Level 5**, and crosses out the extra squares [*see Group 1A Sample 2 Log Form S: Base Schedule*]. She continues to evaluate her workout at the end of each day using **Worksheet 3G1: Evaluate Log Form S for Self-Paced Plan (Levels 1 through 5)**.

Friday 4/21: On her first day of 50-minute glides, Sarah has no trouble completing her 15 glide drills with good form. However, in her enthusiasm to clear Phase Three, she lost her mental focus and increased her glide pace, and her maximum pain level has increased from 1 (on her previous **Log Form S, Level 4**) to 7 (a level at which she would have taken medication for pain if she were not on this program). Although she maintained correct form and symmetry, she cannot

count this day toward her Phase Three clearance because her pain level increased significantly.

Monday 4/24: On her second day of 50-minute glides, Sarah improves her mental focus, and is able to maintain good form, symmetry, and pace throughout her exercise, with no increase in pain. She can count this as her first day toward Phase Three clearance. She does the same on *Wednesday 4/26*.

Friday 4/28: On this day, Sarah achieves her goal of 3 consecutive Base Schedule days with correct form and no increase in symptoms, which meets her requirements for Base Schedule clearance in Phase Three Part Two [*see Sample 2 Worksheet 3G1*]. She enters the clearance date on her Level 5 form.

Sarah checks lines 15.17A through 15.23A on her Course Map, and goes immediately to *Self-Assessment 3H* for clearance to start Phase Four.

Group 1A Sample 2 (Clearance)

Log Form S: Base Schedule
Level 5

	Starting Day/Date: Friday/4/21			Days since *last day you ran* (on starting day): 47		
	Target Days per week (3, 4, 5) 3			Clearance date: Friday 4/28		
	Activity	**Type**		**Repetitions**	**Duration**	**Total Time**
Warmup	Fitness Walk					10 min
Base Schedule **(***Table 15-4E***)**	Glides	50-minute glides				50 min
	15 Glide Drills:	Drill #1		3	15 sec ea	
		Drill #2		3	15 sec ea	
		Drill #3		3	15 sec ea	
		Drill #4		3	15 sec ea	
		Drill #5		3	15 sec ea	
Cooldown	Fitness Walk					5 min

	Day/Date	Day/Date	Day/Date	Day/Date	Day/Date
Week 1	Friday/4/21	Monday/4/24	Wednesday/4/26	/	/
Pain (0-10)	7	1	1		
Drills/Form	15	15	15		
Notes:	Increased pace, increased pain Good form.	Good form, symmetry, and pace.	Good form, symmetry, and pace.		
Week 2	Friday/4/28	/	/	/	/
Pain (0-10)	1				
Drills/Form	15				
Notes:	CLEARED for Phase Four				
Week 3	/	/	/	/	/
Pain (0-10)					
Drills/Form					
Notes:					
Week 4	/	/	/	/	/
Pain (0-10)					
Drills/Form					
Notes:					

~ 161 ~

Worksheet 3G1: Evaluate Log Form S for Self-Paced Plan (Level 0)			
1. Evaluate your ability to fitness-walk your *Base Schedule* according to the instructions in Chapter 15 of *The Running Injury Recovery Program*:	Did you have any increase in pain or break in form during your 60-minute fitness walk?	Yes	No
2. Evaluate your notes:	A. Did you note any weakness, asymmetry, or problem with your stride?	Yes	No
	B. Are you aware of any other problem that you need to work on before progressing to Walk/Glide sets?	Yes	No

Worksheet 3G1: Evaluate Log Form S for Self-Paced Plan (Levels 1 through 5)			
1. Evaluate your ability to perform each part of your *Base Schedule* according to the instructions in Chapter 15 of *The Running Inujry Recovery Program*:	A. *Warmup:* Did you have any increase in pain or break in form during your 10-minute fitness walk?	Yes	(No)
	B. *Walk/glide sets:* Did you have any increase in pain or break in form during walk/glide sets?	Yes	(No)
	C. *Glide drills:* Did you have any difficulty performing any of the drills with correct form (as described in the instructions for that drill)?	Yes	(No)
	D. *Cooldown:* Did you have any increase in pain or break in form during your 5-minute fitness walk?	Yes	(No)
2. Evaluate completion of all drills:	A. Were you *unable* to complete the required time (*duration*) for any drill?	Yes	(No)
	B. Were you *unable* to complete the required number of sets (*repetitions*) for any drill?	Yes	(No)
3. Evaluate your notes:	A. Did you note any weakness, asymmetry, or problem with your stride?	Yes	(No)
	B. Are you aware of any other problem that you need to work on before progressing to the next level?	Yes	(No)
4. Level 5 only: Continue until the two numbers on the right match:	Write your number of *Target Days per Week* (3, 4, or 5).		3 ✔
	Write the number of consecutive days you have cleared your Base Schedule at Level 5 with no break in form and no increase in symptoms.		3 ✔

Self Assessment 3H:
Phase Three Clearance and Preparation for Phase Four

Sarah is now on lines 15.24A, 15.25A, and 15.26A of her Course Map. She cleared all six of her Regional Closed-Chain Exercises (Stage 1) on 4/5 (in *Self-Assessment 3F*), while she was still working on her Base Schedule, Level 2. She continued to practice all of her Regional Closed-Chain Exercises at the *Final Target* level while working to complete her Base Schedule through Level 5 as quickly as possible.

Following the Self-Paced Plan, Sarah cleared her Base Schedule at Level 5 on Friday 4/28 [*see Self-Assessment 3G1*], which was 47 days after her last regular training run . Sarah can now complete *Self Assessment 3H Part 1*, **Worksheet 3H1: Phase Three Clearance.**

Sarah answers "Yes" to both questions in **Worksheet 3H1** and is cleared to enter Phase Four. She now follows the instructions in *Self-Assessment 3H Part 2* to prepare her first **Log Form R** and **Log Form S** for Phase Four:

(1) Sarah prepares her first Stage 2 **Log Form R** for Phase Four [*see Sample 4 Log Form R*]:

- On her **Log Form R**, Sarah enters the date for her first P.T. day in Phase Four (Tuesday 5/2), the number of days since her last training run on that date (51), and Phase Four (Stage 2). She enters #1 for the first day in Phase Four.

- She copies her six Regional Closed-Chain Exercises to her log form. Since all Regional Closed-Chain Exercises are now at *Final Target* levels, she does not enter *Symmetry Targets* for those six exercises. She checks to make sure she has entered the correct *Symmetry Goals* for her *Final Target* times.

- She goes to *Appendix Z* and copies the information for Hill CC#1 and Hill CC#2 to her log form (after her Regional Closed-Chain exercises). She copies both the *Symmetry Target* (for clearance) and the *Final Target* for Fitness Runners.

Worksheet 3H1: Phase Three Clearance		
1. Have you cleared all of your Regional Closed-Chain Exercises through Stage 1 (*Self-Assessment 3F*)?	No	(Yes)
2. Have you cleared your Base Schedule through Level 5 (*Self-Assessment 3G1 or 3G2*)?	No	(Yes)

Specific Mental Focus Statement:

"I will control my body to run with a straight and strong kickback."

Sample 4 **Log Form R: Regional Closed-Chain** (Phase Four)

DAY/DATE: Tuesday 5-2		Days since *last day you ran:* 51	
PHASE (3 or 4): 4 (Stage 2)		Days in this Phase: 1	
Injury Region(s) and Side:			

Regional Closed-Chain Exercise (number and name)	CC# 2 Side Step-Down		CC# 7 weighted kickback		CC# 8 Box step up and over		CC# 12 1-leg armswing, 2 pillows	
Symmetry Target								
Rest Between Sets	0		0		0		0	
Final Target	30 sec		2.5 min		2.5 min		30 sec	
Build pace as:	glide (A)		glide		glide (A)		acceleration	
Set Times	Left	Right	Left	Right	Left	Right	Left	Right
1								
2								
3								
4								
5								
Total								
Avg Set Time								
L/R Difference								
Symmetry Goal	2 sec		8 sec		8 sec		2 sec	
Max Pain (0-10)	L:	R:	L:	R:	L:	R:	L:	R:
NOTES:								

FOOTNOTES: (A) *See instructions to build box height [Box 14-2].*

DAY/DATE: Thursday 5-4		Days since *last day you ran:* 53	Days in this Phase: 2

Regional Closed-Chain Exercise (number and name)	CC# 14 1-leg armswing, double weights		CC# 20 Theraband kickback		CC# Hill 1 Uphill Incline		CC# Hill 2 Downhill Incline	
Symmetry Target					20 sec		20 sec	
Rest Between Sets	0		0		0		0	
Final Target	30 sec		60 sec		(30 sec)		(30 sec)	
Build pace as:	acceleration		acceleration		acceleration		acceleration	
Set Times	Left	Right	Left	Right	Left	Right	Left	Right
1								
2								
3								
4								
5								
Total								
Avg Set Time								
L/R Difference								
Symmetry Goal	2 sec		3 sec		1 sec		1 sec	
Max Pain (0-10)	L:	R:	L:	R:	L:	R:	L:	R:
NOTES:								

FOOTNOTES: *Achieve symmetry in Hill Closed-Chain before beginning Hill Drills.*

(2) Sarah now prepares her first **Log Form S** for Level 6, Level 7, and Level 8 [*see Sample 3 Log Form S: Level 6*]:

- Sarah takes one **Log form S** for each remaining Level (6, 7, and 8) and writes in her *Target Days per Week* (3). She crosses out the last two boxes in each week, leaving three boxes per week.

- In the guidelines at the top of the form, she crosses out the target time in column B for *Racers* and circles the target time in column A for *Fitness Runners*.

- She goes to *Appendix R* and finds the *Specific Mental Focus Statement* for Region 8 (hamstring): *"I will control my body to run with a straight and strong kickback,"* and writes it in the box for *Mental Focus Statement*.

- On **Log Form S Level 6** only, Sarah enters the *Starting Day/Date* for her first Base Schedule day in Phase Four (Monday 5/1), and the number of *Days since last training run* on that date (50).

Sarah is now prepared to enter Phase Four. She checks line 15.26A on her Course Map, and continues to the **Checkpoint to Enter Phase Four**.

Self-Assessment 4A:
Base Schedule Level 6 Clearance

Sarah has entered Phase Four of her Recovery Program, and has reached lines 16.5 through 16.12 on her Course Map. She has studied the instructions for Acceleration Drills and for Hill Closed-Chain Exercises. Sarah alternates between her Base Schedule (Monday, Wednesday, and Friday) and her P.T. Time (Tuesday and Thursday). She cleared Phase Three (*Self-Assessment 3H*) on Friday 4/28, and begins Phase Four on Monday 5/1.

Monday 5/1: In her Base Schedule, Sarah uses the **Log Form S Level 6** that she prepared in *Self-Assessment 3H* [*see Sample 4 Log Form S Level 6*]. She is anxious to begin her first day of Acceleration Drills, but she is careful to follow the instructions and not over-exert herself. She follows the timing guidelines for Fitness Runners in *Table 16-2A* for inserting Acceleration Drills into her glide program, and she is able to complete all glides and drills smoothly and continuously for 50 minutes, with no break in form and only a very slight increase in pain (level 1) which she considers insignificant. She writes *"Cleared"* on her **Log Form S: Base Schedule Level 6**.

Log Form S: Base Schedule
Level 6

Starting Day/Date: Monday 5-1				Days since *last day you ran* (on starting day): 50			
Target Days per week (3, 4, 5) 3				Clearance date:			
	Activity	Type	Reps	A. Fitness Runners	B. Racers		Total Time
Warmup	Fitness Walk						10 min
Base Schedule (*Table 16-2*)	Glides	50-min. glides					
	9 Acceleration Drills:	Drill #1	3		Build to		
		Drill #2	3	30 sec each	90 sec each		50 min
		Drill #3	3				
Cooldown	Fitness Walk						5 min
Mental Focus Statement:	I will control my body to run with a straight and strong kickback						

	Day/Date	Day/Date	Day/Date	Day/Date	Day/Date
Week 1	/	/	/	/	/
Pain (0-10)					
Drills/Form					
Notes:					
Week 2	/	/	/	/	/
Pain (0-10)					
Drills/Form					
Notes:					
Week 3	/	/	/	/	/
Pain (0-10)					
Drills/Form					
Notes:					
Week 4	/	/	/	/	/
Pain (0-10)					
Drills/Form					
Notes:					

Log Form S: Base Schedule
Level 6

	Activity	Type	Reps	A. Fitness Runners	B. Racers	Total Time
Starting Day/Date: Monday 5-1				**Days since *last day you ran* (on starting day):** 50		
Target Days per week (3, 4, 5) 3				**Clearance date:**		
Warmup	Fitness Walk					10 min
Base Schedule (*Table 16-2*)	Glides	50-min. glides				
	9 Acceleration Drills:	Drill #1	3		Build to	
		Drill #2	3	30 sec each	90 sec each	
		Drill #3	3			50 min
Cooldown	Fitness Walk					5 min
Mental Focus Statement:	I will control my body to run with a straight and strong kickback					

	Day/Date	Day/Date	Day/Date	Day/Date	Day/Date
Week 1	Monday 5-1	/	/	/	/
Pain (0-10)	1				
Drills/Form	9				
Notes:	Cleared glides and drills with good form				
Week 2	/	/	/	/	/
Pain (0-10)					
Drills/Form					
Notes:					
Week 3	/	/	/	/	/
Pain (0-10)					
Drills/Form					
Notes:					
Week 4	/	/	/	/	/
Pain (0-10)					
Drills/Form					
Notes:					

Tuesday 5/2: In her P.T. Time, Sarah is using **Log Form M: Maintain Mobility** and the **Log Form R: Regional Closed-Chain** that she prepared in *Self-Assessment 3H*.

Sarah has been working on her six Regional Closed-Chain Exercises since she reached Stage 1 clearance on 4/5, so by now she is perfect in these exercises. At this point, Sarah only needs to clear the new Hill Closed-Chain Exercises at the *Symmetry Target* level [*see Sample 5 Log Form R*]. On this date, she does Hill Closed-Chain Exercises 1 and 2, plus two Regional Closed-Chain Exercises (CC#14 and CC#20) to bring her total up to four exercises. She limits herself to her *Final Target* goals during her Regional Closed-Chain Exercises, so she doesn't have to calculate her *Total* to figure out her *Average Set Time* for these exercises. At the end of P.T. Time, she calculates her *Average Set Times* for Hill Closed-Chain Exercises 1 and 2, and compares them to their *Symmetry Goals*. She finds that she has met her clearance requirements for both Hill Closed-Chain Exercises, and she writes "Cleared" on these exercises.

Sarah then fills in her **Worksheet 4A1: Level 6 Clearance.** She answers "yes" to all four questions in and is cleared to progress to Level 7 in her Base Schedule. She will continue with all of her regional and hill closed-chain exercises at the *Final Target* level during her P.T. Time. She checks lines 16.5 through 16.12 on her Course Map, and continues to the next line.

Self-Assessment 4B:
Base Schedule Level 7 Clearance

Sarah is now on lines 16.14 through 16.18 in her Course Map. She was cleared to start Base Schedule Level 7 on Tuesday 5/2, when she cleared her Hill Closed-Chain Exercises, and she progresses to Hill Training Drills on her next Base Schedule day (Wednesday 5/3).

Sarah uses the **Log Form S: Base Schedule Level 7** that she prepared in *Self Assessment 3H*, and follows the guidelines for Fitness Runners for inserting Hill Training drills into her glide program (*Table 16-3A*). Using her *Mental Focus Statement*, she is able to complete all glides and Hill Drills smoothly and continuously for 50 minutes, with no break in form and no increase in pain [*see Sample 6 Log Form S: Base Schedule Level 7*]. She writes "*Cleared*" on her log form, and fills out Worksheet **4B1: Level 7 Clearance.**

Sarah answers "yes" to the questions in **Worksheet 4B1** and is cleared to progress to Level 8 in her Base Schedule. There is no clearance requirement for P.T. Time at this level, but Sarah wants to be well-rested and mobilized for plyometric exercises, so she sticks with her schedule and does her P.T. Time on Thursday 5/4.

Sarah checks lines 16.14 through 16.18 on her Course Map and continues to the next line.

Sample 5 **Log Form R: Regional Closed-Chain** (Hill Clearance)

DAY/DATE: Tuesday 5-2	Days since *last day you ran*: 51
PHASE (3 or 4): 4 (Stage 2)	Days in this Phase: 1
Injury Region(s) and Side:	

Regional Closed-Chain Exercise (number and name)	CC# 14 1-leg armswing, double weights		CC# 20 Theraband kickback		CC# Hill 1 Uphill Incline		CC# Hill 2 Downhill Incline	
Symmetry Target					(20 sec)		(20 sec)	
Rest Between Sets	0		0		0		0	
Final Target	(30 sec)		(60 sec)		(30 sec)		(30 sec)	
Build pace as:	acceleration		acceleration		acceleration		acceleration	
Set Times	Left	Right	Left	Right	Left	Right	Left	Right
1	30	30	60	60	20	20	20	20
2	30	30	60	60	20	20	20	20
3	30	30	60	60	20	19	20	19
4	30	30	60	60	20	19	20	18
5	30	30	60	60	20	19	20	18
Total					100	97	100	95
Avg Set Time	30	30	60	60	20	19	20	19
L/R Difference	0 sec		0 sec		(1 sec)		(1 sec)	
Symmetry Goal	2 sec		3 sec		(1) sec		(1) sec	
Max Pain (0-10)	L: 0	R: 0	L: 0	R: 0	L: 0	R: 0	L: 0	R: 0
NOTES:					(CLEARED)		(CLEARED)	
FOOTNOTES:	Achieve symmetry in Hill Closed-Chain before beginning Hill Drills.							

Worksheet 4A1: Level 6 Clearance				
Log Form S Level 6:	1. Are you able to perform all nine of your acceleration drills for the time required for your group (Fitness Runner or Racer), with no break in form and no increase in pain?		No	(Yes)
	2. Are you able to complete your Base Schedule (glides and acceleration drills) continuously for 50 minutes, with no break in form or significant increase in pain?		No	(Yes)
Log Form R (Stage 2)	3. Are you maintaining symmetry in all of your Regional Closed-Chain Exercises, with no significant increase in pain?		No	(Yes)
	4. Have you reached your *Symmetry Target* for Hill Closed-Chain Exercises 1 and 2?		No	(Yes)

Log Form S: Base Schedule
Level 7

Starting Day/Date:	Wednesday 5-3			Days since *last day you ran* (on starting day):		52
Target Days per week (3, 4, 5)	3			Clearance date:	Wednesday 5-3	

	Activity	Type	Reps	A. Fitness Runners	B. Racers	Total Time
Warmup	Fitness Walk					10 min
Base Schedule (*Table 16-3*)	Glides	50-min. glides				
	6 Hill Drills:	Uphill Drill	3	(90 sec each)	Build to 4.5 min each	50 min
		Downhill Drill	3	(90 sec each)	Build to 4.5 min each	
Cooldown	Fitness Walk					5 min
Mental Focus Statement:	I will control my body to run with a straight and strong kickback					

	Day/Date	Day/Date	Day/Date	Day/Date	Day/Date
Week 1	Wednesday 5-3	/	/	/	/
Pain (0-10)	0				
Drills/Form	6				
Notes:	Cleared glides and Hills with good form				
Week 2	/	/	/	/	/
Pain (0-10)					
Drills/Form					
Notes:					
Week 3	/	/	/	/	/
Pain (0-10)					
Drills/Form					
Notes:					
Week 4	/	/	/	/	/
Pain (0-10)					
Drills/Form					
Notes:					

Worksheet 4B1: Level 7 Clearance			
Log Form S Level 7:	1. Are you able to perform all six of your Hill Training drills for the time required for your group (Fitness Runner or Racer), with no break in form and no increase in pain?	No	(Yes)
	2. Are you able to complete your Base Schedule (glides and Hill-Training drills) continuously for 50 minutes, with no break in form or significant increase in pain?	No	(Yes)

Self-Assessment 4C:
Base Schedule Level 8 Clearance

Sarah has studied the instructions for each of the four Plyometric Drills, and has carefully practiced the unfamiliar "Bounding" movement, following the positions shown in the illustrations. She has also studied *Table 17-1A* and understands how she will insert 12 plyometric drills, followed by 10 glide drills, into her 50-minute glide program.

Sarah has now reached lines 17.5 through 17.10 on her Course Map, and is using the **Log Form S: Base Schedule Level 8** that she prepared in *Self Assessment 3H*. On Friday 5/5, Sarah follows the instructions and does her Base Schedule for Plyometric Drills on the street, not on a treadmill. She uses her Mental Focus Statement, and remembers to perform her plyometric drills in a smooth, controlled manner (submaximal). She then finishes her Base Schedule by alternating glides with 15-second glide drills. She records a pain level of 1, which she considers insignificant [*see Sample 7 Log Form S: Base Schedule Level 8*].

Sarah has now successfully completed her 12 plyometric drills and 10 glide drills with no break in form and no significant increase in pain. She writes "Cleared" on her log form and fills out **Worksheet 4C1: Level 8 Clearance.**

Sarah answers "yes" to both questions in **Worksheet 4C1.** She checks lines 17.5 through 17.10 on her Course Map and continues to the next line.

Sample 7 (Level 8 Clearance)

Log Form S: Base Schedule
Level 8

Starting Day/Date: Friday 5-5				Days since *last day you ran* (on starting day): 54		
Target Days per week (3, 4, 5) 3				Clearance date: Friday 5-5		
	Activity	Type	Reps	A. Fitness Runners	B. Racers	Total Time
Warmup	Fitness Walk					10 min
Base Schedule (*Table 17-1*)	Glides	50-min. glides				
	12 Plyometric Drills:	Drill #1	3	⟨15 sec each⟩	Build to 45 sec each	
		Drill #2	3			50 min
		Drill #3	3			
		Drill #4	3			
	10 Glide Drills	5 glide drills	2 each	⟨15 sec each⟩	15 sec each	
Cooldown	Fitness Walk					5 min
Mental Focus Statement:	I will control my body to run with a straight and strong kickback					

	Day/Date	Day/Date	Day/Date	Day/Date	Day/Date
Week 1	Friday 5-5	/	/	/	/
Pain (0-10)	1				
Drills/Form	12				
Notes:	Cleared plyometric drills	RETURN TO RUNNING!!!			
Week 2	/	/	/	/	/
Pain (0-10)					
Drills/Form					
Notes:					
Week 3	/	/	/	/	/
Pain (0-10)					
Drills/Form					
Notes:					
Week 4	/	/	/	/	/
Pain (0-10)					
Drills/Form					
Notes:					

Worksheet 4C1: Level 8 Clearance			
Log Form S Level 8:	1. Are you able to perform all twelve of your Plyometric Drills for the time required for your group (Fitness Runner or Racer), with no break in form and no increase in pain?	No	(Yes)
	2. Are you able to complete your Base Schedule (glides and Plyometric Drills and Glide Drills) continuously for 50 minutes, with no break in form or significant increase in pain?	No	(Yes)

Self-Assessment 4D:
Clearance for Post-Recovery Running

Sarah has completed lines 18.1 through 18.7 on her Course Map. In her Phase Four plyometric drills, she has demonstrated her ability to put excess force through her injury region with no increase in symptoms, and she is physically prepared to return to running.

In post-recovery running, Sarah's goal is to run smarter as well as stronger. She considers what she has learned about her running habits during her *Recovery Program* and fills in **Worksheet 4D1: Habits for Post-Recovery Running.**

Sarah can now check line 18.8 and the **Checkpoint to Return to Running** on her Course Map. She has completed her *Running Injury Recovery Program*, and is free to design her own post-recovery training plan.

Following the guidelines in her **Worksheet 4D1**, Sarah can now return to running as a stronger, smarter, and safer runner.

Worksheet 4D1: Habits for Post-Recovery Running		
Post-Recovery Running Habits Checklist:	1. I will make a plan, and train consistently.	X
	2. I will set realistic running goals.	X
	3. I will start each run with a proper warmup.	X
	4. I will pay close attention to my equipment, particularly my footwear.	X
	5. I will focus on functional running.	X
	6. I will manage my running injuries early, before they become severe.	X

The most important lessons I have learned from my *Running Injury Recovery Program* that I will use when I return to regular training are:

1. I will train more consistently – at least five miles, three times per week.

2. I will not push myself to a pace that is too hard or too fast – I will warm up, then gradually build up to a smooth, easy training pace, then cool down. This will keep me from getting too sore and help me train more consistently.

Example #2:
Complex Injury ("Karl")

"Karl" has been running for many years without a serious running injury, but he doesn't train consistently, and his weekly mileage frequently drops below 10 miles.

When he and his friends decide to try a local triathlon, Karl greatly increases his training time and effort. He develops a pain in his right arch, but he is determined to run through the pain. One of his friends tells him that a barefoot style of running will fix his problem, so he buys a pair of minimalist shoes and keeps on running.

Soon the pain in his arch is going up his entire leg, but he doesn't want to let his friends down, so he takes medication for the pain and keeps on running. It's not long until Karl is crippled with red-hot pain all around his right foot and leg. In the morning when he first tries to stand, his foot is crippling him. When he walks up stairs, his knee is crippling him. The pain is so widespread that he can't tell exactly where it's coming from.

Karl finally admits that he needs help. He begins self-management, following his Course Map and the Guidelines for Phase One. Since Karl is not a big fan of filling out lots of forms, he just reads *Self-Assessments 1A thorough 1C*, and determines that he has a running

injury with no pre-existing medical conditions. He stops running, stops taking medication for his pain, and fills out **Worksheets 1D1 through 1D5.**

Karl sees that he will enter Phase One injury management in treatment Group 2 for complex injuries. He must now start to ICE all six of the areas that he has identified as *possible affected regions*, which will require some planning. He reads the instructions for ICE in Chapter 5 of *The Running Injury Recovery Program*, and finds that his combination of *possible injury regions* covers three icing positions [Box 5-2], so he compromises on Icing Position 5-2, which will still elevate all of his injury regions.

Karl follows the instructions in Box 5-1, makes lots of ice packs, and does his icing at home for 20 minutes, three times a day: once in the morning before he goes to work, once when he gets home from work, and once in the evening before he goes to bed. While icing, he wraps his arch, calf, knee, band, and hamstring with Ace bandages until he looks like half a mummy, and he places the ice pack for his right buttock inside his biking shorts. He records his icing sessions on **Log Form I**, and rates his maximum symptoms before each icing session on a scale of 1 to 10.

Worksheet 1D:
Document Your Injury and Phase One Treatment Group

Last day you ran: _Saturday July 7_   **Today's date:** _Tuesday July 10_

Worksheet 1D1: Pain Pattern

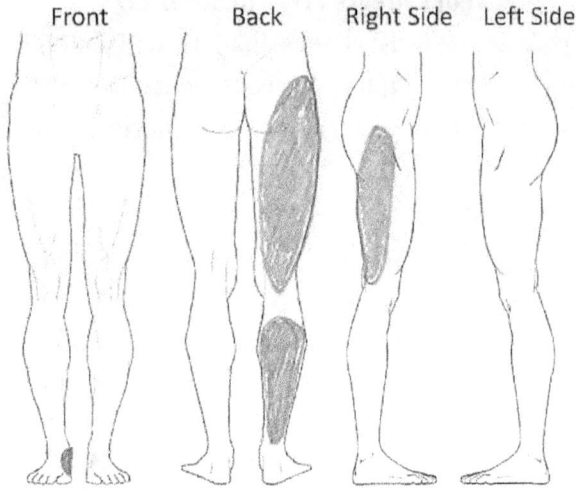

Front   Back   Right Side   Left Side

Compare to *Appendix A* and list your *possible affected regions* and side here:

Right Side:

Region 2: Arch

Region 5: Calf

Region 7: Band

Region 8: Hamstring

Region 10: Butt

Worksheet 1D2: Swelling Within Past 2 Weeks

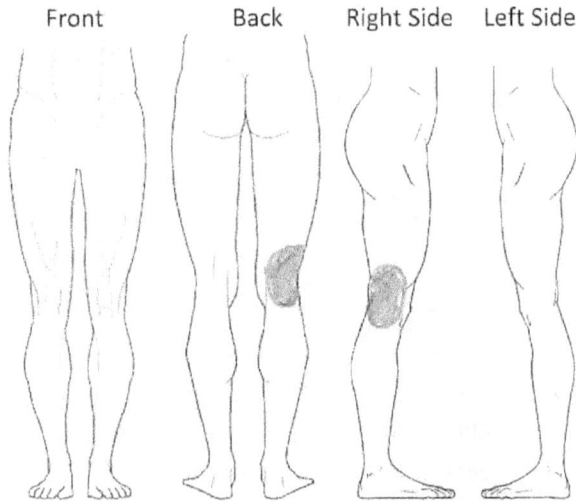

Front   Back   Right Side   Left Side

Compare to *Appendix A* and list your *possible affected regions* and side here:

Right Side:

Region 6: Knee

Region 7: Band

Region 8: Hamstring

Worksheet 1D3: Injury Stage

Injury Side and *possible affected region(s)*: <u>right arch, calf, band, hamstring, butt, knee</u>

Table A: Maximum Symptoms *within the past 2 weeks*

Injury Stages	Emerging Symptoms	Red Flags	Which region(s)?
Stage 1	Pain while running	Pain that alters your stride	
Stage 2	Pain at rest (after running)	Pain that disturbs your rest	
(Stage 3)	Pain during your normal daily activities	Pain that interferes with or makes you avoid ADLs	*All 6 regions*
(Stage 4)	Running injury pain that you take medication for	Being in Stage 4	*All 6 regions*
(Stage 5)	Pain that cripples you	Being in Stage 5	*Arch & Knee*

Table B: Maximum Symptoms *from more than 2 weeks ago*

Injury Stages	Emerging Symptoms	Red Flags	Which region(s)?
(Stage 1)	Pain while running	Pain that alters your stride	*Arch*
(Stage 2)	Pain at rest (after running)	Pain that disturbs your rest	*Arch*
(Stage 3)	Pain during your normal daily activities	Pain that interferes with or makes you avoid ADLs	*Arch*
Stage 4	Running injury pain that you take medication for	Being in Stage 4	
Stage 5	Pain that cripples you	Being in Stage 5	

Worksheet 1D4: Summary of Original Injury

Refer to:	Worksheet 1D1: Pain Pattern	Worksheet 1D2: Swelling	Worksheet 1D3: Table A Injury Stage in Past 2 Weeks	
Right Leg Circle *Possible Affected Regions*	**Pain Severity (1-10)**	**Swelling in past 2 weeks (yes/no)**	**Injury Stage Scale (1-5)**	**Red Flag (yes/no)**
1 Toe				
2 Arch	10		5	Yes
3 Heel				
4 Shin				
5 Calf	6		4	Yes
6 Knee	6	Yes	5	Yes
7 Band	8	Yes	4	Yes
8 Hamstring	8		4	Yes
9 Hip				
10 Buttock	8		4	Yes

Worksheet 1D5: Phase One Treatment Group

Circle ONE of the two statements below:

I will enter Phase One injury management in treatment Group 1, and I do not have to ICE.	I will enter Phase One injury management in treatment Group 2, and I will now begin to ICE (**Log Form I**).

Log Form I: Group 2 ICE Log

Phase # ONE	Starting DAY/DATE: Tuesday July 10	Number of ICE Days: 3

Week 1 (Day/Date/Phase)	ICE#	Symptoms (0 to 10)	Week 2 (Day/Date/Phase)	ICE#	Symptoms (0 to 10)
Day: Tuesday	(1)	10	Day:	1	
Date: 7/10	(2)	10	Date:	2	
Phase: 1	(3)	8	Phase:	3	
Day: Wednesday	(1)	8	Day:	1	
Date: 7/11	(2)	8	Date:	2	
Phase: 1	(3)	6	Phase:	3	
Day: Thursday	(1)	6	Day:	1	
Date: 7/12	(2)	6	Date:	2	
Phase: 1	(3)	4	Phase:	3	
Day:	1		Day:	1	
Date:	2		Date:	2	
Phase:	3		Phase:	3	
Day:	1		Day:	1	
Date:	2		Date:	2	
Phase:	3		Phase:	3	
Day:	1		Day:	1	
Date:	2		Date:	2	
Phase:	3		Phase:	3	
Day:	1		Day:	1	
Date:	2		Date:	2	
Phase:	3		Phase:	3	

In Phase One, Karl is following the PRICE method. Following the instructions in *The Running Injury Recovery Program*, he examines his new minimalist running shoes, and compares them to his regular training shoes. He discovers that his original shoes met all his requirements, but his new minimalist shoes do not. Since his original training shoes are still fairly new and don't have much mileage on them, he can do his post-injury training in those shoes. He takes out the elastic laces he was using and, when he laces his shoes up properly, he finds that his training shoes fit

better and hold his foot firmly to the platform.

By reading the sections about habits in *The Running Injury Recovery Program*, Karl figures out the most likely cause of his injury. He had increased his speed and mileage too quickly without a proper running base. When he starts his Base Schedule, he will start with the mileage he was able to run without injury.

After three days of PRICE and education, Karl's symptoms are reduced. He still has some pain in his foot when he gets out of bed in the morning, and some pain when he climbs stairs, but he is able to do it and he is not limping. His pain level is below 5 and he has no more Red Flag symptoms or visible swelling. He consults the Guidelines for Group 2 in *Table 5.1* **Guidelines for Phase One Treatment Groups**, and finds that he can now enter Phase Two.

In Phase Two, Karl follows the Guidelines for Group 2 in *Table 11-1*: **Guidelines for Phase Two Treatment Groups**, and the Guidelines for complex injuries in *Table 11-2*: **Phase Two Guidelines for Simple and Complex Injuries.** He is very happy to see that he no longer has to go through his icing routine three times a day. However, he must continue to ICE once a day for another two weeks, so he starts a new **Log Form I** on Friday 7/13.

At this point, Karl is looking forward to figuring out which of his *possible affected regions* is the real source of his problem. Karl follows the instructions for *Self-Assessment 2A*, and fills in **Worksheet 2A1**. At the top, he circles all six of his *possible affected regions* on the right side. He looks down the columns for each *possible affected region* that he has circled, finds the shaded boxes, and circles the matching stretch numbers. Because he has so many *possible affected regions*, he circles all of the stretches except stretches 11-1 and 11-12.

Karl does all 13 stretches, left and right, and fills in his mobility numbers. After he has filled out his worksheet, Karl returns to *Self-Assessment 2A* to rank his stretches in order of difficulty. He sees that he has asymmetry in every stretch except stretches 11-6 and 11-12. He circles all the asymmetrical pairs in the columns for his *possible affected regions*. Looking at all the pairs he has circled, he has the greatest asymmetry (left-right difference) and stiffness in stretch number 11-8. He ranks this stretch number 1 on the right side only. Next in order of left-right difference and stiffness are stretches 11-2 and 11-9. He ranks these stretches as numbers 2 and 3 on the right side only. Stretches number 11-3, 11-4, 11-5, 11-7, and 11-11 are next in order of left-right difference and stiffness, and they are numbered 4 through 8 on the right side only. Stretch numbers 11-10 and 11-13, with the least asymmetry, are numbered 9 and 10 on the right side only.

He goes back to each of the stretches he has numbered 1 through 10 on the right side, and numbers the left sides 11 through 20, but he does not circle the left side. The three remaining stretches are either for unaffected region or have symmetry. He numbers them 21/22, 23/24, and 25/26. Karl now has the order he will do his stretches in Phase Two.

Karl then continues to **Worksheet 2A2: Ranking Affected Regions**, and fills in the information for his right side. Since he has six *possible affected regions*, and they are all very stiff and asymmetrical, Karl ranks his regions based on maximum pain (arch is #1) and swelling (band and knee are #2 and #3). At this point, Karl really can't tell much difference between the six *possible affected regions*, so he is making an educated guess. He knows his unaffected regions also have problems, but he decides to worry about them later.

Worksheet 2A1: Mobility Self-Assessment

Circle *Possible Affected Region* and Side →

(Circled regions in header: 2: Arch, 5: Calf, 7: Band, 10: Butt. Circled "Right" under: Arch, Calf, Knee, Band, Hams, Hip, Butt.)

Stretch	SIDE / Rank #	1: Toe	2: Arch	3: Heel	4: Shin	5: Calf	6: Knee	7: Band	8: Hams	9: Hip	10: Butt
11-1	Left: 21	2									
	Right: 22	5									
Notes:											
(11-2)	Left: 12			1	1	1					
	(Right:) 2			4	4	4					
Notes:											
(11-3)	Left: 14								3		
	(Right:) 4								5		
Notes:											
(11-4)	Left: 15								3	3	3
	(Right:) 5								5	5	5
Notes:											
(11-5)	Left: 16	3	3	3	3	3	3		3		
	(Right:) 6	5	5	5	5	5	5		5		
Notes:											
(11-6)	Left: 23			1	1	1			1		
	Right: 24			1	1	1			1		
Notes:											
(11-7)	Left: 17			3	3	3		3	3		
	(Right:) 7			5	5	5		5	5		
Notes:											
(11-8)	Left: 11							2			2
	(Right:) 1							5			5
Notes:											
(11-9)	Left: 13							1			1
	(Right:) 3							4			4
Notes:											
(11-10)	Left: 19					1				1	
	(Right:) 9					2				2	
Notes:											
(11-11)	Left: 18									3	3
	(Right:) 8									5	5
Notes:											
11-12	Left: 25									1	
	Right: 26									1	
Notes:											
(11-13)	Left: 20		3	3	3	3					
	(Right:) 10		4	4	4	4					
Notes:											

Worksheet 2A2: Ranking Affected Regions								
SIDE: Right	From Worksheet 2A1			From Worksheet 1D4			Summary	
Possible Affected Regions	Maximum Stiffness		Maximum Asymmetry (left/right)	Pain (0-10)	Swelling yes/no	Injury Stage (1-5)	Assessment	Rank #
	Left	Right						
1 Toe								
2 Arch	3	5	3/5	10		5	Possible affected	1
3 Heel								
4 Shin								
5 Calf	3	5	1/4	6		4	Possible affected	6
6 Knee	3	5	3/5	6	yes	5	Possible affected	3
7 Band	3	5	1/4	8	yes	4	Possible affected	2
8 Hams	3	5	3/5	8		4	Possible affected	5
9 Hip								
10 Butt	3	5	1/4	8		4	Possible affected	4

Karl enters all of the stretches in order of rank from his **Worksheet 2A1** to his first **Log Form C**, and circles the *rank number* for all the "affected" stretches on the right side. At the top of **Log Form C**, he writes all six of his *possible affected regions*.

Karl then consults ***Table 2A2: Injury Regions and Stretches***, and adds self-mobilizations for all his *possible affected regions* to his first **Log Form C**. Note that, although he ranked his arch region #1, the first stretch on his list that is associated with the arch is stretch number 11-5, which is sixth on his list. Since stretches 11-1 and 11-12 are not associated with any of his six possible affected regions, he lists no self-mobilization for those exercises. He checks to make sure he has listed at least one self-mobilization for each of his six *possible affected regions*.

Karl completes his mobility self-assessment on the same day that he clears Phase One, and is ready to start his Phase Two P.T. Time on Friday 7/13. He reads **Self-Assessment 2B*: *Phase Two Treatment Group and Complexity Subgroup**, and confirms that he will enter Phase Two in Group 2, in the subgroup for complex injuries. For the next two weeks, he will ICE 20 minutes a day (**Log Form I**) and do his stretch/mobilization cycles 40 minutes a day (**Log Form C**).

On his first day of Phase Two, Karl checks ***Table 2C1:* Clearance Goals for Phase Two** and sees that the goal for complex injuries is to exactly match the positions in the illustrations for each stretch on both sides, and to have 0 stiffness. Since Karl is so stiff and so asymmetrical in every stretch, he doesn't feel like filling out all those high numbers every day. He follows the order of stretches in his **Log Form C**, and pays attention to the stretch/mobilization cycles for affected and unaffected regions [Box 11-1], and he just records the tenderness levels in the self-mobilizations on his **Log Form C**.

Karl has read all of his instructions, and he knows that it is very important for him to evaluate the tenderness in his self-mobilizations *on both sides* so that he can pinpoint the location of his actual injury region among all his *possible injury regions*. He records his maximum tenderness levels for each self-mobilization on his **Log Form C**, left and right, then he goes to *Self-Assessment 2D: Evaluate Log Form C for Regional Tenderness* and fills in **Worksheet 2D1: Regional Tenderness**.

Log Form C: Stretch/Mobilization Cycles

DAY/DATE:	Days since *last day you ran*:
PHASE #	Days in this Phase:
AFFECTED SIDE: Right	AFFECTED REGION(S): *Arch, calf, knee, band, hams, butt*

Circle affected side →		Left		Right	Symmetry	
Enter your exercise list from *Worksheets 2A1* and *2A2*	Rank #	**Stretches: Stiffness (0-5)** / **Self Mobs: Tenderness (0-5)**	Rank#	**Stretches: Stiffness (0-5)** / **Self Mobs: Tenderness (0-5)**	No	Yes
Stretch # 11- 8 / *Self-Mob: band 1*	11	1	①1	5		
Stretch # 11- 2 / *Self-Mob: calf 1*	12	2	②2	3		
Stretch # 11- 9 / *Self-Mob: band 2*	13	1	③3	5		
Stretch # 11- 3 / *Self-Mob: hams 1*	14	1	④4	3		
Stretch # 11- 4 / *Self-Mob: hams 2*	15	1	⑤5	3		
Stretch # 11- 5 / *Self-Mob: arch 1*	16	1	⑥6	5		
Stretch # 11- 7 / *Self-Mob: calf 2*	17	2	⑦7	3		
Stretch # 11- 11 / *Self-Mob: butt 1*	18	2	⑧8	5		
Stretch # 11- 10 / *Self-Mob: knee 1*	19	1	⑨9	3		
Stretch # 11- 13 / *Self-Mob: arch 2*	20	1	⑩10	5		
Stretch # 11- 1 / *Self-Mob: none*	21		22			
Stretch # 11- 6 / *Self-Mob: hams 1*	23	1	24	3		
Stretch # 11- 12 / *Self-Mob: none*	25		26			

~ 184 ~

Worksheet 2D1: Regional Tenderness				
List *possible affected regions* from **Log Form C**	Max tenderness on *more affected* side: Right	Max tenderness on *less affected* side: Left	Left/Right Difference	Assessment (affected or not)
Arch	5	1	4	Yes
Calf	3	2	1	No
Knee	3	2	1	No
Band	5	1	4	Yes
Hams	3	1	2	Maybe?
Butt	5	2	3	Maybe?

Based on his **Worksheet 2D1**, Karl decides that he definitely has running injuries in his right arch and band, and that he can drop the right calf and knee from his list of *possible affected regions*. He still is not sure about his right hamstring and right butt. He no longer has to ice his right calf and knee during his P.T. Time; but he continues icing the arch, band, hamstring and butt.

After 14 days of ICE and stretching, Karl's symptoms have greatly improved. He no longer has pain when going up or down steps, or when he stands up in the morning, and he only has pain when he does his stretching exercises. Karl has met the requirements for clearance in *Self-Assessment 2C: Phase Two Clearance*, and he can now progress to Phase Three Part One.

Karl exercises at a gym that has all of the equipment he needs for his injury-management program. In Phase Three Part One, he follows the instructions for Basic-Closed Chain Exercises, but he doesn't have anyone to help him time every set to the exact second and record it on his **Log Form B**. Instead, he watches his timer and estimates his average on each leg, then he fills in his results at the end of each exercise. He completes his first two days of Basic Closed-Chain Exercises and evaluates his **Log Form B** for initial difficulty and clearance of individual exercises.

Karl clears his quick steps, weighted kickback, and step up/step over exercises immediately. For all of his other exercises, he is cleared on the left side, but not on the injured right side. He has a lot of trouble on his right side with balance and keeping his hip stable while doing square hops and side step-downs. He also has pain in his right leg and foot during side step-down and barefoot push-up. In his two barefoot armswings, he has balance problems on the right side.

On day 3, he repeats his day 1 exercises, and improves in each exercise but still does not reach clearance. On day 4, he clears barefoot push-ups and one-leg armswings, barefoot; then works on his square hops and side-steps. On day 5, he clears square hops and side-steps, and repeats his one-leg armswings to keep four exercises in his P.T. Time. He has now cleared all Basic Closed-Chain Exercises, and he fills in his **Worksheet 3A1**.

Log Form B: Basic Closed-Chain

DAY/DATE Fri 7/27		Days since *last day you ran:*	
PHASE 3, Part# 1		Days in this Phase 1	
AFFECTED SIDE and REGION(S) Right Arch, band, hams?, butt?			

Basic Closed-Chain Exercise	CC#1 Square Hops		CC#2 Side Step-Down		CC#3 One-Leg Armswings, Barefoot		CC#4 One-Leg Armswings, 1 Pillow	
Target Time	20 sec		20 sec		15 sec		30 sec	
Rest Between Sets	10 sec		0		0		0	
Set Times	Left	Right	Left	Right	Left	Right	Left	Right
1	20	5	20	10	15	10	20	10
2		5		10		10		
3		10		10		10		
4		10		15				
5		15		15				
Total								
Avg Set Time								
L/R Difference								
Symmetry Goal	1 sec		1 sec		1 sec		2 sec	
Max Pain (0-10)	L:	R:	L:	R:	L:	R:	L:	R:
NOTES:	Weakness in right hip		Whole right leg is weak		Balance problem		Balance problem	

DAY/DATE Sat 7/28		Days since *last day you ran:*	Days in this Phase 1

Basic Closed-Chain Exercise	CC#5 Barefoot Push-Up		CC#6 Quick Steps		CC#7 Weighted Kickback		CC#8 Box Step Up and Over	
Target Time	15 sec		20 sec		60 sec		60 sec	
Rest Between Sets	0		10 sec		0		0	
Set Times	Left	Right	Both Legs [(A)]		Left	Right	Left	Right
1	15	10	20					
2								
3								
4								
5								
Total								
Avg Set Time								
L/R Difference								
Symmetry Goal	1 sec				3 sec		3 sec	
Max Pain (0-10)	L:	R:	L:	R:	L:	R:	L:	R:
NOTES:	Pain in rt foot and arch		(Pass)		(Pass)		(Pass)	

[(A)] See instructions line 9: *Special Instructions for Quick Steps*

Worksheet 3A1: Evaluation of Basic Closed-Chain Exercises

1. Based on your daily assessments, list all eight Basic Closed-Chain Exercises **in order of difficulty**:

1. CC# _____ 1 Square hops _____

2. CC# _____ 2 Side step-down _____

3. CC# _____ 5 Barefoot push-up _____

4. CC# _____ 4 one-leg armnswing, pillow _____

5. CC# _____ 3 one-leg armnswing, barefoot _____

6. CC# _____ 6 quick steps _____

7. CC# _____ 7 weighted kickback _____

8. CC# _____ 8 box step _____

2. Count the number of days since you started your Basic Closed-Chain exercises, and **circle** the statement below that applies to you:

I was *able* to clear all Basic Closed-Chain Exercises in 7 days or less, and I am progressing to Regional Closed-Chain Exercises.	I was *unable* to clear all Basic Closed-Chain Exercises in 7 days or less, and I am continuing with Basic Closed-Chain Exercises.

In *Self-Assessment 3B*, Karl compares all of his symptoms and worksheets to the descriptions in **Worksheet 3B1: Regional Self-Assessment Tables.** He fills in the tables for four *possible affected regions* (arch, band, hamstring, and buttock) and stress fracture.

Karl checks all of the symptoms in the tables for the arch and band regions. In the tables for hamstring and buttock regions, Karl can check some of the symptoms, such as stiffness and wobbling, but his kickback in closed-chain exercises was okay, and his tenderness is not in the right place for these regions. In the table for stress fracture he doesn't check any symptoms.

Karl eliminates the hamstring, buttock, and stress fracture as *possible affected regions*. He identifies the right arch and right band as separate Injury Regions, and enters both of them on **Worksheet 3B2: Injury Regions in Order of Severity.**

In *Self-Assessment 3C*, Karl copies the Regional Closed-Chain Exercises for the arch and band regions from ***Table 3C1*: Closed-Chain Exercises by Region** to **Worksheet 3C1: Regional Closed-Chain Exercises in Order of Severity**, and crosses out the duplicated exercises in the 2nd Region (numbers 2, 8, and 12).

Karl copies his nine remaining closed-chain exercises, in order, from **Worksheet 3C1** to his first **Log Form R**. Because **Log Form R** has only eight spaces, he has to use one additional form. He then goes to *Appendix Z: Regional Closed-Chain Tables for Fitness Runners and Racers* and copies the Fitness Runner times for *Rest Between Sets*, *Final Target*, and *Build Pace*. He also copies footnote A (from exercises 2 and 8) and footnote B (from exercise 16) to the line for *Notes*.

Karl now has his Regional Closed-Chain program for Phase Three Part Two. He will do his *Initial Assessments* on the first three days of P.T. Time to calculate his *Symmetry Targets* and *Symmetry Goals*.

Worksheet 3B1: Regional Self-Assessment Tables

Region 2: Arch

Activity	Self-Assessment		Left	Right
Self - mobilization	I have **tenderness** in or around the bottom of my foot; or under and/or to the outside of the heel and arch.			X
Stretches	I have reduced range of motion (**stiffness**) in the ankle region, *resulting in* difficulty flexing the foot upward.			X
Closed-Chain Exercises	I have **weakness** in the toe-flexing muscles, *resulting in* rolling the foot to the inside or outside when standing on one leg.			X
Pre-Injury Stride Tendency	While running, I have a tendency to:	A. Turn the leg excessively out or in.		X
		B. Overstrike and foot-slap into an overpronated foot.		X

Region 7: Band

Activity	Self-Assessment		Left	Right
Self - mobilization	I have **tenderness** on the outside of the knee, with or without visible swelling.			X
Stretches	I have reduced range of motion (**stiffness**) from the hip and buttock down to the upper leg.			X
Closed-Chain Exercises	I have **weakness** in the band region, *resulting in*:	A. Difficulty staying balanced on one leg.		X
		B. Difficulty kicking out to the side.		X
Pre-Injury Stride Tendency	While running, I have a tendency to:	A. Wobble side-to-side at the hip.		X
		B. Lean to the outside with my foot sticking out, causing my knee to go to the inside.		X

Region 8: Hamstring

Activity	Self-Assessment		Left	Right
Self - mobilization	1. I have **tenderness** in the back of the leg between the knee and buttock.			
Stretches	I have reduced range of motion (**stiffness**) in the Straight Leg Raise.			X
Closed-Chain Exercises	I have **weakness** in the hamstring region, *resulting in* asymmetrical weakness and inflexibility in the hamstring area during kickback.			
Pre-Injury Stride Tendency	While running, I have a tendency to:	A. Push off from the inner side of the big toe.		X
		B. Have a kickback that is short, asymmetrical, or twists.		

Region 10: Buttock
(Secondary Region: Lateral hip)

Activity	Self-Assessment		Left	Right
Self-mobilization	I have **tenderness** and swelling to the rear and side of the hip.			
Stretches	I have reduced range of motion (**stiffness**) in any hip stretching exercise.			X
Closed-Chain Exercises:	I have **weakness** in the hip and buttock region that affects symmetrical kickback and overall balance.			
Pre-Injury Stride Tendency	While running, I have a tendency to:	A. Wobble side-to-side at the hip.		X
		B. Be unable to kick back straight and/or fully.		
		C. Have asymmetrical rotation of the pelvis.		X

Region 11: Regional Injury with Stress Fracture

Activity	Self-Assessment	Left	Right
Self-mobilization	I have **tenderness** in any weight-bearing bone in my injury region (anywhere from the foot to the pelvis), with or without pain in the associated soft tissues.		
Stretches	I have reduced range of motion (**stiffness**) in the region where I have bone tenderness.		
Closed-Chain Exercises:	After icing *and* not running for at least 3 weeks, I can *still* **reproduce my injury pain** when I hop on the injured leg (unable to clear CC#1 Square Hop Exercise).		
Pre-Injury Stride Tendency	While running, I feel pain in the region where I have bone tenderness.		

Worksheet 3B2: Injury Regions in Order of Severity			
Rank #	Side (left/right)	Injury Region	
1.	Right	Region #	2 Arch
2.	Right	Region #	7 Band
3.		Region #	
4.		Region #	

Worksheet 3C1: Regional Closed-Chain Exercises in Order of Severity

1st Injury Region and Side: right arch	
Box 1: Regional Closed-Chain Exercises	
CC# 2	Side Step-Down
CC# 3	One-Leg Armswings, Barefoot
CC# 8	Box Step Up and Over
CC# 11	Straight-Leg Raise with Theraband
CC# 12	One-Leg Armswings, Double Pillows
CC# 16	Barefoot Push-Through

2nd Injury Region and Side: right band	
Box 2: Regional Closed-Chain Exercises	
CC# 2	Side Step-Down
CC# 8	Box Step Up and Over
CC# 9	Hip Abduction with Theraband
CC# 12	One-Leg Armswings, Double Pillows
CC# 13	One-Leg Armswings, Side Incline
CC# 20	Theraband Kickback

3rd Injury Region and Side:	
Box 3: Regional Closed-Chain Exercises	
CC#	
CC#	
CC#	
CC#	
CC#	
CC#	

Stress Fracture, Side:	
Box 4: Regional Closed-Chain Exercises	
CC# 1	
CC# 2	
CC# 8	

Log Form R: Regional Closed-Chain

DAY/DATE:	Days since *last day you ran:*
PHASE (3 or 4):	Days in this Phase:
Injury Region(s) and Side: Right arch & band	

Regional Closed-Chain Exercise (number and name)	CC# 2 Side Step-Down		CC# 3 One-Leg Armswings, Barefoot		CC# 8 Box Step Up and Over		CC# 11 Straight-Leg Raise with Theraband	
Symmetry Target								
Rest Between Sets	0		0		0		0	
Final Target	30 sec		30 sec		2.5 min		60 sec	
Build pace as:	glide (A)		glide		glide (A)		glide	
Set Times	Left	Right	Left	Right	Left	Right	Left	Right
1								
2								
3								
4								
5								
Total								
Avg Set Time								
L/R Difference								
Symmetry Goal		sec		sec		sec		sec
Max Pain (0-10)	L:	R:	L:	R:	L:	R:	L:	R:
NOTES:								

FOOTNOTES: (A) See instructions to build box height [Box 14-2].

DAY/DATE:	Days since *last day you ran:*	Days in this Phase:

Regional Closed-Chain Exercise (number and name)	CC# 12 One-Leg Armswings, Double Pillows		CC# 16 Barefoot Push-Through (B)		CC# 9 Hip Abduction with Theraband		CC# 13 One-Leg Armswings, Side Incline	
Symmetry Target								
Rest Between Sets	0		30 sec		0		0	
Final Target	30 sec		4.5 min		60 sec		30 sec	
Build pace as:	acceleration		glide		glide		acceleration	
Set Times	Left	Right	Left	Right	Left	Right	Left	Right
1								
2								
3								
4								
5								
Total								
Avg Set Time								
L/R Difference								
Symmetry Goal		sec		sec		sec		sec
Max Pain (0-10)	L:	R:	L:	R:	L:	R:	L:	R:
NOTES:								

FOOTNOTES: (B) Box 14-3: Special Instructions for Push-Through

DAY/DATE:			Days since *last day you ran:*				Days in this Phase:	

Regional Closed-Chain Exercise (number and name)	CC#20 Theraband Kickback		CC#		CC#		CC#	
Symmetry Target								
Rest Between Sets	0							
Final Target	60 sec							
Build pace as:	acceleration							
Set Times	Left	Right	Left	Right	Left	Right	Left	Right
1								
2								
3								
4								
5								
Total								
Avg Set Time								
L/R Difference								
Symmetry Goal		sec		sec		sec		sec
Max Pain (0-10)	L:	R:	L:	R:	L:	R:	L:	R:
NOTES:								
FOOTNOTES:								

In *Self-Assessment 3D*, Karl writes his *Impairment Statements* and determines his group for Phase Three Part Two.

Karl looks at his list of Basic Closed-Chain Exercises in **Worksheet 3A1: Evaluation of Basic Closed-Chain Exercises**, then finds his two main balance problems in *Table 3D1*: **Basic Closed-Chain Balance Problems**. The first two Basic Closed-Chain Exercises on his list are #1 Square Hops and #2 Side Step-down, which have the same Basic Balance Problem: "Difficulty maintaining balance over a straight foot." He combines this statement with his two Injury Regions to write his first Impairment Statement: "*I was unable to balance my body on my right foot due to wobbling in my hip.*"

The next Basic Closed-Chain Exercises on his list is #5 Barefoot Push-up, which has this Basic Balance Problem:

"Difficulty maintaining balance while pushing off straight through the big toe." Combining this statement with his two Injury Regions, Karl writes his second Impairment Statement: "*I was unable to push off straight through my right big toe because my arch was collapsing and my hip wobbled.*"

Karl completes **Worksheet 3D1** to determine his treatment group for Phase Three Part Two. Since he didn't write down his last day of regular training in *Self-Assessment 1B: Running History*, he has to go back to his calendar to find the number of days since the "*last day you ran.*" He completes Phase Three Part One on Tuesday 7/31, and his last day of regular training was Sunday 7/8, so he counts 23 days. Based on his answers, he finds that he will enter Phase Three Part Two in Group 2A.

Worksheet 3D1: Treatment Groups for Phase Three Part Two

1. Which of the following statements applies to you?

    (A.) I have cleared all eight Basic Closed-Chain Exercises in 7 Days or less.

    B. I have completed Day 7 of Basic Closed-Chain Exercises, and I still have *not* cleared one or more of the eight Basic Closed-Chain Exercises.

2. Based on your **Self-Assessment 2B**, which complexity subgroup are you in?

    A. *Simple Injuries.*

    (B.) *Complex Injuries.*

3. How many Injury Regions did you list in **Worksheet 3B2: Injury Regions in Order of Severity**?

    A. One

    (B.) More than one

4. Look at the top section of today's **Log Form B: Basic Closed-Chain**, and find the box for "Days since *last day you ran*." Which of the following statements applies to you?

    (A.) Today is 42 days or less (6 weeks or less) since the last day I ran.

    B. Today is 43 days or more (more than 6 weeks) since the last day I ran.

5. Based on questions 1 through 4, find your Treatment Group for Phase Three Part Two:

You are in:	If your answers to questions 1 though 4 are:
GROUP 1A	"A" to ALL FOUR questions
GROUP 1B	"B" to question 1 AND "A" to ALL of questions 2, 3 and 4
(**GROUP 2A**)	"A" to question 1 AND "B" to ONE OR MORE of questions 2, 3, and 4
GROUP 2B	"B" to question 1 AND "B" to ONE OR MORE of questions 2, 3, and 4

In *Self-Assessment 3E*, Karl determines his Base Schedule. Since he had not been running very regularly before his injury, and his weekly mileage often fell below 10 miles per week, he chooses the minimum times for Fitness Runners in *Table 3E1*: **Base Schedules for Fitness Runners and Racers**. Due to his work schedule, the best time for him to do his P.T. Time and Base Schedule is on the weekends. He can now fill in his **Worksheet T: Training Plan for Phase Three Part Two**, and begin his Base Schedule.

Karl does the first day of his Base Schedule on the treadmill at his gym on Wednesday 8/1, using **Log Form S Level 0** for fitness walking. He follows the Guidelines for Group 2 in *Table 13-3*, and evaluates his Base Schedule using *Self-Assessment 3G2 for Two-Week-Interval Plan*. He completes 2 weeks (6 Base Schedule sessions) at Level 0 with no difficulty, and begins his fist day of walk/glides at Level 1 on Wednesday 8/15.

By now, Karl understands that his original running problem was a lack of balance. To compensate for the lack of balance, he had been running too fast, with too long a stride. The higher speed helped him balance better, but it contributed to his foot injury because it caused him to land badly. In his walk/glides, Karl's new goal is to slow down his pace while taking shorter, faster strides (a higher turnover rate) to create balance. The shorter strides and reduced effort will keep him balanced and prevent him from coming down too hard on his foot.

On his first day in the walk/glide program [See **Log Form S Level 1**], Karl keeps his pace very slow to practice his new stride, so he does not count that day toward his goal. On his second day, Saturday 8/18, he gets impatient and really wants to run. He lengthens his stride and starts running too fast – falling onto his old pattern. He blows up his foot, his pain increases from level 1 to level 8, and he doesn't finish his drills.

He gets through his P.T. Time with only a slight increase in pain, and checks his Running Injury Stage the next day. He knows that if he has any Stage 3 symptoms he has to go back a step, so he is relieved when he feels better the next morning. On Sunday 8/19 he is very careful – he slows his pace and shortens his stride to remain balanced throughout his walk/glides – then he works on his P.T. Time.

Karl starts counting his Base Schedule Level 1 days again on Wednesday 8/22, and this time he is more careful. He clears Level 1 on Sunday 9/2.

Karl completes the remainder of his Phase Three Base Schedule (Levels 2 through 5) without any problems, and clears *Self-Assessment 3G2 for Two-Week-Interval Plan* and *Self Assessment 3H: Phase Three Clearance and Preparation for Phase Four* on Sunday 10/28.

He prepares his log forms for Phase Four, and writes two Specific Mental Focus Statements: *(1) I will use my hip and arch to balance my body on a straight foot,* and *(2) I will use my band and foot to push off straight through my big toe.*

Worksheet T: Training Plan for Phase Three Part Two

1. I am a (Fitness Runner or Racer): ____Fitness Runner____.

2. I plan to do my P.T. Time (**Log Form M** and **Log Form B** or **Log Form R**) 60 minutes per day, two days per week, on these days: ____Saturday____ and ____Sunday____.
(*Note:* P.T. Time may be done on the same days as your Base Schedule, or on different days).

3. I plan to do my Base Schedule (**Log Form S**) 60 minutes per day, __3__ days per week, on these days:

____Saturday, Sunday, and Wednesday____.

4. I am in Treatment Group Number (1A, 1B, 2A, or 2B) __2A__.

5. I am following the (*Self-Paced Plan* or *Two-Week-Interval Plan*):
____2 week____.

6. I will start my Base Schedule at Level ____0____.

7. My weekly mileage *goal* is ____10____ miles per week.

8. My daily mileage *maximum* is ____3 ½____ miles per day (divide line 7 by line 3).

Write your personalized *Impairment Statements* from *Self-Assessment 3D* here:

1. I was unable to balance my body on my right foot due to wobbling in my hip.

2. I was unable to push off straight through my right big toe because my arch was collapsing and my hip wobbled.

Log Form S: Base Schedule
Level 1

	Activity	Type	Repetitions	Duration	Total Time
Starting Day/Date: Wed 8/15			**Days since *last day you ran* (on starting day):**		
Target Days per week (3, 4, 5) 3			**Clearance date:** Sun 9/2		
Warmup	Fitness Walk				10 min
Base Schedule (*Table 15-4A*)	Walk/glide sets	Glide 1min/walk 4 min	10		
	10 Glide Drills:	Drill #1	2	15 sec	50 min
		Drill #2	2	15 sec	
		Drill #3	2	15 sec	
		Drill #4	2	15 sec	
		Drill #5	2	15 sec	
Cooldown	Fitness Walk				5 min

	Day/Date	Day/Date	Day/Date	Day/Date	Day/Date
Week 1	Wed/ 8-15	Sat/ 8-18	Sun/ 8-19	/	/
Pain (0-10)	1	8	2		
Drills/Form	10	5	10		
Notes:	Very slow but good	Too fast Bad landing Hurt foot	Very slow and careful		
Week 2	Wed/ 8-22	Sat/ 8-25	Sun/ 8-26	/	/
Pain (0-10)	0	0	0		
Drills/Form	10	10	10		
Notes:	Good New Day 1	good	good		
Week 3	Wed/ 8-29	Sat/ 9-1	Sun/ 9-2	/	/
Pain (0-10)	0	0	0		
Drills/Form	10	10	10		
Notes:	good	good	Day 6- Cleared!		
Week 4	/	/	/	/	/
Pain (0-10)					
Drills/Form					
Notes:					

Worksheet 3G2: Evaluate Log Form S for Two-Week-Interval Plan (Level 0)

1. Evaluate your ability to fitness-walk your Base Schedule according to the instructions in Chapter 15 of *The Running Injury Recovery Program*:	Did you have any increase in pain or break in form during your 60-minute fitness walk?	Yes	(No)
2. Evaluate your notes:	A. Did you note any weakness, asymmetry, or problem with your stride?	Yes	(No)
	B. Do you have any other problem that you need to work on before progressing to Walk/Glide sets?	Yes	(No)
3. Level 0: Continue until the two numbers on the right match:	Multiply your number of *Target Days per Week* (3, 4, or 5) times two.		(6)
	Write the number of consecutive days you have cleared your Base Schedule at Level 0 with no break in form and no increase in symptoms.		(6)

Worksheet 3G2: Evaluate Log Form S for Two-Week-Interval Plan (Levels 1 through 5)

1. Evaluate your ability to perform each part of your Base Schedule according to the instructions in Chapter 15 of *The Running Injury Recovery Program*:	A. *Warmup:* Did you have any increase in pain or break in form during your 10-minute fitness walk?	Yes	(No)
	B. *Walk/glide sets:* Did you have any increase in pain or break in form during walk/glide sets?	Yes	(No)
	C. *Glide drills:* Did you have any difficulty performing any of the drills with correct form (as described in the instructions for that drill)?	Yes	(No)
	D. *Cooldown:* Did you have any increase in pain or break in form during your 5-minute fitness walk?	Yes	(No)
2. Evaluate completion of all drills:	A. Were you *unable* to complete the required time (*duration*) for any drill?	Yes	(No)
	B. Were you *unable* to complete the required number of sets (*repetitions*) for any drill?	Yes	(No)
3. Evaluate your notes:	A. Did you note any weakness, asymmetry, or problem with your stride?	Yes	(No)
	B. Do you have any other problem that you need to work on before progressing to the next level?	Yes	(No)
4. Levels 1 through 5: Continue until the two numbers on the right match.	Multiply your number of *Target Days per Week* (3, 4, or 5) times two.		(6)
	Write the number of consecutive days you have cleared your Base Schedule at this level with no break in form and no increase in symptoms?		(6)

Worksheet 3H1: Phase Three Clearance		
1. Have you cleared all of your Regional Closed-Chain Exercises through Stage 1 (*Self-Assessment 3F*)?	No	Yes
2. Have you cleared your Base Schedule through Level 5 (*Self-Assessment 3G1 or 3G2*)?	No	Yes

---

Specific Mental Focus Statement:

(1) I will use my hip and arch to balance my body on a straight foot.

(2) I will use my band and foot to push off straight through my big toe.

When Karl starts Phase Four, he is finally done with the two-week-interval plan. He completes all of his Phase Four exercises (*Self-Assessments 4A through 4C*) in one week with no problems, and is ready to return to running.

In *Self-Assessment 4D*, Karl fills in his **Worksheet 4D1**, and returns to his regular training. It is 17 weeks since his injury, but now he feels stronger and more balanced.

Worksheet 4D1: Habits for Post-Recovery Running		
Post-Recovery Running Habits Checklist:	1. I will make a plan, and train consistently.	X
	2. I will set realistic running goals.	X
	3. I will start each run with a proper warmup.	X
	4. I will pay close attention to my equipment, particularly my footwear.	X
	5. I will focus on functional running.	X
	6. I will manage my running injuries early, before they become severe.	X

The most important lessons I have learned from my *Running Injury Recovery Program* that I will use when I return to regular training are:

1. I need to train regularly and consistently – at least 3 times per week, for a total of 10 miles per week.

2. I need to pay attention to my stride and cadence.

3. I need to continue doing stretches for mobility and closed-chain exercises for balance, and to check up on my injury status.

Example #3:
Simple Injury with Other Running Dysfunctions ("Erica")

"Erica" is a strong, competitive long-distance runner who runs two to three marathons each year. On her current training schedule, she trains early in the morning, 5 days a week. She listens to music with earphones on, especially when she's on the treadmill, and she doesn't really pay attention to her foot-sounds.

About 20 miles into her long runs, she started developing a pain in her right foot, near her outside toes. She continued running thorough the pain, but now she is starting to get the pain earlier and earlier in each of her runs, and it's really bothering her. She realizes that she needs to address the problem before it gets any worse. She reads *The Running Injury Recovery Program* and finds that her music may be an *extrinsic factor* that is distracting her during her runs. Before deciding between self-management and professional management, Erica goes for a run without her music, and can actually hear that she is slapping her right foot.

Phase One

Erica decides to start self-management to correct her bad habits and fix her running injury. She reads through *Self-Assessments 1A, 1B,* and *1C*, and writes down the last day that she ran. In *Self-Assessment 1D*, she fills in **Worksheet 1D parts 1 through 5**.

Erica finds that she has a Stage 1 injury in one region on her right side. Since she has had no swelling and no Red Flags in any region during the past 2 weeks, she enters Phase One in Group 1.

Looking at **Worksheet 1E1: Phase One Clearance**, she finds she can answer "yes" to all questions. She immediately checks off the requirements for Phase One on her Course Map, and continues to Phase Two on the same day.

***

Worksheet 1D:
Document Your Injury and Phase One Treatment Group

Last day you ran: _Saturday January 5_   **Today's date**: _Sunday January 6_

Worksheet 1D1: Pain Pattern

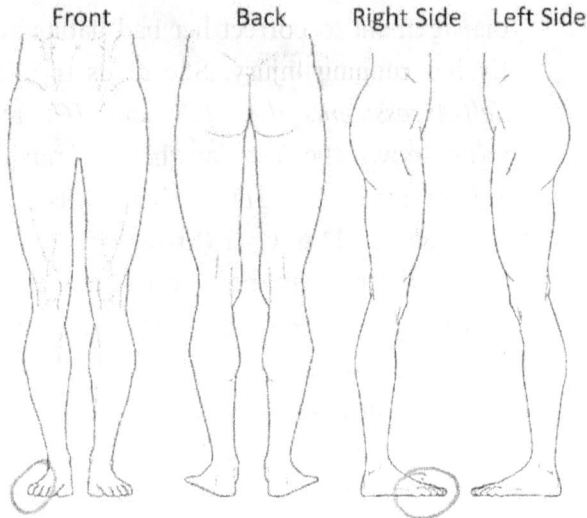

Front   Back   Right Side   Left Side

Compare to *Appendix A* and list your *possible affected regions* and side here:

_____

Outer Toes on Right Side

_____

_____

_____

_____

Worksheet 1D2: Swelling Within Past 2 Weeks

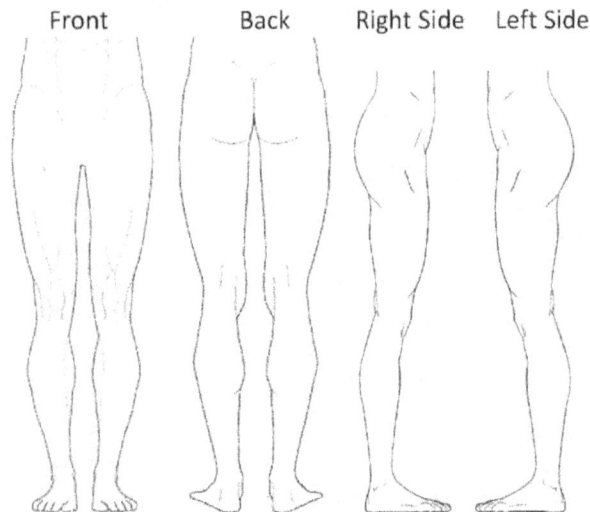

Front   Back   Right Side   Left Side

Compare to *Appendix A* and list your *possible affected regions* and side here:

_____

_____

_None_____

_____

_____

_____

Worksheet 1D3: Injury Stage

Injury Side and *possible affected region(s)*: _____ *Right Outer Toes*_____

Table A: Maximum Symptoms *within the past 2 weeks*

Injury Stages	Emerging Symptoms	*Red Flags*	Which region(s)?
Stage 1	Pain while running	Pain that alters your stride	*Outer Toes*
Stage 2	Pain at rest (after running)	Pain that disturbs your rest	
Stage 3	Pain during your normal daily activities	Pain that interferes with or makes you avoid ADLs	
Stage 4	Running injury pain that you take medication for	Being in Stage 4	
Stage 5	Pain that cripples you	Being in Stage 5	

Table B: Maximum Symptoms *from more than 2 weeks ago*

Injury Stages	Emerging Symptoms	*Red Flags*	Which region(s)?
Stage 1	Pain while running	Pain that alters your stride	
Stage 2	Pain at rest (after running)	Pain that disturbs your rest	
Stage 3	Pain during your normal daily activities	Pain that interferes with or makes you avoid ADLs	
Stage 4	Running injury pain that you take medication for	Being in Stage 4	
Stage 5	Pain that cripples you	Being in Stage 5	

Worksheet 1D4: Summary of Original Injury

Refer to:	Worksheet 1D1: Pain Pattern	Worksheet 1D2: Swelling	Worksheet 1D3: Table A Injury Stage in Past 2 Weeks	
Left Leg Circle *Possible Affected Regions*	Pain Severity (1-10)	Swelling in past 2 weeks (yes/no)	Injury Stage Scale (1-5)	Red Flag (yes/no)
1 Toe				
2 Arch				
3 Heel				
4 Shin				
5 Calf				
6 Knee				
7 Band				
8 Hamstring				
9 Hip				
10 Buttock				

Refer to:	Worksheet 1D1: Pain Pattern	Worksheet 1D2: Swelling	Worksheet 1D3: Table A Injury Stage in Past 2 Weeks	
Right Leg Circle *Possible Affected Regions*	Pain Severity (1-10)	Swelling in past 2 weeks (yes/no)	Injury Stage Scale (1-5)	Red Flag (yes/no)
1 Toe	8	No	1	No
2 Arch				
3 Heel				
4 Shin				
5 Calf				
6 Knee				
7 Band				
8 Hamstring				
9 Hip				
10 Buttock				

Worksheet 1D5: Phase One Treatment Group

Circle ONE of the two statements below:

I will enter Phase One injury management in treatment Group 1, and I do not have to ICE.	I will enter Phase One injury management in treatment Group 2, and I will now begin to ICE (**Log Form I**).

***

Worksheet 1E1: Phase One Clearance

I have *no* Red Flag symptoms or visible swelling.	No	Yes
All of the emerging symptoms I recorded in Worksheets 1D1 through 1D4 have improved.	No	Yes
My sleep is not disturbed by pain due to this injury.	No	Yes
I can perform my activities of daily living (ADLs) normally, with less pain.	No	Yes
I do not need to take medication for pain and inflammation due to my running injury.	No	Yes
I have checked lines 5.1 through 9.4 on my Course Map.	No	Yes
I have followed all of the instructions in chapters 5 through 9 to implement protection and recovery for my running injury.	No	Yes
Group 2 ONLY: I have Iced 3 times a day, and the symptoms I have recorded on **Log Form I** have improved.	No	Yes

Phase Two

In Phase Two, Erica follows the instructions for *Self-Assessment 2A: Mobility Self-Assessment and Phase Two Recovery Plan*, and completes her **Worksheet 2A1**.

Erica has only one *possible affected region*, the right outer toes. When she evaluates her **Worksheet 2A1**, she finds two stretches associated with that region. She ranks stretches 11-1 and 11-5 as numbers 1 and 2 on the right side, and numbers 3 and 4 on the left side.

Now Erica looks at her stretches for *unaffected* regions. She finds some asymmetry with greater stiffness on her injury side (the right side) in stretch 11-13, particularly in her right arch. She ranks this stretch with numbers 5 and 6 on the right and left sides.

Erica also finds a great deal of stiffness and asymmetry in certain stretches on her left side for Region 10: buttock, even though she has no injury on her left side. This problem comes as a surprise to Erica, and means that she also has a weakness on her left side that might affect her running. Since the left butt is *not* a region affected by this injury, she places these stretches on her *unaffected* list (following the instructions for Stretch/ Mobilization Cycles for unaffected regions). She ranks stretches 11-4, 11-11, 11-8, and 11-9, left and right, at numbers 7 through 14.

All of Erica's remaining stretches are at level 0 for "no stiffness." She can number these stretches for unaffected regions in any order she likes.

Erica now fills in her **Worksheet 2A2: Ranking Affected Regions** for the affected right side. She ranks the affected right outer toes region #1, and the unaffected right arch region #2. She fills in a second **Worksheet 2A2** for the left side, and ranks the left buttock as region #3.

Erica copies all 13 stretches, in order of rank, from her **Worksheet 2A1: Mobility Self Assessment** to her first *Log Form C:* **Stretch/Mobilization Cycles.** She consults *Table 2A2:* **Injury Regions and Stretches** to select her self-mobilizations for each stretch.

For her first two stretches for *possible affected regions*, she chooses self-mobilizations for the toe region. For stretch 11-13, she writes in an arch self-mobilization.

For stretches 11-4, 11-11, 11-8, and 11-9, she chooses mobilizations for the butt region.

Stretches number 11-2, 11-6, and 11-7 are all associated with mobilizations for the heel, shin, and calf. Although Erica did not list any of these regions in her **Worksheet 2A2: Ranking Affected Regions**, she did have some tightness in these regions when she did her back incline stretch (CC#13), so she chooses one self-mobilization for each of these regions.

Stretches 11-3, 11-10 and 11-12 are not associated with any region of concern, so she has no self-mobilizations for these stretches.

Erica's **Log Form C** is now ready for Phase Two.

Worksheet 2A1: Mobility Self-Assessment

Circle *Possible Affected Region* and Side → / Stretch	SIDE / Rank #	1: Toe	2: Arch	3: Heel	4: Shin	5: Calf	6: Knee	7: Band	8: Hams	9: Hip	10: Butt
11-1	Left: 3	(1)									
11-1	Right: 1		5								
Notes:	Wall toe stretch with rope										
11-2	Left:			0	0	0					
11-2	Right:			0	0	0					
Notes:											
11-3	Left:								0		
11-3	Right:								0		
Notes:											
11-4	Left: 7								1	1	(4)
11-4	Right: 8								1	1	(1)
Notes:	Ankle knee wall stretch – stiff left butt										
11-5	Left: 4	(0)	(0)	0	0	0	0		0		
11-5	Right: 2	(2)	(2)	0	0	0	0		0		
Notes:	Toes to nose stretch										
11-6	Left:			0	0	0			0		
11-6	Right:			0	0	0			0		
Notes:											
11-7	Left:			0	0	0		0	0		
11-7	Right:			0	0	0		0	0		
Notes:											
11-8	Left: 11							0			(1)
11-8	Right: 12							0			(0)
Notes:	SLR belt stretch to side										
11-9	Left: 13							0			(1)
11-9	Right: 14							0			(0)
Notes:	Cross leg side bend										
11-10	Left:						0			0	
11-10	Right:						0			0	
Notes:											
11-11	Left: 9									1	(4)
11-11	Right: 10									1	(1)
Notes:	Ankle knee diagonal stretch – stiff left butt										
11-12	Left:									0	
11-12	Right:									0	
Notes:											
11-13	Left: 6		(1)	(1)	(1)	(1)					
11-13	Right: 5		(4)	(2)	(2)	(2)					
Notes:	Incline stretch -- General stiffness on right										

Worksheet 2A2: Ranking Affected Regions

SIDE: (RIGHT)		From Worksheet 2A1			From Worksheet 1D4			Summary	
Possible Affected Regions		Maximum Stiffness		Maximum Asymmetry (left/right)	Pain (0-10)	Swelling yes/no	Injury Stage (1-5)	Assessment	Rank #
		Left	Right						
1	Toe	1	5	1/5	8	No	1	affected region	1
2	Arch	1	4	1/4				Work on stiffness	2
3	Heel								
4	Shin								
5	Calf								
6	Knee								
7	Band								
8	Hams								
9	Hip								
10	Butt								

Worksheet 2A2: Ranking Affected Regions

SIDE: (LEFT)		From Worksheet 2A1			From Worksheet 1D4			Summary	
Possible Affected Regions		Maximum Stiffness		Maximum Asymmetry (left/right)	Pain (0-10)	Swelling yes/no	Injury Stage (1-5)	Assessment	Rank #
		Left	Right						
1	Toe								
2	Arch								
3	Heel								
4	Shin								
5	Calf								
6	Knee								
7	Band								
8	Hams								
9	Hip								(No injury)	
10	Butt	4	1	4/1				Tender in stretches	3

In *Self-Assessment 2B*, Erica fills in her **Worksheet 2B1: Phase Two Treatment Group and Sub-Group.** She finds that, since she has only one set of symptoms on her injury side, she will continue in Group 1 and follow the guidelines for a simple injury. Although the found some problems with her balance on the left side, this is not a part of her injury and does not make her injury complex.

On her first day of Phase Two, Erica performs all of her Stretch/Mobilization Cycles for affected and unaffected regions, and records her stiffness in the stretches, and her tenderness in the self-mobilizations. In *Self-Assessment 2C*, she compares the left/right numbers for stiffness only (not tenderness in self-mobilizations) and checks "no" for symmetry in her first seven stretches.

Erica fills in one **Log Form C** each day for three days, at which time she can finally check "yes" for symmetry for each stretch. Because she has a simple injury, she only has to achieve symmetry – she does not have to record a "0" for each stretch.

Erica then fills in her **Worksheet 2D1: Regional Tenderness** based on her first **Log Form C**.

At this point, Erica still has only one *possible affected region* on her right side, plus some unexplained tenderness in the left buttock region. Erica has now completed all of her requirements for Phase Two clearance, and she is done with **Log Form C**. In Phase Three, Erica will record her Stretch/Mobilization Cycles on **Log Form M: Maintain Mobility.**

Worksheet 2B1: Phase Two Treatment Group and Subgroup

1. Did you begin Phase One in Group 2 (with *Red Flags* or swelling)?
   A. No
   B. Yes

2. Do you *now* have any *Red Flags* or visible swelling in the injured region?
   A. No
   B. Yes

3. Based on your answers to questions 1 and 2, find your Phase Two treatment group:

Question 1:	Question 2:	Treatment Group
A. No	*and* A. No	*Group 1*
A. No	*and* B. Yes	*Group 2*
B. Yes	*and* A. No	*Group 2*
B. Yes	*and* B. Yes	*Group 2*

4. Go to your completed **Worksheet 2A2: Ranking Affected Regions**. How many regions did you assess as *possibly affected regions*?

A. If you have only one *possible affected region* on one side (no regions on the other side), then count your injury as **one region**.

B. If you have two or three *possible affected regions* on one side (and no regions on the other side), AND your *possible affected regions* are in closely associated areas (such as 1, 2, 3 or 6, 7, 8), AND you have decided, based on the guidelines in this book, that your symptoms are due to one simple injury, then count your injury as **one region**.

C. If you circled one or more *possible affected region* on the left side AND one or more *possible affected region* on the right side, count your injury as **two or more regions**.

D. If you circled two or more *possible affected regions* on one side, and they are NOT all closely associated with each other (such as 2, 3 and 7), count your injury as **two or more regions**.

5. Go to your **Self-Assessment 1C: Medical History**.

A. If you answered NO to *all* questions in **Self-Assessment 1C**, you have **NO pre-existing condition** that might affect your running.

B. If you answered YES to *any* question in **Self-Assessment 1C**, you have a **pre-existing condition** that might affect your running.

6. Based on your answers to questions 4 and 5 above, find your complexity subgroup below:

Question 4:	Question 5:	Subgroup
A or B (One region)	*and* A. NO pre-existing condition	Simple Injury
A or B (One region)	*and* B. Pre-existing condition	Complex Injury
C or D (Two or more regions)	*and* A.NO pre-existing condition	Complex Injury
C or D (Two or more regions)	*and* B. Pre-existing condition	Complex Injury

7. Fill in your Phase Two Recovery Group and Complexity Subgroup here:

Entering Phase Two, I am in recovery group (*1 or 2*) __Group 1__ , and I will follow the guidelines for (*simple or complex*) __Simple__ injuries.

Log Form C: Stretch/Mobilization Cycles

DAY/DATE: Sun 1/6	Days since *last day you ran*: 1
PHASE # 2	Days in this Phase: 1
AFFECTED SIDE: Right	AFFECTED REGION(S): Outer Toes

Circle affected side →		Left		Right		Symmetry	
Enter your exercise list from *Worksheets 2A1* and *2A2*	Rank #	Stretches: Stiffness (0-5) / Self Mobs: Tenderness (0-5)	Rank#	Stretches: Stiffness (0-5) / Self Mobs: Tenderness (0-5)		No	Yes
Stretch # 11-1	3	1	(1)	4		X	
Self-Mob: Toe 1		1		5			
Stretch # 11-5	4	1	(2)	4		X	
Self-Mob: Toe 2		1		5			
Stretch # 11-13	6	1	5	2		X	
Self-Mob: Arch 2		1 .		2			
Stretch # 11-4	7	3	8	1		X	
Self-Mob: Butt 1		3		0			
Stretch # 11-11	9	3	10	1		X	
Self-Mob: Butt 2		3		0			
Stretch # 11-8	11	1	12	0		X	
Self-Mob: Butt 1		3		0			
Stretch # 11-9	13	1	14	0		X	
Self-Mob: Butt 2		3		0			
Stretch # 11-2		0		0			X
Self-Mob: heel 1		0		0			
Stretch # 11-3		0		0			X
Self-Mob: none		--		-			
Stretch # 11-6		0		0			X
Self-Mob: shin 1		0		0			
Stretch # 11-7		0		0			X
Self-Mob: calf 1		0		0			
Stretch # 11-10		0		0			X
Self-Mob: none		-		-			
Stretch # 11-12		0		0			X
Self-Mob: none		-		-			

Worksheet 2D1: Regional Tenderness				
List *possible affected regions* from **Log Form C**	Max tenderness on *more affected* side:	Max tenderness on *less affected* side:	Left/Right Difference	Assessment (affected or not)
Right Toe	5	1	4	affected region
Right arch	2	1	1	Not affected
Left butt	1 (left)	3 (right)	2	No injury

Phase Three Part One

In Phase Three Part One, Erica does her Basic Closed-Chain Exercises and evaluates her **Log Form B** for clearance (*Self-Assessment 3A*).

Erica is working out at home with the alternative equipment listed in ***Table 14-2: Equipment for Closed-Chain Exercises***. She does her step exercises (CC#2 and CC#8) on the stairs in her apartment building, and her quicksteps (CC#6) on a curb in the parking lot. She completes her first four exercises on Day 1, and the second four exercises on Day 2.

On her first day, Erica has trouble with hopping on her left side (CC#1) because her balance is off – her left hip wobbles. When she hops on her injured right foot she has a little pain, but her shoes support her and she can finish this exercise with no problem. In side step-downs (CC#2), she wobbles on her left hip, but performs better on her injured right side.

In her barefoot armswings (CC#3), Erica's hip wobbles on the left side, and her arch tends to collapse on the right side. She does better on the left than on the right. When she does armswings in her shoes (CC#4), her shoes support her injured foot, and she does better on the right than on the left.

On her second day, Erica again has difficulty with the barefoot exercise. In barefoot push-ups (CC#5), her right foot has no support and she has some pain. She clears this exercise on the left but not on the right.

Erica follows the special instructions for timing quicksteps (CC#6) and rest between sets. However, she is unable to finish her quicksteps (CC#6) because she keeps landing on the outside of her injured foot, and her injury pain returns at a level 8. She learns that she has to focus on placing her weight through her big toe, not the outside of her foot.

She clears weighted kickback (CC#7) with no problem. For box step up and over (CCD#8), she steps up two stairs at a time for 60 seconds with one leg, then switches to the other leg. She passes this exercise with just a little pain left over from her quicksteps.

Erica works hard to achieve balance and push off through her right big toe. She passes Basic Closed-Chain Exercises CC#1 through CC#4 on day 3, and exercises CC#5 and CC#6 on day 4.

She has now met all the requirements for clearance in *Self-Assessment 3A*. When she fills in her **Worksheet 3A1**, she is careful to evaluate her difficulty on the injured right side only, not the balance problem on her left side.

In *Self-Assessment 3B*, Erica completes **Worksheet 3B1: Regional Self-Assessment Tables** for Region 1 Toe and Region 11 Stress Fracture. She checks almost all of the lines on the right side in the table for Region 1, and identifies her primary injury as the outer toes on the right foot. She checks one stride problem on the left side, which is associated with her unaffected left hip. She doesn't check any lines on the table for stress fracture.

When she fills in her **Worksheet 3B2: Injury Regions in Order of Severity**, it has only one region: the right outer toes. She does not list the problem in her left buttock region as an injury region. However, she does make a note that she wants to work on her balance in that region.

Erica now completes *Self-Assessment 3C*. She copies the Regional Closed-Chain Exercises for the toe region from *Table 3C1:* **Closed-Chain Exercises by Region** to **Worksheet 3C1**. For extra credit, she also lists the exercises for her unaffected left butt region.

Erica is ready to prepare her first **Log Form R** [See Erica's **First Log Form R: Regional Closed-Chain**]. She copies the six Regional Closed-Chain Exercises for the toe region from her **Worksheet 3C1** to **Log Form R**. She also wants to try some of the exercises for the butt region in her spare time, but she doesn't have to evaluate these for clearance, so she doesn't copy them to her **Log Form R**.

She goes to *Appendix Z* and copies the times for "Racers" for *Rest Between Sets*, *Final Target*, and *Build Pace*. For the push-through exercises CC#16 and CC#18, she copies footnote B: "See Special Instructions" to the line for *"Notes."* Following the special instructions in *Self Assessment 3C, Part 2, line 7*, Erica crosses out one of the left/right columns on **Log Form R**, and writes "both legs." These exercises will have no "left/right difference."

Erika also copies the footnote for box step-up (CC#19) about building up box height to the 90/90 position. Since Erica is not using a box, she will step up two stairs at a time, as she did in box step-up-and-over (CC#8).

She will fill in the date and calculate her *Symmetry Target* and *Symmetry Goal* for each exercise when she does her Initial Assessment (in the **Instructions for Log Form R**).

Erica then completes *Self-Assessment 3D*. Her two most difficult Basic Closed-Chain Exercises from **Worksheet 3A1: Evaluation of Basic Closed-Chain Exercises** are CC#5 and CC#3, so she looks those numbers up in *Table 3D1:* **Basic Closed-Chain Balance Problems**, and writes two Impairment Statements for her outer toe region.

Log Form B: Basic Closed-Chain

DAY/DATE	Wed 1/9	Days since *last day you ran:*	4
PHASE 3, Part#	1	Days in this Phase	1
AFFECTED SIDE and REGION(S)		Right outer toes	

Basic Closed-Chain Exercise	CC#1 Square Hops		CC#2 Side Step-Down		CC#3 One-Leg Armswings, Barefoot		CC#4 One-Leg Armswings, 1 Pillow	
Target Time	20 sec		20 sec		15 sec		30 sec	
Rest Between Sets	10 sec		0		0		0	
Set Times	Left	Right	Left	Right	Left	Right	Left	Right
1	10	20	15	20	10	5	10	30
2	5	"	10	15	5	5	15	"
3	10	"	10	15	15	5	10	"
4	10	"	10	15	10	5	12	"
5	5	"	5	10	10	5	18	"
Total								
Avg Set Time	8	20	10	15	10	5	10	30
L/R Difference	12 sec		5 sec		5 sec		20 sec	
Symmetry Goal	1 sec		1 sec		1 sec		2 sec	
Max Pain (0-10)	L: 0	R: 2	L: 0	R: 0	L: 0	R: 0	L: 0	R: 0
NOTES:	wobbly left hip		left hip		left hip & rt toes		left hip	

DAY/DATE		Days since *last day you ran:*	Days in this Phase:

Basic Closed-Chain Exercise	CC#5 Barefoot Push-Up		CC#6 Quick Steps	CC#7 Weighted Kickback		CC#8 Box Step Up and Over	
Target Time	15 sec		20 sec	60 sec		60 sec	
Rest Between Sets	0		10 sec	0		0	
Set Times	Left	Right	Both Legs [A]	Left	Right	Left	Right
1	Left	Right	Both Legs [2]	Left	Right	Left	Right
2	15	12	10	60	60	60	60
3	"	10	10	"	"	"	"
4	"	10	8	"	"	"	"
5	"	10	10	"	"	"	"
Total	"	8	8	"	"	"	"
Avg Set Time							
L/R Difference	5 sec		Stopped at 5 min	0 sec		0 sec	
Symmetry Goal	1 sec			3 sec		3 sec	
Max Pain (0-10)	L: 0	R: 4	L: 0 R: 2	L: 0	R: 0	L: 0	R: 2
NOTES:	Right toes		Hurt Right toes	Cleared		Cleared on stairs - Pain in rt foot stepping up	

[A] See instructions line 9: *Special Instructions for Quick Steps*

Worksheet 3A1: Evaluation of Basic Closed-Chain Exercises

1. Based on your daily assessments, list all eight Basic Closed-Chain Exercises **in order of difficulty**:

1. CC# _____5_____ _Barefoot push up -- rt foot_

2. CC# _____3_____ _one leg armswings barefoot -- rt foot_

3. CC# _____6_____ _quicksteps – pain in rt foot_

4. CC# _____8_____ _Box step up (stairs) pain in rt foot_

5. CC# _____2_____ _side step down_

6. CC# _____1_____ _square hops_

7. CC# _____4_____ _one leg armswings – 1 pillow_

8. CC# _____7_____ _weighted kickback_

2. Count the number of days since you started your Basic Closed-Chain exercises, and **circle** the statement below that applies to you:

I was *able* to clear all Basic Closed-Chain Exercises in 7 days or less, and I am progressing to Regional Closed-Chain Exercises.	I was *unable* to clear all Basic Closed-Chain Exercises in 7 days or less, and I am continuing with Basic Closed-Chain Exercises.

Phase Three Part Two

In **Worksheet 3D1: Treatment Groups for Phase Three Part Two**, Erica confirms that she has a simple injury and will enter Phase Three Part Two in Group 1A, which follows the *Self-Paced Plan*.

Erica is now ready to determine her Base Schedule. In *Self-Assessment 3E*, Erica consults the guidelines for "Racers" (*Table 3E1*: **Base Schedules for Fitness Runners and Racers**) and finds that she can continue training 5 days per week, but she must lower her mileage to a total of 25 miles per week.

She finds Group 1A in *Table 3E2*: **Starting Your Self-Paced Plan**, and is referred to *Table 3E3*: **Group 1 Self-Paced Plan: Where to Begin Your Base Schedule**. Since she had been able to run 10 miles on her injury before her pain started, she finds that she will begin her Base Schedule at Level 5.

Erica enters all this information on her **Worksheet T: Training Plan for Phase Three Part Two.**

Erica cleared her Basic Closed-Chain on Saturday 1/12, so she is ready to begin Phase Three Part Two on Monday1/14. During her P.T. Time, Erica follows the **Instructions for Log Form R** and the **Guidelines for Regional Closed-Chain [Box 14-4]**, and clears her Regional Closed Chain Exercises, Stage 1, in two days of P.T. Time *(Self-Assessment 3F: Regional Closed-Chain Clearance)*.

Following the plan in her Worksheet T, Erica begins her Base Schedule with **Log Form S Level 5**. She concentrates on pushing through the big toe of her injured right foot, and on controlling her balance in her wobbly left hip. Because she is a long-time competitive athlete, she has no difficulty with the glide drills. She follows the instructions in *Self-Assessment 3G1 for Self-Paced Plan*: **Base Schedule Clearance (Levels 0 through 5)** and is able to clear Level 5 in one week.

Phase Four

Erica completes *Self Assessment 3H: Phase Three Clearance and Preparation for Phase Four*, on Saturday 1/19, and continues to Phase Four the following Monday. She clears her Phase Four exercises (*Self-Assessments 4A, 4B, and 4C*) in three days with no problem. Erica has completed her Recovery Program in 18 days, and is now running better than she did before her injury.

In reading the sections in *The Running Injury Recovery Program* about running habits and shoes, Erica realized that the foot pain she had when she wore her dress shoes probably had something to do with the way they function. She uses what she has learned about training shoes to buy some well-made, flat dress shoes that break easily at the forefoot, not in the middle; and some comfortable heels that allow her to push off straight through her big toe when she walks.

Erica fills in what she has learned on her **Worksheet 4D1**, and is ready to return to regular training.

Worksheet 3B1: Regional Self-Assessment Tables

Region 1: Big Toe (1st Ray)
(Secondary Region: Outer Toes)

Activity	Self-Assessment		Left	Right
Self-mobilization	I have **tenderness** and/or bruising on the ball of the foot.			X
Stretches	I have reduced range of motion **(stiffness)** in the toe region, *resulting in* difficulty flexing the toes up or down.			X
Closed-Chain Exercises	I have **weakness** in the toe region, *resulting in:*	A. Difficulty flexing the toes during push off.		X
		B. Difficulty flexing the toes during step-up.		X
Pre-Injury Stride Tendency	While running, I have a tendency to:	A. Rotate the leg outward.	X	
		B. Push off from the inner or outer side of the big toe.		X

Region 11: Regional Injury with Stress Fracture *NO*

Activity	Self-Assessment	Left	Right
Self-mobilization	I have **tenderness** in any weight-bearing bone in my injury region (anywhere from the foot to the pelvis), with or without pain in the associated soft tissues.		
Stretches	I have reduced range of motion **(stiffness)** in the region where I have bone tenderness.		
Closed-Chain Exercises:	After icing *and* not running for at least 3 weeks, I can *still* **reproduce my injury pain** when I hop on the injured leg (unable to clear CC#1 Square Hop Exercise).		
Pre-Injury Stride Tendency	While running, I feel pain in the region where I have bone tenderness.		

Worksheet 3B2: Injury Regions in Order of Severity

Rank #	Side (left/right)	Injury Region
1.	*right*	Region # *1 outer toes*
2.		Region #
3.		Region #
4.	** left*	Region # *10 buttock – not an injury – balance problem in hip*

Worksheet 3C1: Regional Closed-Chain Exercises in Order of Severity

1st Injury Region and Side:	Region 1: right outer toes

Box 1: Regional Closed-Chain Exercises	
CC# 3	One-Leg Armswings, Barefoot
CC# 5	Barefoot Push-Up
CC# 11	Straight-Leg Raise with Theraband
CC# 16	Barefoot Push-Through
CC# 18	Shod Push-Through with Ankle Weights
CC# 19	Box Step-Up

2nd Injury Region and Side:	Also work on Region 10: left butt (unaffected region)

Box 2: Regional Closed-Chain Exercises	
CC# 6	Quick Steps
CC# 7	Weighted Kickback
CC# 8	Box Step Up and Over
CC# 9	Hip Abduction with Theraband
CC# 13	One-Leg Armswings, Side Incline
CC# 14	One-Leg Armswings, Double Weights

3rd Injury Region and Side:	

Box 3: Regional Closed-Chain Exercises	
CC#	
CC#	
CC#	
CC#	
CC#	
CC#	

Stress Fracture, Side:	

Box 4: Regional Closed-Chain Exercises	
CC# 1	
CC# 2	
CC# 8	

(First) Log Form R: Regional Closed-Chain

DAY/DATE:		Days since *last day you ran:*	
PHASE (3 or 4): Phase Three Part Two, Stage 1		Days in this Phase: *1*	
Injury Region(s) and Side: *Region 1: right outer toes*			

Regional Closed-Chain Exercise (number and name)	CC# 3 Barefoot One-Leg Armswings,		CC# 5 Barefoot Push-Up		CC# 11 Straight-Leg Raise with Theraband		CC# 16 (B) Barefoot Push-Through	
Symmetry Target								
Rest Between Sets	0		0		0		0	
Final Target	90 sec		90 sec		2.5 min		10 min	
Build pace as:	glide		glide		glide		glide	
Set Times	Left	Right	Left	Right	Left	Right	Left	Right
1								
2								
3								
4								
5								
Total								
Avg Set Time								
L/R Difference							BOTH LEGS	
Symmetry Goal		sec		sec		sec		sec
Max Pain (0-10)	L:	R:	L:	R:	L:	R:	L:	R:
NOTES:								
FOOTNOTES: CC#16: See Special Instructions for Push-Through								

DAY/DATE:		Days since *last day you ran:*		Days in this Phase:	

Regional Closed-Chain Exercise (number and name)	CC# 18 (B) Shod Push-Thru w/ Ankle Weights		CC# 19 Box Step-Up		CC#		CC#	
Symmetry Target								
Rest Between Sets	0		0					
Final Target	10 min		10 min					
Build pace as:	glide		Glide (A)					
Set Times	Left	Right	Left	Right	Left	Right	Left	Right
1								
2								
3								
4								
5								
Total								
Avg Set Time								
L/R Difference	BOTH LEGS							
Symmetry Goal		sec		sec		sec		sec
Max Pain (0-10)	L:	R:	L:	R:	L:	R:	L:	R:
NOTES								
FOOTNOTES: #18:Instructions for Push-Through; CC#19 Instructions to build box height (Box 14-2).								

Worksheet T: Training Plan for Phase Three Part Two

1. I am a (Fitness Runner or Racer): _____ Racer _____ .

2. I plan to do my P.T. Time (**Log Form M** and **Log Form B** or **Log Form R**) 60 minutes per day, two days per week, on these days: Saturday A.M __ and Wednesday P.M.__ . (*Note:* P.T. Time may be done on the same days as your Base Schedule, or on different days).

3. I plan to do my Base Schedule (**Log Form S**) 60 minutes per day, __5__ days per week, on these days:

_____ Monday through Friday mornings _____

4. I am in Treatment Group Number (1A, 1B, 2A, or 2B) __1A__ .

5. I am following the (*Self-Paced Plan* or *Two-Week-Interval Plan*):

_____ Self-Paced Plan _____

6. I will start my Base Schedule at Level __5__ .

7. My weekly mileage *goal* is __25__ miles per week.

8. My daily mileage *maximum* is __5__ miles per day (divide line 7 by line 3).

Write your personalized *Impairment Statements* from *Self-Assessment 3D* here:

1. I have difficulty maintaining balance while pushing off straight through my right big toe.

2. I have difficulty with my outer right toes when I use armswings to balance on one leg.

Worksheet 4D1: Habits for Post-Recovery Running		
Post-Recovery Running Habits Checklist:	1. I will make a plan, and train consistently.	X
	2. I will set realistic running goals.	X
	3. I will start each run with a proper warmup.	X
	4. I will pay close attention to my equipment, particularly my footwear.	X
	5. I will focus on functional running.	X
	6. I will manage my running injuries early, before they become severe.	X

The most important lessons I have learned from my *Running Injury Recovery Program* that I will use when I return to regular training are:

1. I have to use my whole body (both sides) to balance in order to push off straight through my right big toe.

2. I will use what I have learned about training shoes to choose my regular shoes, and I will push off correctly when I am wearing them.

Section 4: Instructions for Post-Injury Training

This section duplicates the Figures and Instructions for P.T. Time and Base Schedules found in *The Running Injury Recovery Program*. They are repeated here in the *Workbook* because you will need to refer to these instructions and photographs while you are doing your exercises in order to do them correctly and to fill out your Log Forms.

However, the information contained in this section is just a summary of what you need to know to do these exercises correctly. **Do not attempt to perform any of these exercises unless you have already read *The Running Injury Recovery Program* and have familiarized yourself with all of the instructions**. To prepare yourself for these exercises, follow your Course Map and check off all of the lines in order.

Remember that each of these exercises is paired with a particular Log Form that you must fill out, which is in turn linked to a particular recovery phase and a series of Self-Assessments and Worksheets. As you do your exercises, it's important to follow the instructions, to complete all of the Self-Assessments, and to fill out your Log Forms to the best of your ability.

Most of these exercises are performed in a progressive manner which means that they will increase in duration or in difficulty as you move through the phases. Your Course Map and Self-Assessments will guide you through everything you need to do, and the Clearance Checkpoints will allow you to progress to the next level when you are ready.

At each Clearance Checkpoint, you may have to revise certain Log Forms, or change to a new Log Form (*see Tables W1A and W1B*). Before starting any exercise session, always double check to make sure that you understand your goals for that day, and that you are working at the correct level and with the correct forms.

BOX 5-1

The Proper Way to ICE

To ice at home, you'll need one or more ice packs with enough surface area to completely cover and wrap around the injured structure, a pillowcase or thin toweling, small ice cubes or crushed ice, some water, some stretchy wrap such as an Ace bandage or Velcro wrap, clips or tape, and a place to lie down and elevate your injured body-part after you've iced it.

1. Prepare your ice packs:
   • For convenience and no worries about leakage, I recommend professional, gel-filled ice packs that you can buy from your pharmacy or on the Internet.
   • To make your own ice packs, you'll need several large, heavy-duty, zip-top bags (quart or gallon size). I recommend freezer bags with strong zippers to reduce the chance of leaking cold water all over yourself and your house. Use enough zip-top bags to completely cover and surround the injured region(s). Fill each zip-top bag about half full with a 50/50 mixture of ice and water. The water is important – don't reduce it. There should be enough ice and water to distribute evenly all the way around the injured structure. Get all the air out and seal the bag securely. Put some pressure on the bag to check for leaks, then put the first bag in a second bag as insurance against leakage.

2 Use the cover that came with your gel ice pack, or put your zip-top bag(s) in the pillowcase or lightweight towel to keep the plastic off your skin.

3. Wrap the ice pack completely around the injured structure (360 degrees) so that the gel or ice is evenly distributed.

4. Wrap the stretchy bandage all the way around the ice pack to completely enclose and compress it against the injury. Secure the bandage with clips or tape.

5. Elevate and support the injured structure so the ice pack is higher than your heart. For a running injury, that means you'll be lying down [Box 5-2].

6. Leave the ice pack on for 20 minutes with the structure elevated. It will be cold and you will feel a burning sensation for about 5 minutes; then it will start to feel numb. The water and pillowcase are there to keep it from getting too cold. While your leg is elevated, you can pump the muscles in the parts that aren't wrapped (for example, moving the foot or lower leg) to help bring the swelling down.

BOX 5-2

ICE Positions

ICE Position 5-1

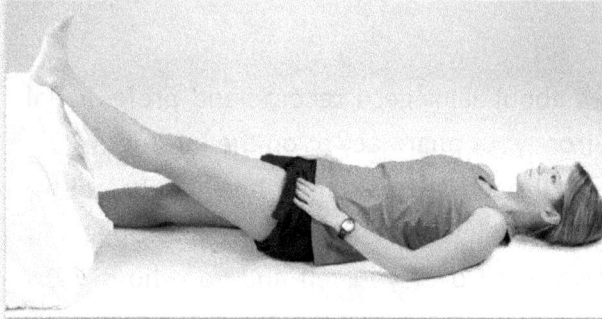

Regions:
Toe, arch, heel, calf, knee, shin, hamstring

Compression	Compress the ice pack around the injured region.
Elevation	Lie on your back and elevate the injured leg above heart level.

ICE Position 5-2

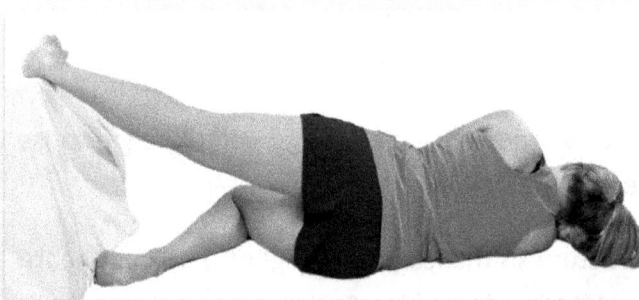

Region:
Band

Compression	Compress the ice pack around the knee region.
Elevation	2. Lie on your side with the lower knee bent and the upper knee straight. 3. Elevate the upper leg above heart level.

ICE Position 5-3

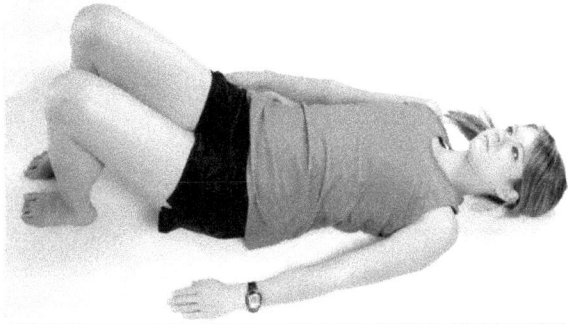

Region:
Hip

Compression	Place the ice pack next to the skin (inside your shorts), along the front side of the hip.
Elevation	Lie on your back with knees bent.

ICE Position 5-4

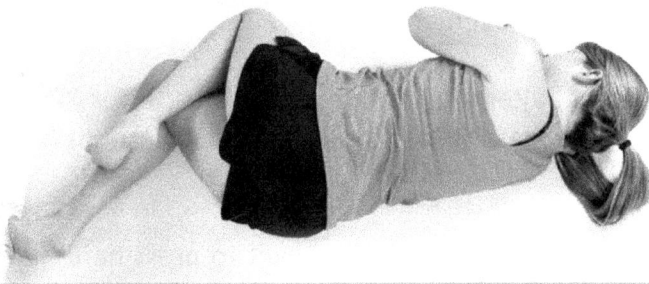

Region:
Buttock

Compression	Place the ice pack next to the skin (inside your shorts), against the back side of the hip.
Elevation	Lie on your side, injury side up, with knees bent and spine straight.

Table 10-1

Tools for Self-Mobilization

Professional Mobilization Tools	Home Mobilization Tools
Small massage ball	Golf ball
Medium massage ball	Tennis ball wrapped in athletic tape
Rubber-tipped massage stick	Plastic vitamin bottle
Roller massage stick	Roller massage stick

Box 10-2   *HOW TO:* Self-Mobilizations

General Instructions:

1. Collect your mobilization tools [*Table 10-1*].

2. Using the mobilization tool, locate one point of tenderness in the affected region. Try different angles to pinpoint the area of restriction.

3. Press deeply into the tender spot with the mobilization tool, and release the restrictions using rolling and strumming movements.

4. While you are rolling and strumming, alternately contract the muscle for 3 seconds and relax it for 7 seconds. Repeat 3 times for a total of 30 seconds for each exercise.

5. Work at a pain threshold of about 5 or 6 out of 10. You want to press hard enough to release the tightness and restriction, but not hard enough to bruise.

6. Start with the tenderest spot in the affected region, then move on to other tender spots in the same region. Do not repeat self-mobilization on the same spot during the same P.T. session.

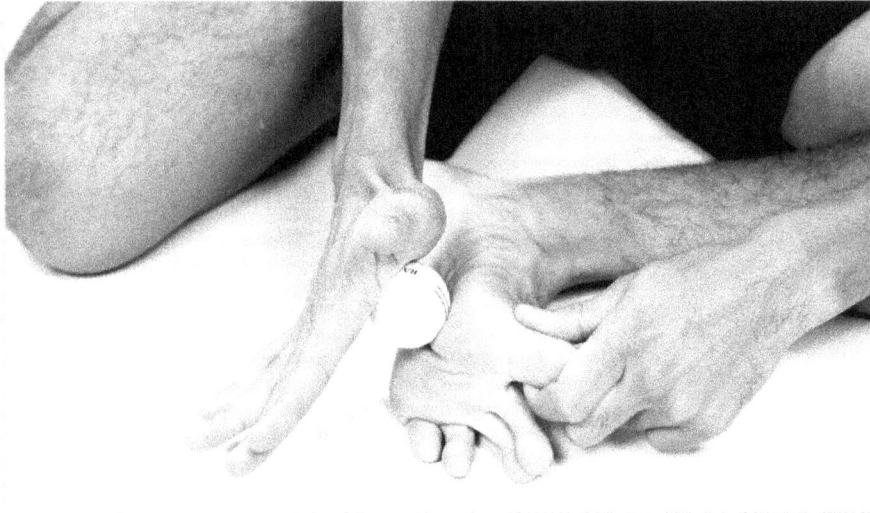

Self-Mob 10-1: Toe 1

Mobilization Tool	Golf ball
Starting Position	Sitting, pull the big toe back until the tendon is exposed.
Action	1. Press the ball into the tender area of the bottom of the toe while extending the big toe up and out. Roll and strum. 2. Contract and relax the muscle by flexing the toe against your hand.

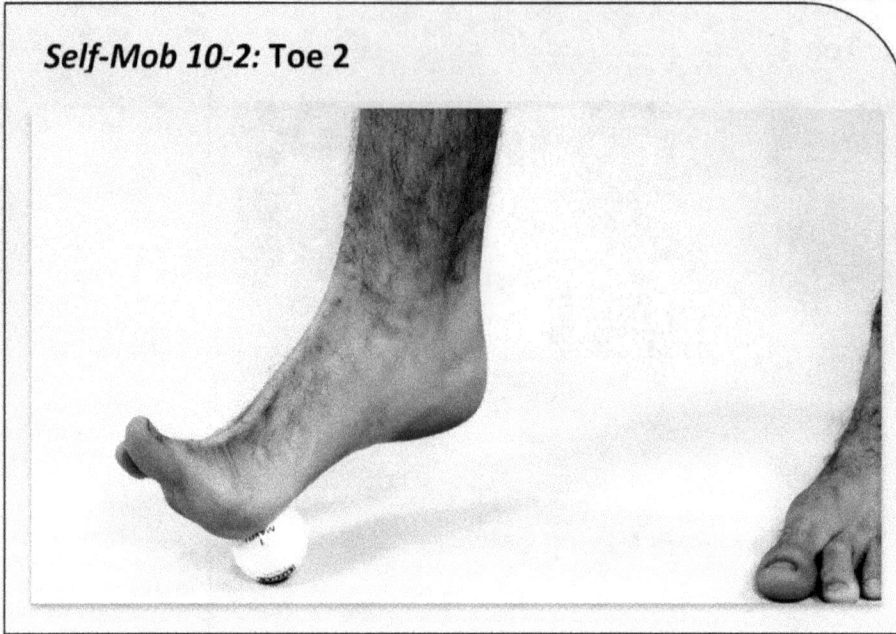

Self-Mob 10-2: Toe 2

Mobilization Tool	Golf ball
Starting Position	Standing, flex the big toe up until the tendon is exposed.
Action	1. Press your foot into the golf ball and roll the ball under the tender spot on the bottom of the big toe while extending the toes. Roll and strum. 2. Contract and relax the muscle by alternately pointing and flexing the toes.

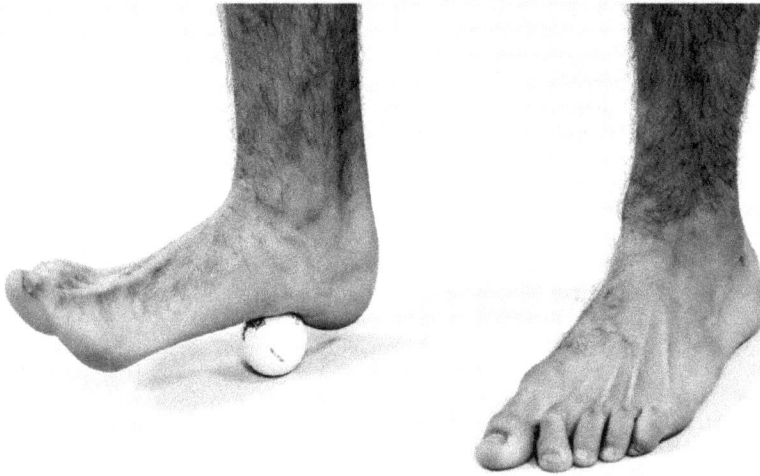

Self-Mob 10-3: Arch 1

Mobilization Tool	Golf ball
Starting Position	Standing, flex toes up and press the arch of your foot into the golf ball.
Action	1. Keeping the foot flexed, press and roll the ball under the tender spot in the arch of the foot. 2. Contract and relax the muscle by alternately pointing and flexing the foot.

Self-Mob 10-4: Arch 2

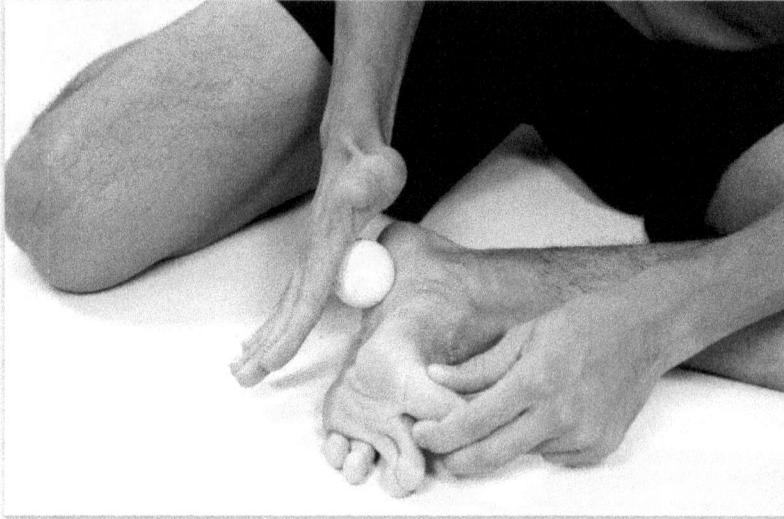

Mobilization Tool	Golf ball
Starting Position	Sitting, flex the foot and pull back on the big toe.
Action	1. Keeping the foot and toe stretched, press and roll the golf ball in circular movements over the tender spot in the arch. 2. Contract and relax the muscle by alternately pointing and flexing the toe.

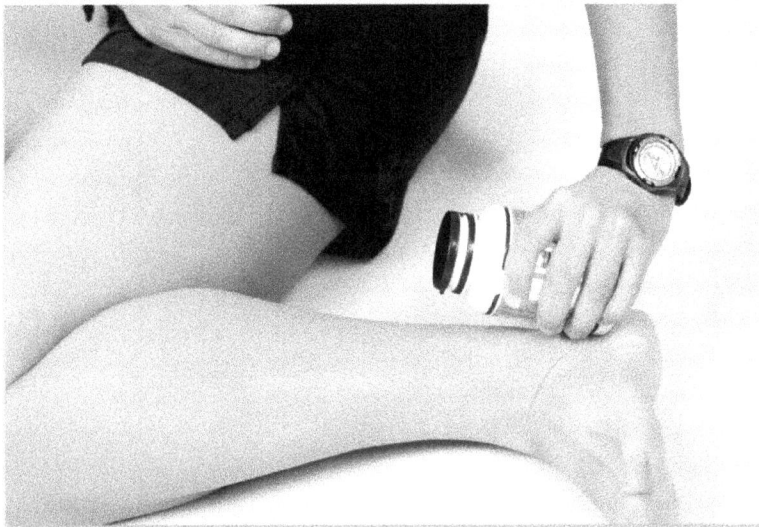

Self-Mob 10-5: Heel 1

Mobilization Tool	Vitamin bottle
Starting Position	Sitting, press the bottom edge of a vitamin bottle into the Achilles tendon.
Action	1. Try different angles and positions to locate the tender part of the heel. 2. Contract and relax the muscle by alternately flexing and extending the foot.

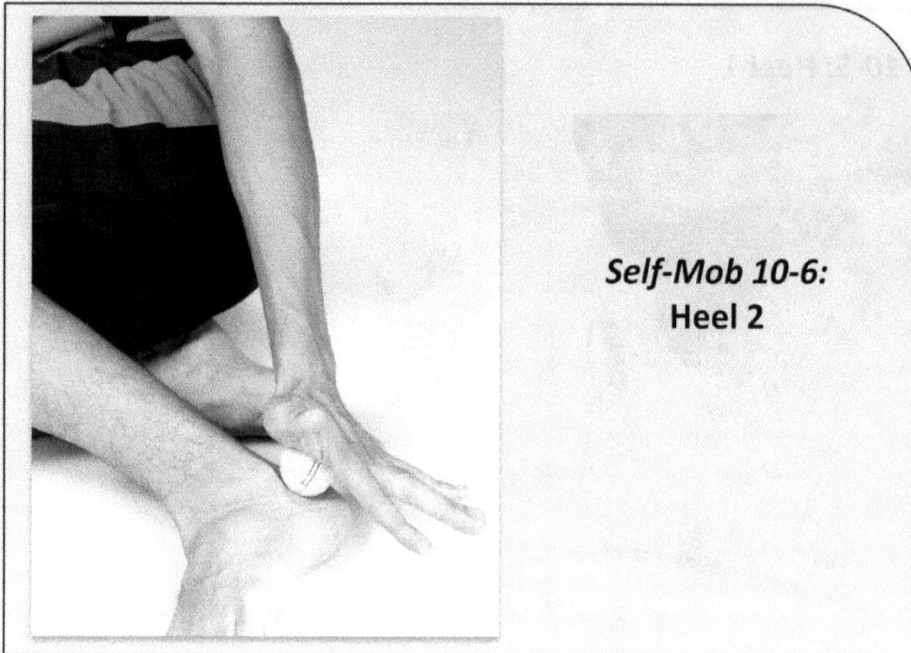

Self-Mob 10-6:
Heel 2

Mobilization Tool	Golf ball
Starting Position	Sitting, press the ball into the Achilles tendon.
Action	1. Roll the ball along the outer border of the heel and Achilles tendon. 2. Contract and relax the muscle by alternately flexing and extending the foot.

Self-Mob 10-7: Shin 1

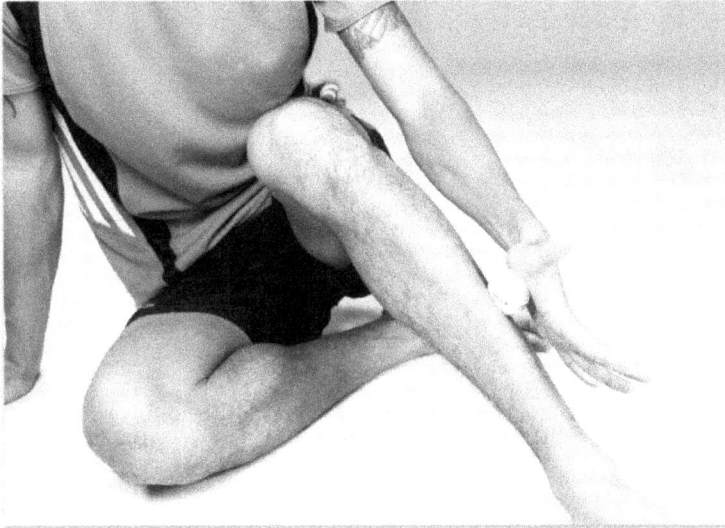

Mobilization Tool	Golf ball
Starting Position	Sitting with legs crossed, press the ball into the muscle along the outer side of the shin.
Action	1. Pressing in, roll the ball up and down alongside the outer shin. 2. Contract and relax the muscle by flexing and extending your foot.

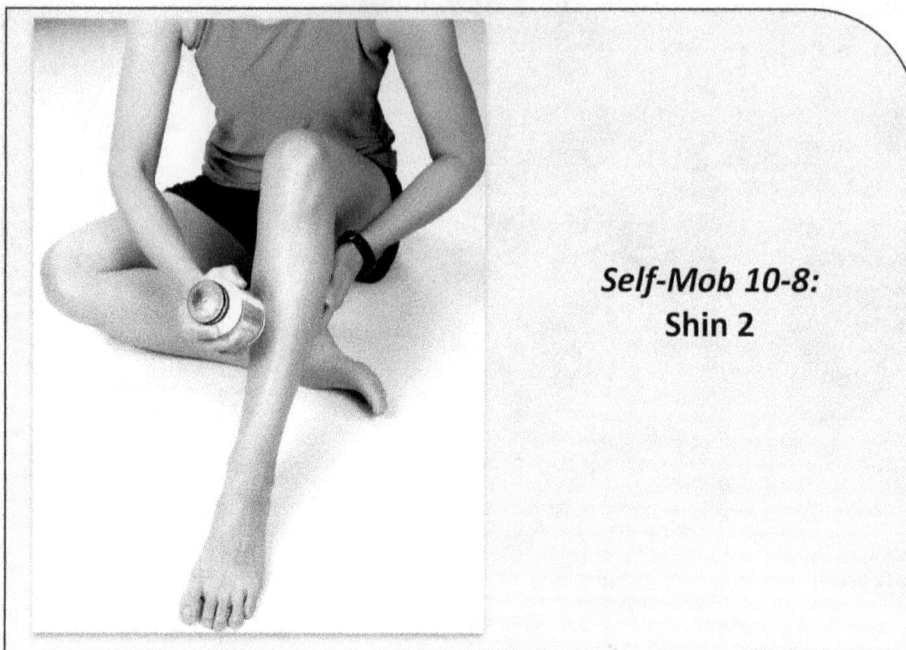

Self-Mob 10-8:
Shin 2

Mobilization Tool	Vitamin bottle
Starting Position	Sitting with legs crossed, press the bottom edge of a vitamin bottle along the muscle along the inner side of the shin.
Action	1. Try different points along the inner side of the shin to find the soreness. 2. Contract and relax the muscle by flexing and extending your foot.

Self-Mob 10-9: Calf 1

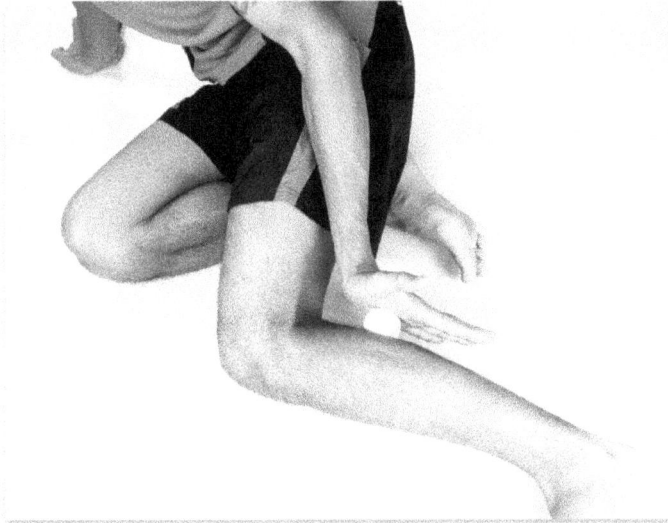

Mobilization Tool	Golf ball
Starting Position	Sitting, flex the foot and press the ball into the calf.
Action	1. Press the ball into the tender spots in the calf muscle. Roll and strum. 2. Contract and relax the muscle by flexing and extending the foot.

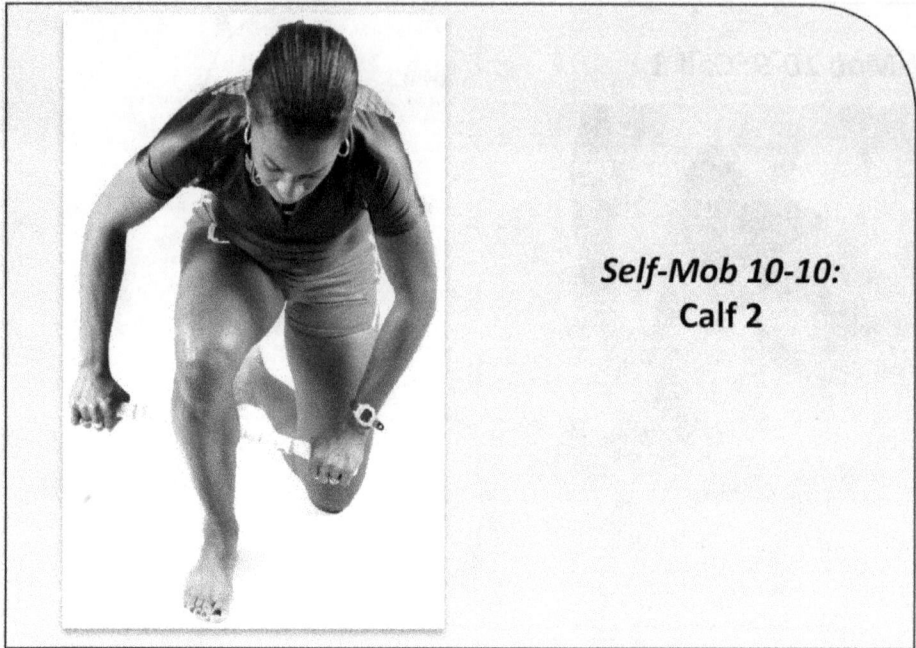

Self-Mob 10-10:
Calf 2

Mobilization Tool	Roller massage stick
Starting Position	1. Kneeling on one knee, press the roller stick into the calf. 2. Place weight on the forward leg and move the knee slightly forward to stretch the calf.
Action	1. Press the knobby edges of the rollers into the tender spots of the calf. Try different angles to find the soreness. Roll and strum. 2. Contract and relax the muscle by alternately flexing and extending the foot.

Self-Mob 10-11: Knee 1

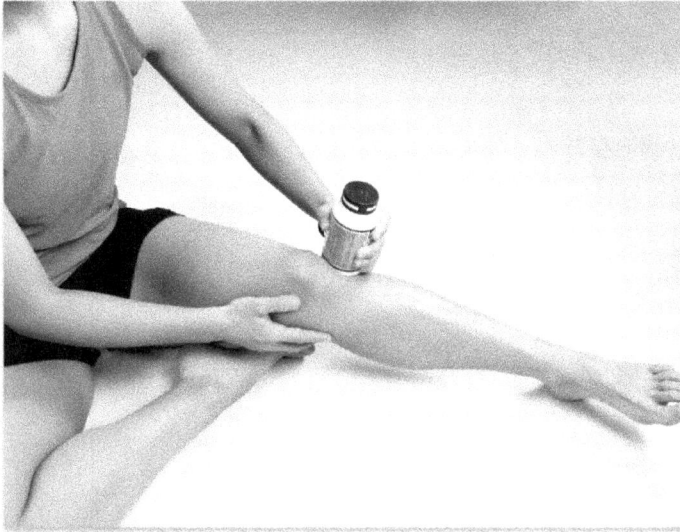

Mobilization Tool	Vitamin bottle
Starting Position	Sitting with your leg extended, press the bottom edge of a vitamin bottle into the tendon on the outer side of the knee and around the kneecap.
Action	1. Try different positions and angles to find the tightness and soreness. 2. Contract and relax the muscle by tightening the knee to straighten it and squeeze the knee tight.

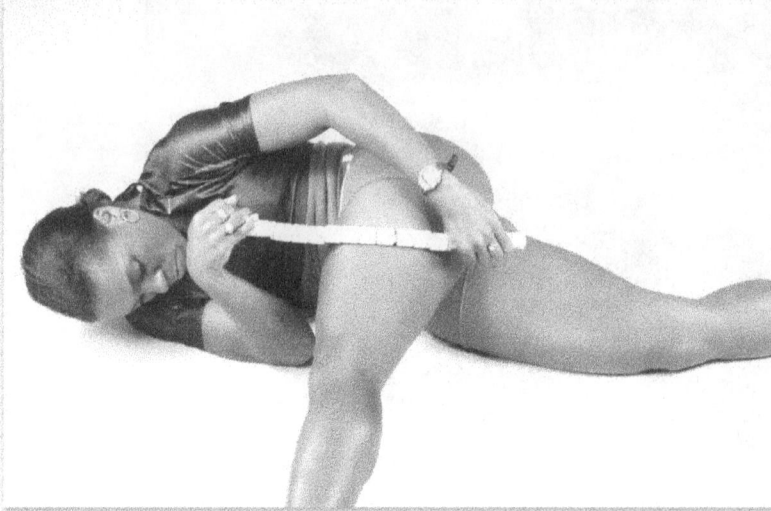

Self-Mob 10-12: Band 1

Mobilization Tool	Roller massage stick
Starting Position	Lying on your back, pull one leg up and across your body, keeping the knee straight.
Action	1. Press the knobby edges of the rollers into the tender spots along the outer thigh from hip to knee. Roll and strum. 2. Contract and relax the muscle by squeezing the buttock, and by straightening the knee and squeezing it tight.

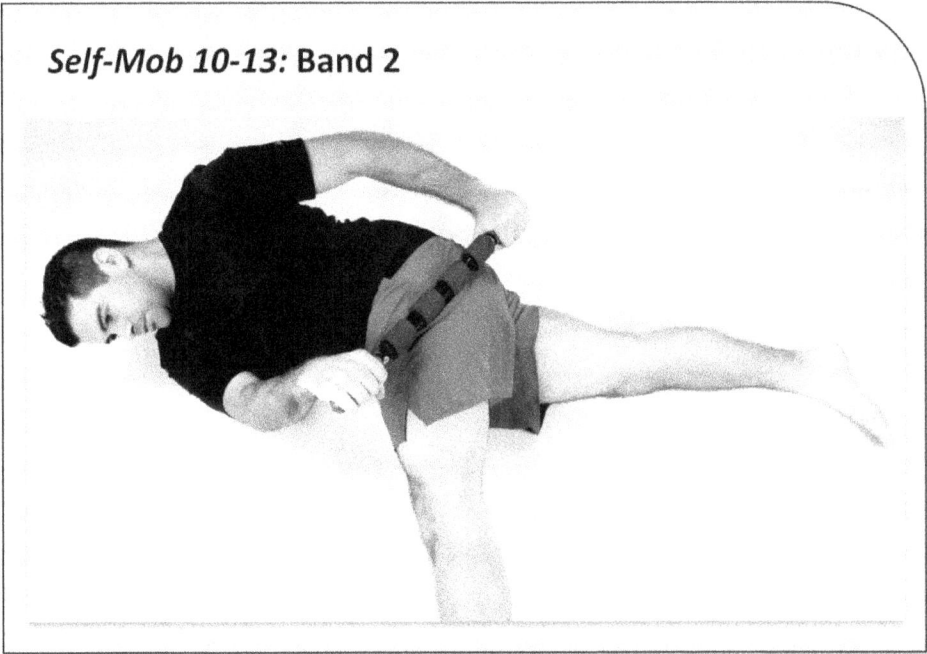

Self-Mob 10-13: **Band 2**

Mobilization Tool	Roller massage stick
Starting Position	Lying on your back, pull one leg up and across your body, keeping the knee straight.
Action	1. Press the knobby edges of the rollers into the tender spots in the gluteal region. Roll and strum. 2. Contract and relax the muscle by squeezing the buttock while bending and straightening the knee in a small range of motion.

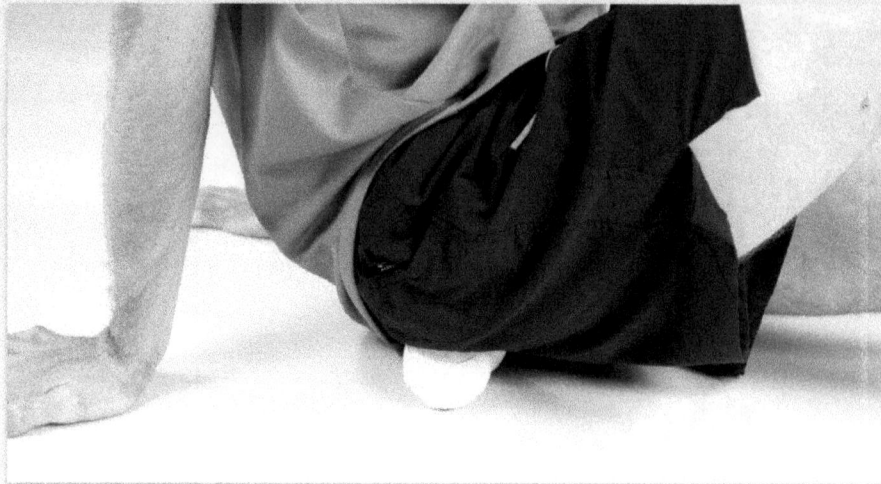

Self-Mob 10-14: Band 3

Mobilization Tool	Tennis ball
Starting Position	Sitting, position the tennis ball under one buttock with your knee bent and the opposite leg straight.
Action	1. Sit on the tennis ball to press it into the areas of soreness in the hip/gluteal region. Roll and strum. 2. Contract and relax the muscle by squeezing the buttock tightly.

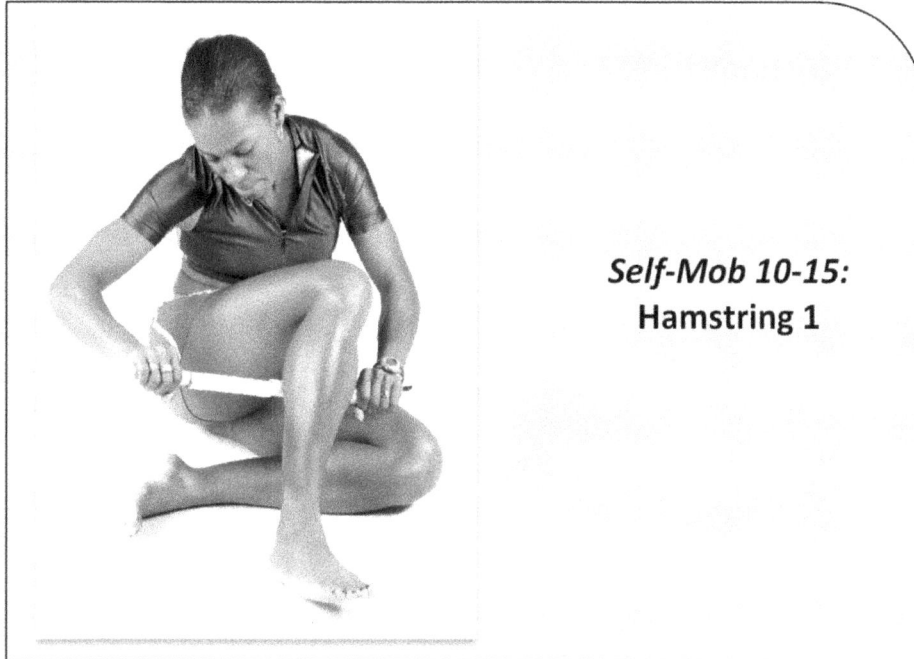

Self-Mob 10-15:
Hamstring 1

Mobilization Tool	Roller massage stick
Starting Position	Sitting, position one foot flat on the floor in front of you and bend the knee until you feel a stretch in the hamstrings.
Action	1. Press the knobby edges of the rollers into the tender spots of the hamstring muscles. Roll and strum. 2. Contract and relax the muscle by alternately flexing and extending the knee with the heel against floor.

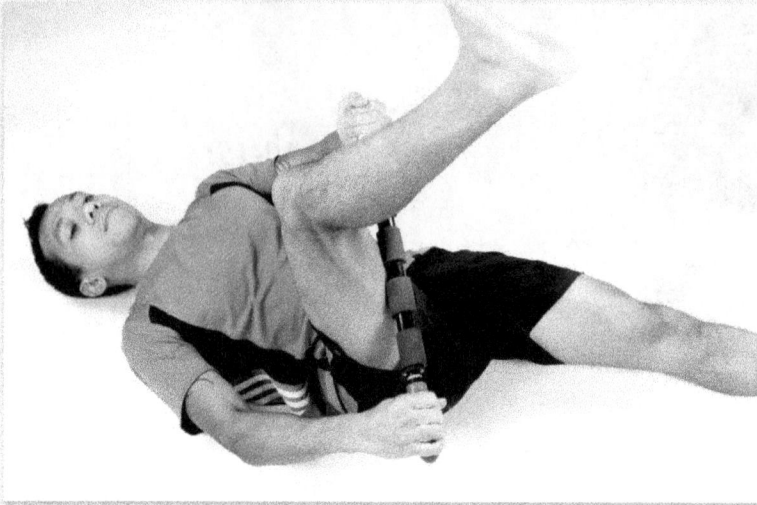

Self-Mob 10-16: Hamstring 2

Mobilization Tool	Roller massage stick
Starting Position	Lying on your back, bend one knee up toward your chest until you feel a stretch in the hamstrings.
Action	1. Press the knobby edges of the rollers into the tender spots of the hamstring muscles. Roll and strum. 2. Contract and relax the muscle by alternately bending and straightening the knee.

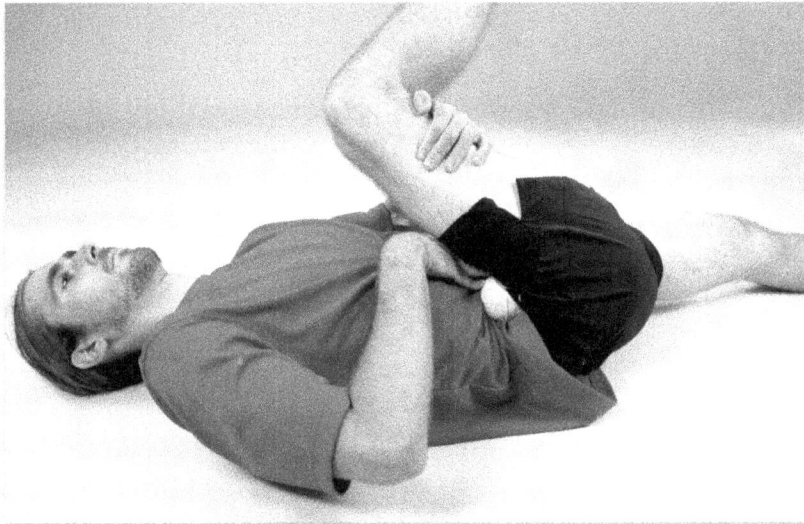

Self-Mob 10-17: Hip

Mobilization Tool	Tennis ball
Starting Position	Lying on your back with one leg straight and the opposite knee bent, place the tennis ball in the crease of the hip.
Action	1. Continue pulling your knee up toward your chest to compress the tennis ball into the hip. Move the tennis ball around a little to find the sore point. 3. Contract and relax the muscle by using hip muscles to squeeze the ball into the pelvis.

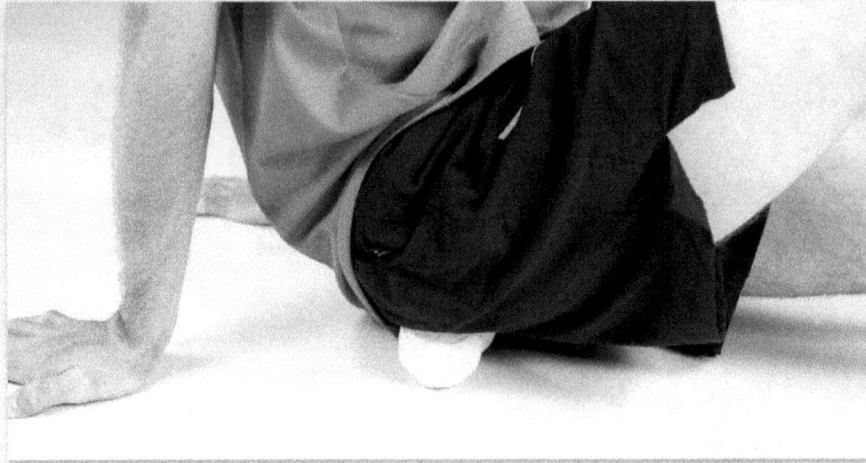

Self-Mob 10-18: Butt 1

Mobilization Tool	Tennis ball
Starting Position	Sitting, position the tennis ball under one buttock with your knee bent and the opposite leg straight.
Action	1. Sit on the tennis ball to press it into the area of soreness in the hip/gluteal region. 2. Contract and relax the muscle by squeezing the buttock tightly.

Self-Mob 10-19: Butt 2

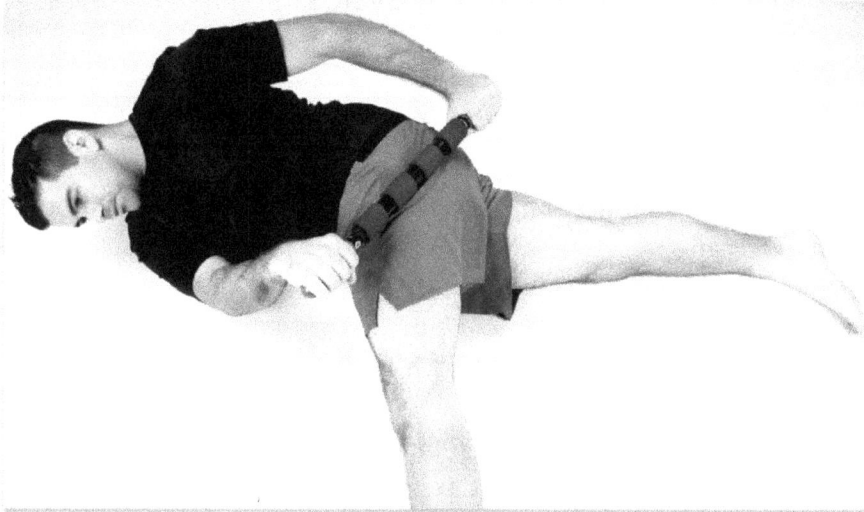

Mobilization Tool	Roller massage stick
Starting Position	Lying on your back, pull one leg up and across your body, keeping the knee straight.
Action	1. Press the knobby edges of the rollers into the tender spots in the gluteal region. Roll and strum. 2. Contract and relax by simultaneously squeezing the buttock tightly and bending and straightening your knee in a small range of motion.

Box 11-1A	Stretch/Mobilization Cycles for *Affected Regions*

1. Stretch
- Begin with the first stretch on your list of *affected regions*, following the instructions for that exercise.
- Perform the stretch for 10 seconds:
  -*Contract* the muscle for 3 seconds.
  -*Relax* the muscle and move deeper into the stretch.
  -*Hold* the stretch for 7 seconds.
- Repeat the *same* stretch (*contract, relax, hold*) 6 times for a total of 1 minute. Move deeper into the stretch each time you relax.

2. Self-Mobilization
- Choose a self-mobilization for your injury region.
- Use the mobilization tool to find the *tenderest* spot in the *affected region*.
- Following the instructions, use your mobilization tool to roll and strum the tender spot.
- While rolling and strumming, *contract* the muscle for 3 seconds, and *relax* the muscle for 7 seconds.
- Repeat 3 times for a total of 1 minute.

3. Repeat
- Repeat *Part 1*, doing the *same* stretch.
- Repeat *Part 2*, but do self-mobilization on a *different* tender spot in the same region.
- Repeat the *same* stretch (*Part 1*) for a total of five times, alternating with four self-mobilizations (begin and end the cycle with the stretch).

4. Start the cycle over with the next stretch on your list of exercises for *affected regions*.

Box 11-1B

Stretch/Mobilization Cycles
for *Unaffected Regions*

1. Stretch
- Begin with the first stretch on your *unaffected regions* list, following the instructions for that exercise.
- Perform the stretch for 10 seconds:
  -*Contract* the muscle for 3 seconds.
  -*Relax* the muscle and move deeper into the stretch.
  -*Hold* the stretch for 7 seconds.
- Repeat the *same* stretch (*contract, relax, hold*) 3 times for a total of 30 seconds. Move deeper into the stretch each time you relax.

2. Self-Mobilization
- Do self-mobilizations on any stretch that you find particularly difficult, or where you find tenderness that corresponds to stiffness.
- Stretch, do 30 seconds of self-mobilizations, then repeat the stretch to see if it has loosened up.

3. Repeat steps 1 and 2 with a *different* stretch. Cycle through the remaining stretches on your *unaffected regions* list until you have completed your P.T. Time.

Table 11-4

Equipment for Stretches

Professional Equipment	Home Alternatives
Incline board	21.5" x 17" x 0.75" plywood propped on a half cinder block
Stretching rope	Belt
Massage stick	Heavy coat-hanger

Box 11-2

HOW TO:
Stretching Exercises

General Instructions:

1. For each session of *P.T. Time*, do all thirteen stretching exercises in the order determined by your *Mobility Self-Assessment* .

2. Combine each stretch with regional self-mobilizations, following the Stretch/Mobilization Cycles for your particular affected and unaffected regions.

3. Follow the instructions for each exercise carefully.

4. For symmetry, repeat each stretching exercise (except incline stretch) with both legs or on both sides.

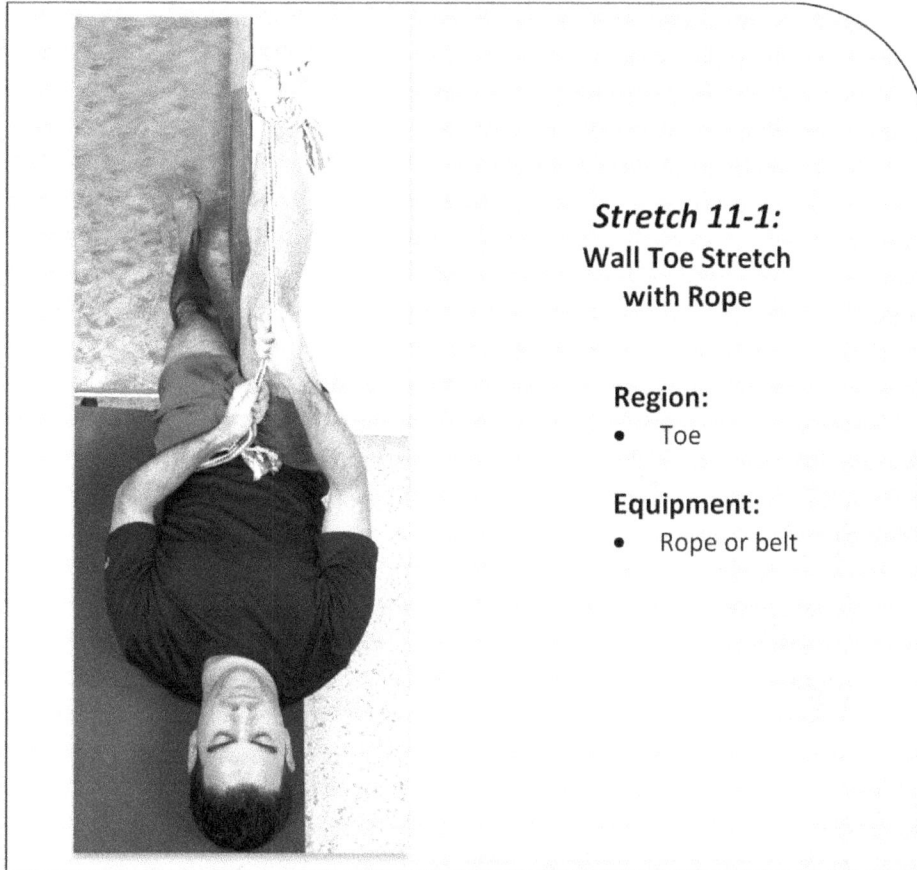

Stretch 11-1:
Wall Toe Stretch with Rope

Region:
- Toe

Equipment:
- Rope or belt

Starting Position	1. Lie on your back in an open doorway, one leg raised straight against the wall, the other leg flat. 2. Tie a loop in the rope and slip it over your big toe.
Action	1. Pull the big toe back with the foot flexed, while slightly bending and straightening your knee. 2. Contract by pointing the toe into the belt. 3. Relax by using the belt to flex the toe and move the leg closer to the wall. Hold the deeper stretch position.

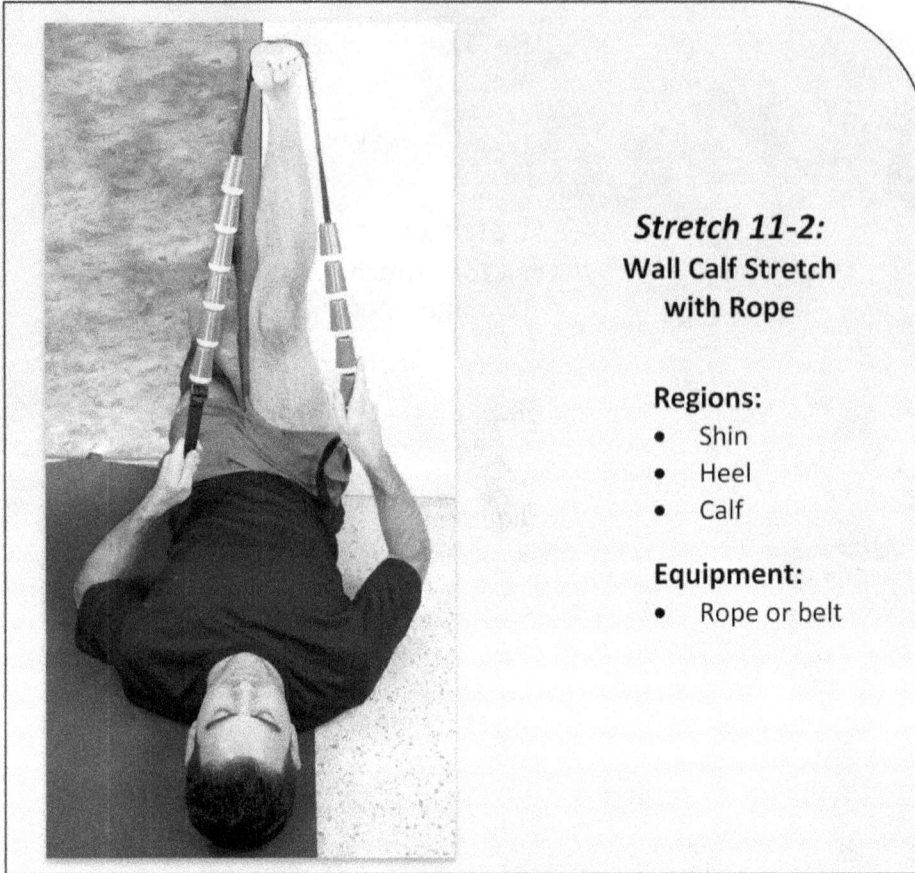

Stretch 11-2:
Wall Calf Stretch with Rope

Regions:
- Shin
- Heel
- Calf

Equipment:
- Rope or belt

Starting Position	1. Lie on your back in an open doorway, one leg raised straight against the wall, the other leg flat. 2. Loop the belt around the ball of the raised foot.
Action	1. Flex the toes while straightening your knee against wall. 2. Contract by pushing your foot into the belt and straightening the knee. 3. Relax and pull the ankle deeper into the flex and your leg closer to the wall. Hold the deeper stretch position.

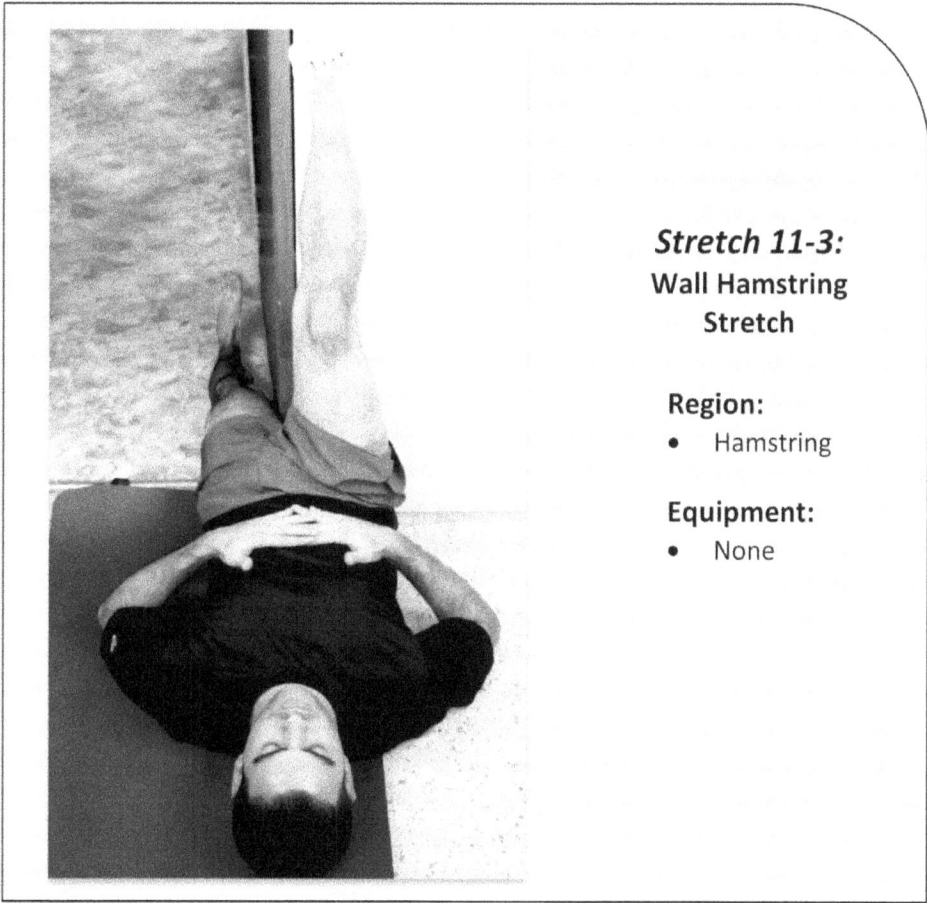

Stretch 11-3:
Wall Hamstring Stretch

Region:
- Hamstring

Equipment:
- None

Starting Position	Lie on your back in an open doorway, one leg raised straight against the wall, the other leg flat.
Action	1. Keeping the leg straight up against the wall, flex your foot (toes toward nose). 2. Contract by pushing your foot against the door frame. 3. Relax and move the leg closer to the wall. Hold the deeper stretch position.

Stretch 11-4: Ankle-Knee Wall Stretch

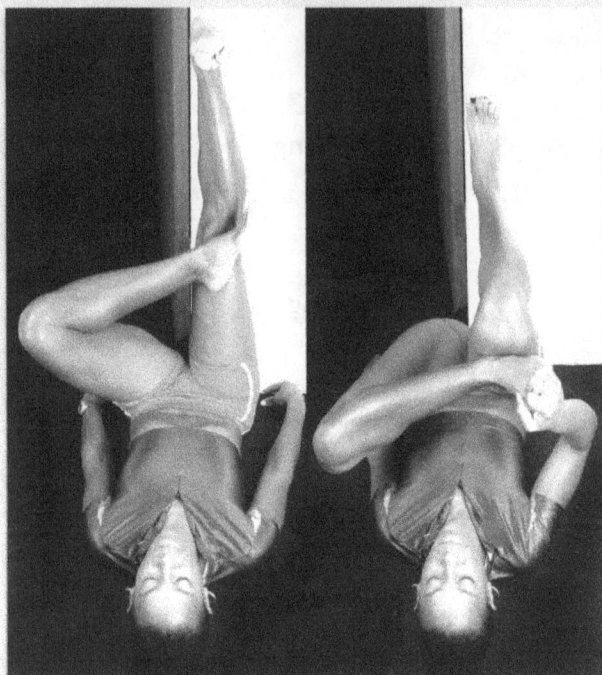

Regions:
- Buttock
- Hip
- Hamstring

Equipment:
- None

Starting Position	1. Lie on your back with your hips close to the wall. 2. Raise one leg straight up against the wall. 3. Cross the opposite ankle over the straight knee.
Action	1. Slowly bend the straight leg so the raised foot slides straight down the wall. Let both knees move toward the chest until you feel a stretch in the opposite hip. 2. Contract using the hip muscles to push the knee against the ankle. 3. Relax, slide the foot down the wall, and hold the deeper stretch position.

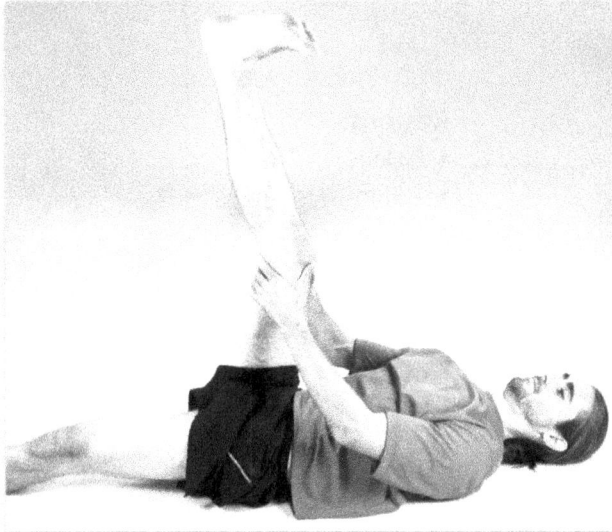

Stretch 11-5: Toes to Nose Stretch

Regions:
- Toe, arch, heel, shin, calf, knee, hamstring

Equipment:
- None

Starting Position	1. Lie on your back with both legs straight. Allow the knees to bend slightly, with the feet relaxed. 2. Grab behind one knee with both hands and raise that leg to a comfortable position, with the foot above your midline, keeping the knee slightly bent.
Action	1. With both hands behind the raised knee, flex the foot and toes toward your nose. 2. Straighten the knee, keeping the foot above your midline, maintaining the flex in your foot and toes. 3. Contract by straightening the knee and flexing the ankle (toes to nose). 4. Relax by bending the knee and relaxing the ankle. Hold the deeper stretch position.

Stretch 11-6: Toes to Nose, Belt Stretch

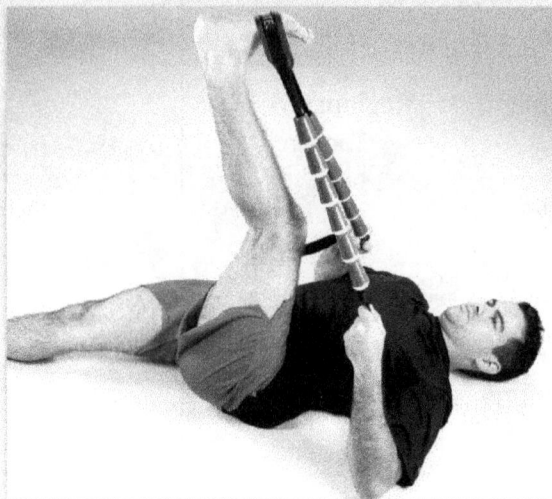

Regions:
- Heel
- Shin
- Calf
- Hamstring

Equipment:
- Rope or belt

Starting Position	1. Lie on your back with both legs straight. Allow the knees to bend slightly, with the feet relaxed. 2. Loop the belt around the ball of one foot and raise that leg to a comfortable position with the foot above your midline, keeping the knee slightly bent.
Action	1. Flex your toes to increase the stretch down the back of the leg. 2. Using the belt to maintain the flex in your foot, straighten the knee, keeping the foot above your midline. 3. Contract by pushing your foot into the belt and straightening your knee. 4. Relax by bending the knee. Hold the deeper stretch position.

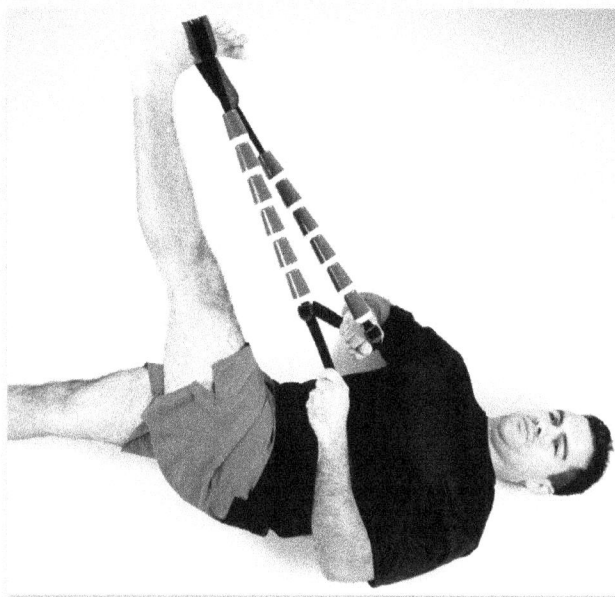

Stretch 11-7: **Straight-Leg Raise, Belt Stretch**

Regions:
- Heel, shin, calf, band, hamstring

Equipment:
- Rope or belt

Starting Position	1. Lie on your back with both legs straight. 2. Loop the belt around one foot and pull the leg up, keeping the knee straight and the ankle flexed.
Action	1. Slightly rotate your hip so your toes point inward to increase the stretch along the side of your leg. 2. Contract by straightening the knee and pushing the foot against the belt. 3. Relax by bending the knee slightly. Hold the deeper stretch position.

Stretch 11-8: Straight-Leg Raise, Belt Stretch to Side

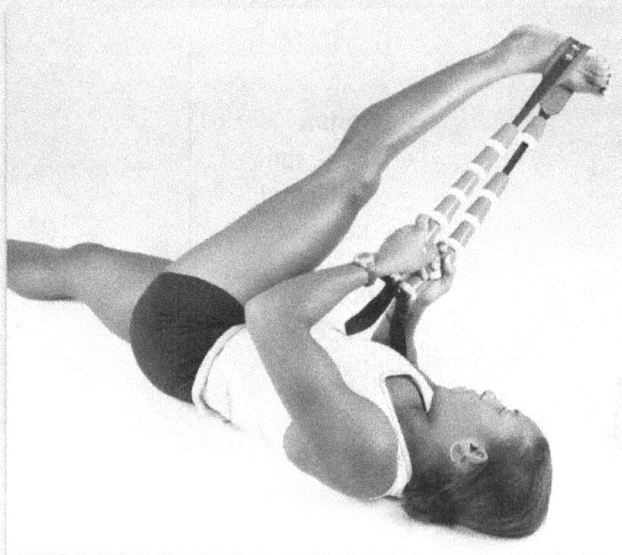

Regions:
- Band
- Buttock

Equipment:
- Rope or belt

Starting Position	1. Lie on your back with both legs straight. 2. Loop the belt around one foot and pull the leg up and across your body, keeping the knee straight and the ankle flexed.
Action	1. Turn your toes down towards the floor with your foot fully flexed. 2. Contract by using your hips to push your foot up into belt. 3. Relax and move the leg farther across your body. Hold the deeper stretch position.

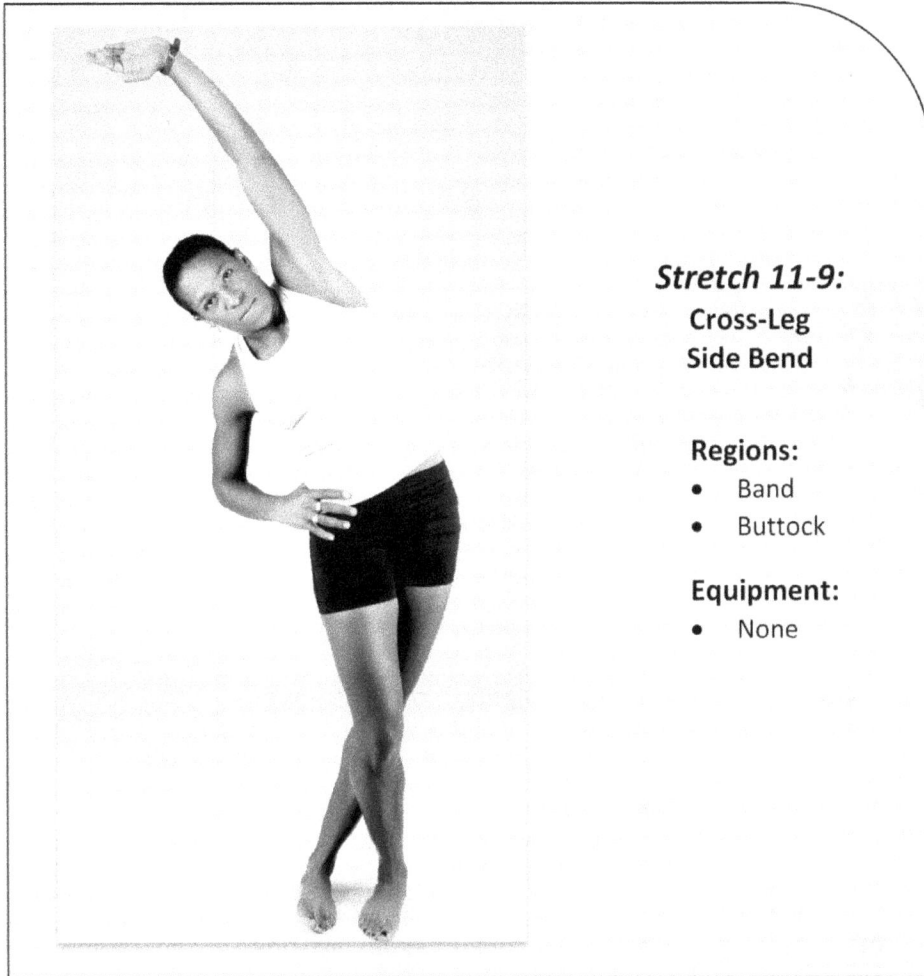

Stretch 11-9:
Cross-Leg
Side Bend

Regions:
- Band
- Buttock

Equipment:
- None

Starting Position	1. Standing, cross one leg to the opposite side, keeping the back leg straight. 2. On the same side as the back leg, raise the arm overhead, keeping the body straight.
Action	1. Stretch to the side while pushing the hip outward. 2. Contract by pushing into the ground with the back leg and tightening the hip muscles. 3. Relax and bend farther sideways. Hold the deeper stretch position.

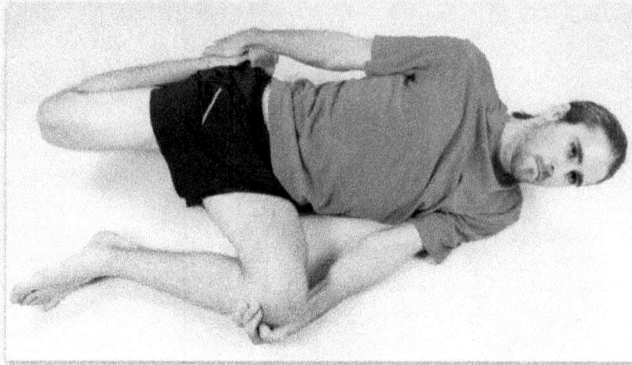

Stretch 11-10: Side Quadriceps Stretch

Regions:
- Knee
- Hip

Equipment:
- None

Starting Position	1. Lying on your side, use your lower hand to pull the lower knee forward, toward your chest. 2. Grasp the ankle of the upper leg with the other hand, flex the foot, and pull the upper leg backwards, toward your butt. 3. Keep your hips in line with your spine, and avoid twisting at the waist.
Action	1. Pull the back leg up toward your butt to stretch the front of the hip and knees. 2. Contract by tightening the knee and pushing the foot against your hand. 3. Relax the knee and pull the back leg farther toward the butt to stretch. Hold the deeper stretch position.

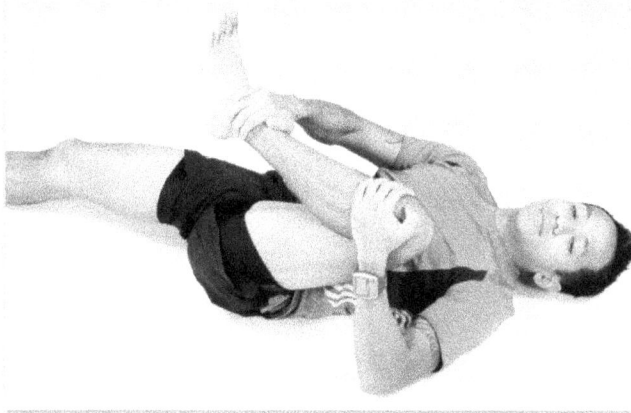

Stretch 11-11: Ankle-Knee Diagonal Stretch

Regions:
- Hip
- Buttock

Equipment:
- None

Starting Position	1. Lie on your back with one leg straight. 2. Hold the bent knee up to your chest with one hand. 3. Grasp the outside of the ankle with the opposite hand.
Action	1. Pull the ankle and knees diagonally across your body, toward the opposite hip, until you feel a stretch in your buttock. 2. While holding the stretch, contract by pushing the ankle and knee against your hands. 3. Relax the leg and bring it up higher. Hold the deeper stretch position.

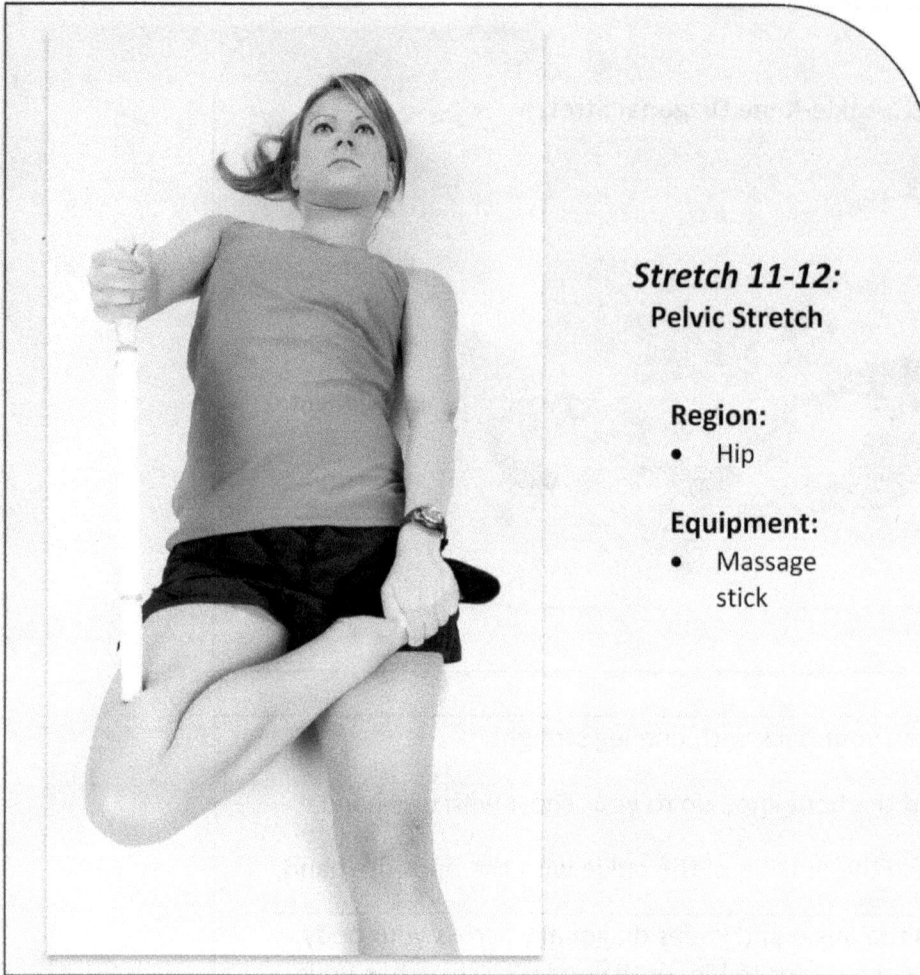

Stretch 11-12:
Pelvic Stretch

Region:
- Hip

Equipment:
- Massage stick

Starting Position	Lying down with one leg straight, pull the ankle of the other leg up to the opposite hip, forming a figure "4."
Action	1. Use the massage stick to push the bent knee down toward the floor to stretch the front of your hip. 2. Contract by lifting the knee upward to push into the massage stick. 3. Relax and use the massage stick to push the leg farther down. Hold the deeper stretch position.

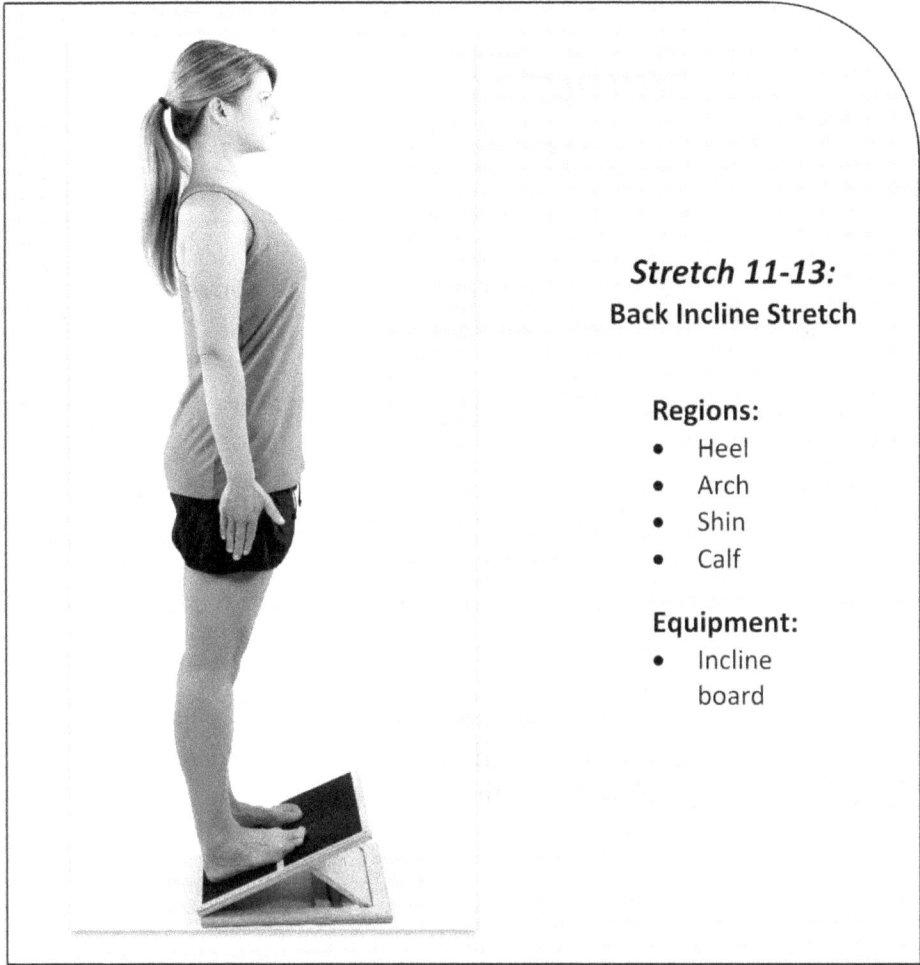

Stretch 11-13:
Back Incline Stretch

Regions:
- Heel
- Arch
- Shin
- Calf

Equipment:
- Incline board

Starting Position	Stand on an incline board, facing uphill, with feet and body straight.
Action	1. Balance your body evenly over both feet. 2. Contract and relax by pushing your feet into the incline board.

Box 14-3	*Guidelines:* Basic Closed-Chain Exercises

1. Assemble the required equipment, including a calculator and a stopwatch or timer (See *Table 14-2:* **Equipment for Closed-Chain Exercises).**

2. In your *Running Injury Recovery Workbook*, complete one **Log Form B: Basic Closed-Chain** for each day.

3. Carefully follow the instructions for each exercise in **Box 14-2**. Note that exercises 1 through 8 have instructions for both *Basic Closed-Chain Clearance* and *Final Target* (for Regional Closed-Chain). While you are using **Log Form B**, skip the instructions for *Final Target*.

4. Do *only* the eight Basic Closed-Chain Exercises (**Box 14-2** *Figures 14-1* through *14-8*) during Phase Three Part One P.T. Time. On your first day, choose four exercises and spend 10 minutes on each one. Do the other four exercises on your second day.

5. Each 10-minute exercise is broken into several **sets**. The maximum number of exercise sets you can complete in 10 minutes will vary, depending upon your fitness and the clearance goal for each Basic Closed-Chain Exercise. The *Target Time* for each exercise varies by exercise, from 15 to 60 seconds, and may or may not include a *Rest Between Sets*. (*Target Times* and *Rest Between Sets* are listed in the instructions on the line for *Basic Closed-Chain Clearance,* and on **Log Form B**.) Once you have reached the *Target Time* on the better leg, you can reduce the sets on that leg to a minimum of 3, and increase your sets on the other leg.

6. For each exercise, start with your least-affected leg and time how long you can maintain correct form without increasing pain. *Example:* Square Hops. Starting on your better leg, hop clockwise around the square, and then counter clockwise. Keep going on the same leg for as long as you can stay balanced and accept load without increasing pain, or up to the *Target Time* of 20 seconds. Then repeat on the more-affected leg for comparison.

(Box 14-3 cont.)

7. While performing each exercise, concentrate on the *Goals* for that exercise. Use the *Focus Statement* to help maintain correct form, create symmetry, and improve body awareness. Correct form means that you are able to hold the *Starting Position* as shown in the figure for that exercise, perform the described *Action*, and achieve the goals listed in the *Focus Statement*.

8. Stop each set when you feel fatigued, break form, or reach the *Target Time* for that exercise. It is better to do an exercise correctly for a shorter time than incorrectly for a longer time. Do not exceed the *Target Time* per set, even if you feel like you can. Record the time for each set on your **Log Form B** for that day.

9. Monitor your maximum pain level in each leg for each exercise, and enter those numbers on **Log Form B.**

10. For each exercise in Basic Closed-Chain, practice more sets on your weaker leg than on your stronger leg, even if the weaker leg in that exercise is not the injured leg. You must achieve **symmetry** in all exercises to clear Basic Closed-Chain before continuing to Regional Closed-Chain.
Average set times on left and right legs are considered equal (symmetrical) if they are within 5% of each other (see *Symmetry Goals* in **Log Form B**).

11. *Special Instructions for CC#6 Quick Steps:* Because this exercise is performed with both legs at the same time, you will not be able to measure a separate time for each leg. Stop each set when you become fatigued or break form, and record that time on your log form. Do not do more than one set every 30 seconds (20 sets in 10 minutes). For this exercise, symmetry is defined as the ability to maintain correct form at glide rhythm, equal weight on both legs, with no increase in pain.

12. When you have completed your daily P.T. Time, complete the calculations on **Log Form B** to check for symmetry and clearance for those exercises (see **Instructions for Log Form B** in the Workbook.)

13. Continue rotating through the eight Basic Closed-Chain Exercises, doing four a day, 10 minutes each, for a total of 40 minutes. When you have cleared a particular Basic Closed-Chain Exercise, you can eliminate that exercise from your next rotation. When you have less than four exercises left to clear, you'll have some extra 10-minute sessions to fill. Select one of the Basic Closed-Chain Exercises you have already cleared at the *Basic* level, and try building your time and/or rhythm up to the *Final Target* level.

| Box 14-4 | *Guidelines:*
Regional Closed-Chain Exercises |

1. In your *Running Injury Recovery Workbook*, fill out one section of **Log Form R: Regional Closed-Chain** for each day of P.T. Time. (See ***Self-Assessment 3B Part 2***, and **Instructions for Log Form R** in the Workbook.)

2. Continue to follow the same general guidelines for exercises that you used in Basic Closed-Chain [**Box 14-3**].

3. Carefully follow the instructions in **Box 14-2** for each individual exercise. Note that exercises 1 through 8 have instructions for both *Basic Closed-Chain Clearance* and *Final Target*. While you are using **Log Form R**, skip the instructions for *Basic Closed-Chain Clearance*.

4. Regional Closed-Chain Exercises progress in two stages. You must clear all of your Regional Closed-Chain Exercises in *Stage 1* (Symmetry and Clearance), before you progress to *Stage 2* (Build to Final Target).

5. On your first day of Regional Closed-Chain Exercises in Stage 1, follow the **Instructions for Log Form R** in the Workbook. Do the first four exercises on **Log Form R** (1st Injury Region), and complete your *Initial Assessment* for those exercises. Enter your Stage 1 *Symmetry Target* and *Symmetry Goal* for each exercise on **Log Form R**, and continue to use those numbers until you have cleared all Regional Closed-Chain Exercises in Stage 1.

6. On your second PT day, continue with the next four exercises on your list, in order (the last two exercises for your 1st Injury Region, and first two exercises for your 2nd Injury Region). Complete your *Initial Assessment* for each exercise, and enter your Stage 1 *Symmetry Target* and *Symmetry Goal* on your **Log Form R.**

7. Continue with four new exercises and *Initial Assessments* in each PT session until you reach the end of your list, then start again at the top of the list with a new rotation.

8. When you begin a new rotation, copy the *Symmetry Target* and *Symmetry Goal* for each exercise from your first **Log Form R**. Do not repeat your *Initial Assessment*. For each exercise, do more repetitions on the more-impaired side, and fewer repetitions on the less-impaired side, until you have achieved symmetry (*Self-Assessment 3F* in the Workbook).

(Box 14-4 cont.)

9. Follow the **Instructions for Log Form R** for Stage 1 and Stage 2. In Stage 1, when you have achieved symmetry in one exercise, you may skip that exercise in your next rotation and go on to the next exercise. As in Basic Closed-Chain, when you have less than 4 exercises remaining on your list, add back exercises that you have already cleared so that you always have 40 minutes of closed-chain exercises in Stage 1.

10. Follow the instructions in *Self-Assessment 3F* in your *Running Injury Recovery Workbook* to clear Stage 1. You must achieve symmetry for all Regional Closed-Chain Exercises on your list before you begin Stage 2.

11. When you have cleared Stage 1, follow the **Instructions for Log Form R, Stage 2** to revise your **Log Form R** for Stage 2. In Stage 2, you must maintain symmetry in all Regional Closed-Chain Exercises, and work to *build* your time and pace toward the goals listed in the *Final Target* for each exercise (for fitness runner or racers). These will be your goals for Phase Four, not clearance requirements.

12. You must clear both Regional Closed-Chain Stage 1 and your Phase Three Part Two *Base Schedule* before you can proceed to Phase Four *(Self-Assessment 3H)* in *The Running Injury Recovery Workbook.*

Weight Guidelines for *Table 14-2*

Your Weight	Hand Weights[1]	Ankle Weights[2]
80-120 lb.	2 pounds	2.5 pounds
120-180 lb.	3 pounds	5.0 pounds
180+ lb.	5 pounds	7.5 pounds

Table 14-2

Equipment for Closed-Chain Exercises

Standard Equipment	Home Alternative
Full-length mirror	Full-length mirror, or window reflection, or someone watching you
Stopwatch	Runner's watch with interval and lap timer
Calculator	Phone with a calculator app
2 Hand weights [1]	2 Hand weights [1]
2 Ankle weights [2]	2 Ankle weights [2]
Low step, adjustable from 6" to 12"	Curb or stair step
Plyometric Box, adjustable from 12" to 24"	Two steps up on a flight of stairs; one step down on a flight of stairs
Square balance foam	2 Bed pillows
Slant board	21.5" X 17" X 0.75" plywood propped on half a cinder block
2.5 feet red (medium-resistance) Theraband tubing, tied in a loop	5 rubber-band loops (1 loop = 5 large rubber bands knotted together)

Box 14-2 *HOW TO:* Closed-Chain Exercises

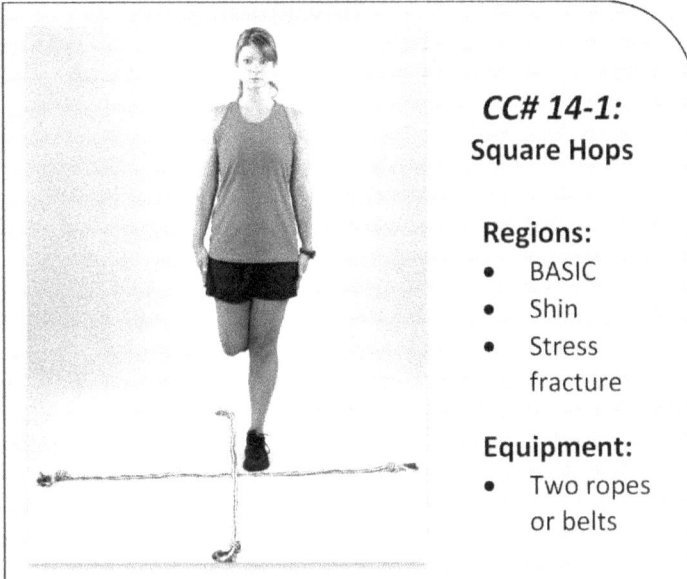

CC# 14-1:
Square Hops

Regions:
- BASIC
- Shin
- Stress fracture

Equipment:
- Two ropes or belts

Starting Position	1. Cross two ropes, belts, or chalk lines on the floor in front of a mirror, forming a 4-square grid. 2. Stand at the center of the grid in "straight" posture, with your feet parallel to the lines, hands down at your sides.
Action	1. Looking in the mirror, balance on one leg. Raise the other leg to "kickback" position. 2. Keeping your toes pointed toward the mirror, hop flat-footed over each of the 4 lines in a clockwise pattern: front, side, back, and side. 3. Staying on the same leg, reverse to counterclockwise and hop side, forward, side, and back. Continue on the same leg until you are fatigued or unable to maintain correct form. 4. Switch legs and repeat.
Goals	Try to maintain your posture and balance as you hop in four directions.
Focus Statement	"I will balance my body on a straight foot."
Basic Closed-Chain Clearance	1. Achieve symmetry at glide pace 2. *Target Time*: 10 repeats of 20 seconds on each leg with 10 second rest in between.
Final Target	Accelerate your pace as you build up to your target time: • Fitness Runners: 30 seconds each leg, with a 10 second rest • Racers: 90 seconds each leg, with a 10 second rest • Total of 10 minutes, with no break in form

CC#14-2: Side Step-Down

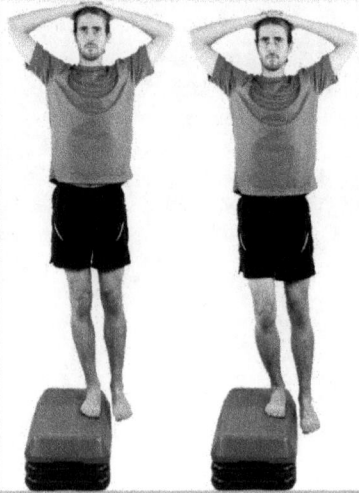

Regions:
- BASIC
- Arch, shin, calf, knee, band, hip, hamstring
- Stress fracture

Equipment:
- Medium step box or stair step

Starting Position	1. Barefoot, stand on one foot, parallel to the edge of a medium-height step. 2. Bend the weightbearing knee slightly, and put your hands on your head. 3. Keep the ankle of the free leg in glide position with the knee straight.
Action	Alternately bend and straighten the knee and ankle of the weightbearing leg slightly, in small controlled movements, keeping the body straight.
Goals	1. Feel your weightbearing foot working while moving up and down, keeping your body straight. 2. Tighten your trunk to maintain your balance.
Focus Statement	"I will balance my body on a straight foot."
Basic Closed-Chain Clearance	1. Create symmetry. 2. *Target Time:* • 20 seconds on each leg • Total of 10 minutes, continuously, on a 6 inch step, with no break in form.
Final Target	Raise your step height as you build up to your glide rhythm and target time: • Fitness Runners: 30 seconds each leg • Racers: 90 seconds each leg • Total of 10 minutes, continuously, on a 12 inch step, with no break in form

CC#14-3:
One-Leg Armswings, Barefoot

Regions:
- BASIC
- Toes
- Arch

Equipment:
- Hand weights

Starting Position	1. Stand barefoot on a level surface, with "straight" posture. 2. Bend one knee 90 degrees to kickback position. 2. Holding a hand weight in each hand, bend elbows to 90 degrees.
Action	1. Slowly swing your arms from the shoulder, keeping the elbows bent and close to the body. As one arm moves forward, the other arm moves backward. Use toes as suction cups to hold balance. 2. Alternate legs before you lose your balance.
Goals	1. Work the ground with your foot while using your arms to help maintain your body straight and balanced over the weight-bearing leg. 2. The only part of your body moving should be the balanced armswings.
Focus Statement	"I will use my arms to balance my body."
Basic Closed-Chain Clearance	1. Create symmetry. 2. *Target Time:* • 15 seconds on each leg with no rest • Total of 10 minutes, continuously, with no break in form.
Final Target	Build up to your glide rhythm and target time: • Fitness Runners: 30 seconds each leg • Racers: 90 seconds each leg • Total of 10 minutes, continuously, with no break in form.

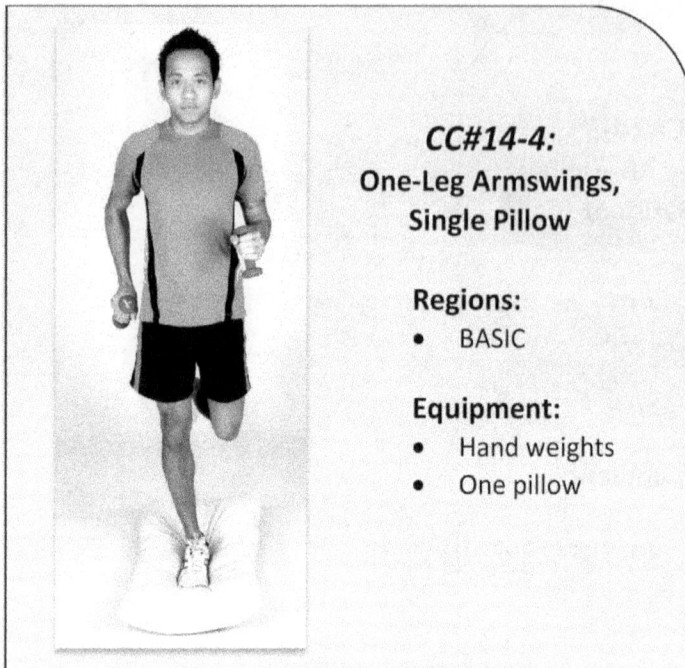

CC#14-4:
One-Leg Armswings,
Single Pillow

Regions:
- BASIC

Equipment:
- Hand weights
- One pillow

Starting Position	1. Wearing shoes, stand on one pillow with "straight" posture. 2. Bend one knee to kickback position. 3. Holding a hand weight in each hand, bend elbows to 90 degrees.
Action	1. Slowly swing your arms from the shoulder, keeping the elbows bent and close to the body. As one arm moves forward, the other arm moves backward. 2. Alternate legs before you lose your balance.
Goals	1. Use your armswings to keep your body straight and balanced over the weight-bearing leg on the unstable surface. Feel your foot inside your shoe working to keep balance. 2. The only part of your body moving is your armswings.
Focus Statement	"I will use my arms to balance my body."
Basic Closed-Chain Clearance	1. Create symmetry. 2. *Target Time:* • 30 seconds on each leg with no rest in between. • Total of 10 minutes, continuously, with no break in form

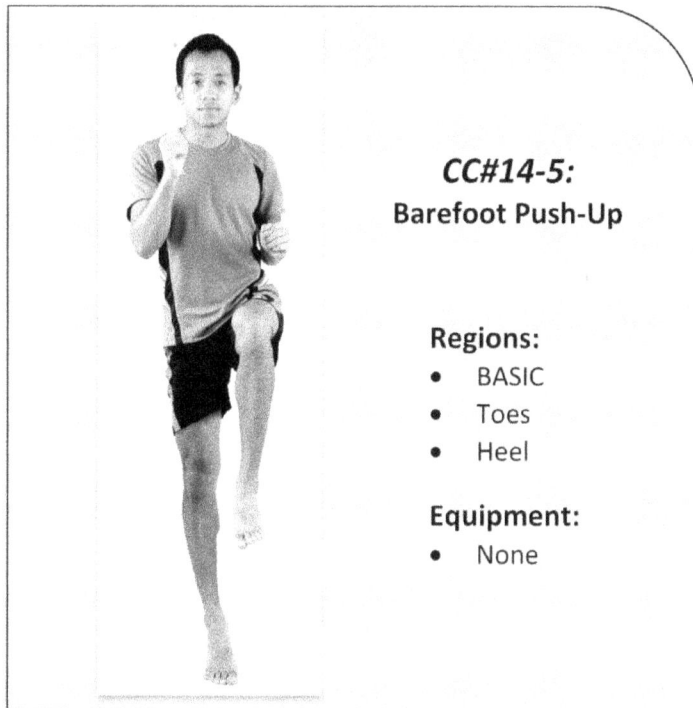

CC#14-5:
Barefoot Push-Up

Regions:
- BASIC
- Toes
- Heel

Equipment:
- None

Starting Position	Barefoot, stand in "straight" posture, elbows bent 90 degrees.
Action	1. Raise one knee to the "high knees" position, keeping your foot aligned under the bent knee, and hold. 2. Move your arms to the coordinated position for balance, and hold. 3. Push up through the big toe, lifting the heel off the ground.
Goals	1. Try to maintain a small, smooth, controlled motion as you transition from the flatfoot position to the big toe, keeping the toes flat. 2. Try to keep your body straight and balanced while your weight moves forward and up into a pushoff position.
Focus Statement	"I will balance my body to push off through the big toe."
Basic Closed-Chain Clearance	1. Create symmetry at glide rhythm. 2. *Target Time:* • 15 seconds on each leg with no rest in between. • Total of 10 minutes, continuously, with no break in form
Final Target	Build up to your target time at glide rhythm: • Fitness Runners: 30 seconds each leg • Racers: 90 seconds each leg • Total of 10 minutes, continuously, with no break in form.

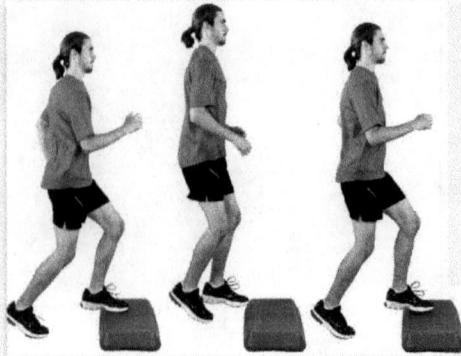

CC#14-6: Quick Steps

Regions:
- BASIC
- Heel, calf, buttock

Equipment:
- Low step box or curb

Starting Position	1. Stand in "straight" posture with a curb-height step in front of you. 2. Place one forefoot on the step, and evenly distribute your weight between both forefeet.
Action	1. Set your timer for 30 seconds. 2. Maintaining equal amounts of weight on the balls of both feet, push up strongly through the toes of both feet. 3. Quickly switch your legs forward and backward, keeping on your forefeet, both feet pointed straight forward. 4. Coordinate your armswings with your leg motion. 5. Note how long you were able to perform each set. Do not exceed 20 seconds. Start your next set when the timer reaches 30 seconds, and repeat.
Goals	Try to keep your motion quick, smooth, and coordinated as you scissor your legs forward in a skipping action.
Focus Statement	"I will balance my body to push off through the big toe."
Basic Closed-Chain Clearance	1. Create symmetry at glide rhythm. 2. *Target Time:* • Sets of 20 seconds with 10 second rest in between • Total of 10 minutes, on a 6 inch step, with no break in form.
Final Target	Build up to your target time, then accelerate your pace: • Fitness Runners: 50-second sets with a 10-second rest • Racers: 1minute-50-second sets with a 10-second rest • Total of 10 minutes, on a 6 inch step, with no break in form.

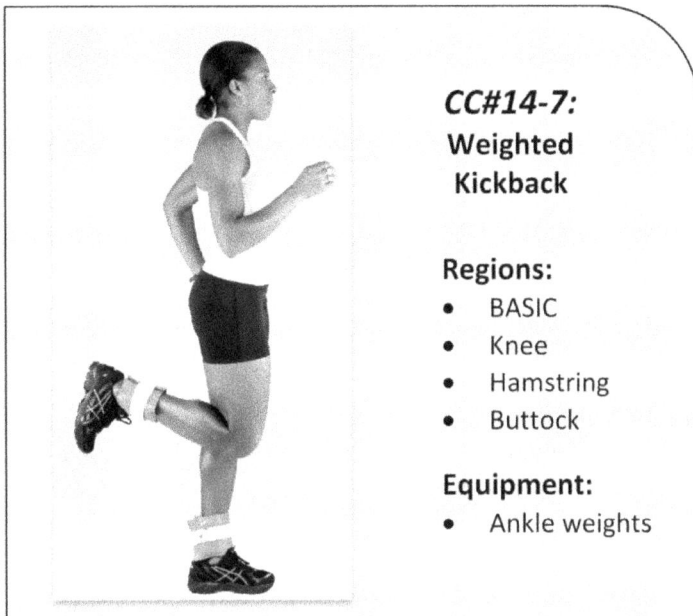

CC#14-7:
Weighted Kickback

Regions:
- BASIC
- Knee
- Hamstring
- Buttock

Equipment:
- Ankle weights

Starting Position	1. Wearing ankle weights, stand in "straight" posture, toes pointed forward, elbows bent 90 degrees. 2. Keeping the knees even, bend the non-weightbearing knee until the toe is just touching down in the "glide" position.
Action	1. Keeping the weightbearing knee straight, slowly bend the non-weightbearing knee to "kickback" position – raising the heel 90 degrees toward the glutes. 2. Continue to alternately bend and straighten the non-weightbearing knee, coordinating your armswings with your leg motion.
Goals	1. Try to maintain a smooth, controlled motion as you kick back. 2. Tighten your trunk to keep your body straight and balanced over the weight-bearing leg.
Focus Statement	"I will balance my body for a straight kickback."
Basic Closed-Chain Clearance	1. Create symmetry. 2. *Target Time:* • 60 seconds on each leg with no rest in between • Total of 10 minutes with no break in form.
Final Target	Build up to your glide rhythm and target time: • Fitness Runners: 2½ minutes each leg • Racers: 5 minutes each leg • Total of 10 minutes, continuously, with no break in form.

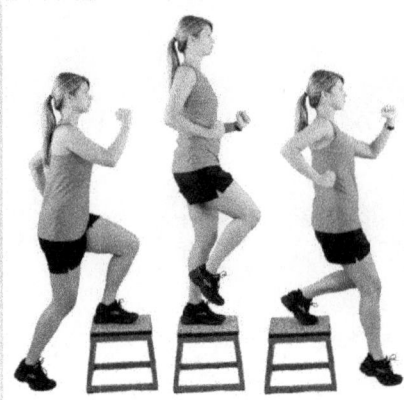

CC#14-8: Box Step Up and Over

Regions:
- BASIC
- Arch, heel, knee, band, hip, buttock, hamstring
- Stress fracture

Equipment:
- 12- to 24-inch plyometric box

Starting Position	Wearing shoes, stand in "straight" posture with a knee-height box in front of you as you face the mirror; arms bent 90 degrees.
Action	1. Place one foot flat on the box, toes pointed forward in "high knees" position. 2. With the lower (second) foot, push up through the big toe. 3. Continuing your motion, step up and over the box, through "kickback" position, and land on the floor in front of you with the big toe of the second foot. 4. Coordinate your armswings with your leg motion. 5. End by bringing the first foot down to the floor, from pushoff to flatfooted. 6. Walk around the box, making a wide turn, and continue in the same direction.
Goals	1. Coordinate your armswings to maintain a smooth, controlled motion. 2. Tighten your trunk to balance your body as you move from the high knees position to kickback position.
Focus Statement	"I will balance my body for a straight kickback."
Basic Closed-Chain Clearance	1. Create symmetry. 2. *Target Time:* • 60 seconds on each leg with no rest in between • Total of 10 minutes, on a 12-inch step, with no break in form.
Final Target	1. Gradually raise step height until hip and knee are at high knees position. 2. Build up to your glide rhythm and target time: • Fitness Runners: 2½ minutes each leg • Racers: 5 minutes each leg • Total of 10 minutes, continuously, with no break in form.

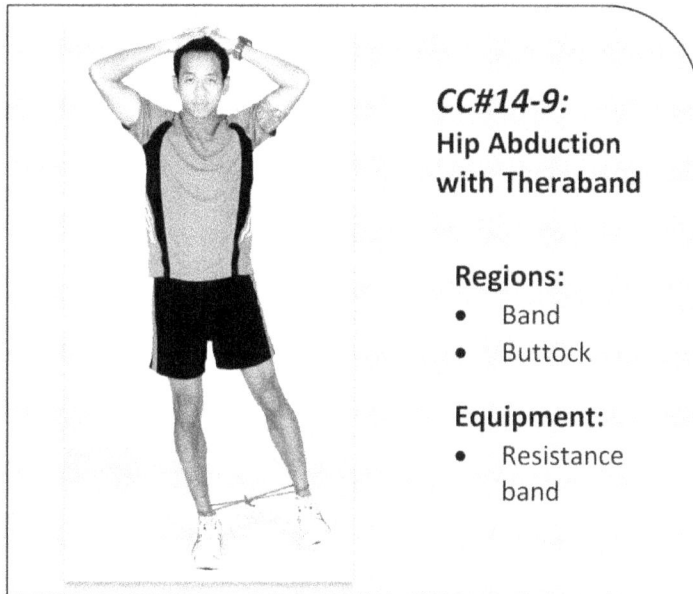

CC#14-9:

Hip Abduction with Theraband

Regions:
- Band
- Buttock

Equipment:
- Resistance band

Starting Position	1. Loop the resistance band around one ankle. Make a half-turn in the loop to form a figure "8," and slip the other end of the loop around the other ankle. 2. Stand with "straight" posture, toes pointed forward, both hands on your head.
Action	1. Keeping both knees straight, slowly raise one leg to the side, keeping the foot in neutral position. 2. Slowly return to the starting position, keeping the foot in neutral position.
Goals	1. Try to maintain a smooth, controlled motion. Keep the arms still, with elbows back. 2. Tighten your trunk to keep your body straight and balanced over the weight-bearing leg. 3. Create symmetry at glide rhythm.
Focus Statement	"I will balance my body on a straight foot."
Final Target	Build up to your target time at glide rhythm: • Fitness Runners: 60 seconds each leg • Racers: 2½ minutes each leg • Total of 10 minutes, continuously, with no break in form.

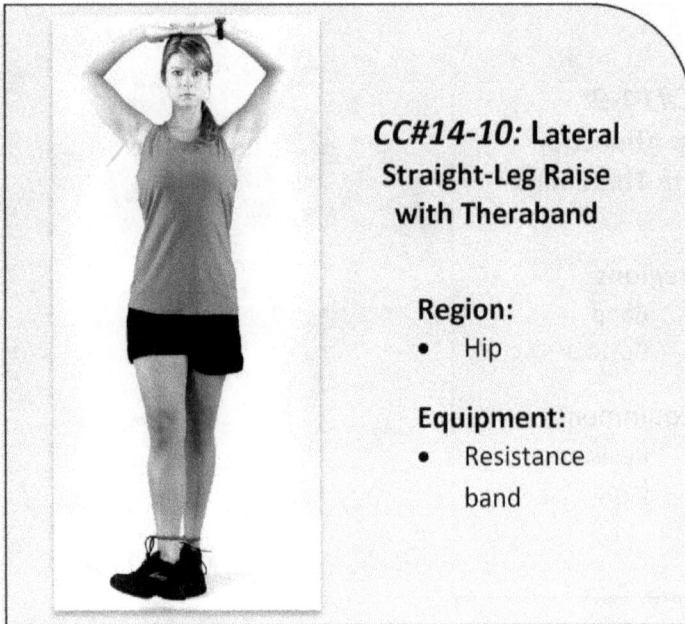

CC#14-10: Lateral Straight-Leg Raise with Theraband

Region:
- Hip

Equipment:
- Resistance band

Starting Position	1. Loop the resistance band around one ankle. Make a half-turn in the loop to form a figure "8," and slip the other end of the loop around the other ankle. 2. Stand with "straight" posture, toes pointed forward. 3. Place both hands on your head, elbows pointing out.
Action	1. Rotate one leg at the hip so the toes point outward. 2. Keeping both knees straight, slowly raise the rotated leg straight forward, keeping the foot in neutral position. 2. Slowly return to the starting position, keeping the foot in neutral position.
Goals	1. Try to maintain a smooth, controlled motion. 2. Tighten your trunk to keep your body straight and balanced over the weightbearing leg without moving your arms. 3. Create symmetry at glide rhythm.
Focus Statement	"I will balance my body on a straight foot."
Final Target	Build up to your target time at glide rhythm: • Fitness Runners; 60 seconds each leg • Racers: 2½ minutes each leg • Total of 10 minutes, continuously, with no break in form.

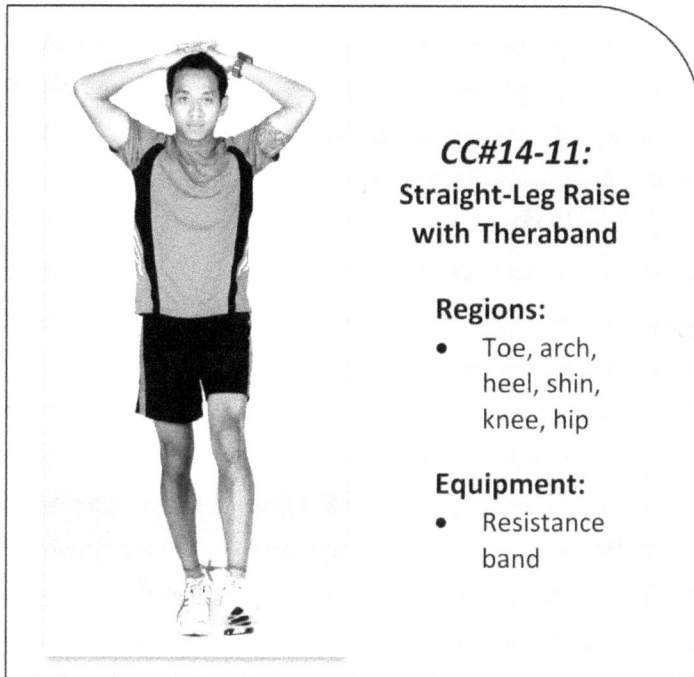

CC#14-11:
Straight-Leg Raise with Theraband

Regions:
- Toe, arch, heel, shin, knee, hip

Equipment:
- Resistance band

Starting Position	1. Loop the resistance band around one ankle. Make a half-turn in the loop to form a figure "8," and slip the other end of the loop around the other ankle. 2. Stand with "straight" posture, toes pointed forward. 3. Place both hands on your head, elbows pointing out.
Action	1. Keeping both knees straight, slowly raise one leg straight forward, keeping the foot in neutral position. 2. Slowly return to the starting position, keeping the foot in neutral position.
Goals	1. Try to maintain a smooth, controlled motion while kicking forward. 2. Tighten your trunk to keep your body straight and balanced over the weight-bearing leg without moving your arms. 3. Create symmetry at glide rhythm.
Focus Statement	"I will balance my body on a straight foot."
Final Target	Build up to your target time at glide rhythm: • Fitness Runners: 60 seconds each leg • Racers: 2½ minutes each leg • Total of 10 minutes, continuously, with no break in form.

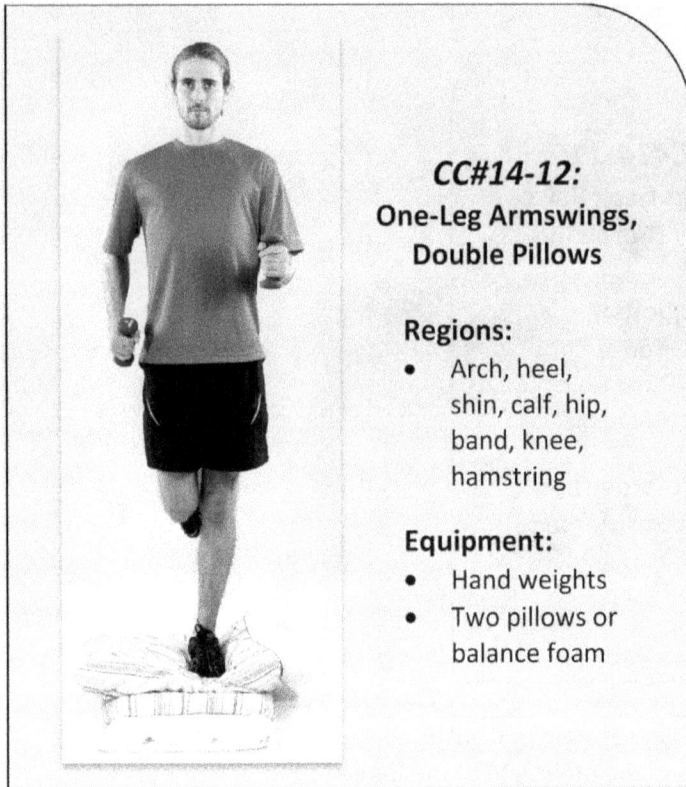

CC#14-12:
One-Leg Armswings, Double Pillows

Regions:
- Arch, heel, shin, calf, hip, band, knee, hamstring

Equipment:
- Hand weights
- Two pillows or balance foam

Starting Position	1. Cross two pillows to form an "X." Wearing shoes, stand on the pillows with "straight" posture. 2. Bend one knee 90 degrees in the kickback position. 3. Holding a hand weight in each hand, bend elbows to 90 degrees.
Action	1. Slowly swing your arms from the shoulder, keeping the elbows bent and close to the body. As one arm moves forward, the other arm moves backward. 2. Work up to progressively faster armswings as you accelerate to glide pace.
Goals	1. Work your arms to keep your body straight and balanced over the weight-bearing leg on this very challenging surface. 2. Achieve symmetry at glide pace.
Focus Statement	"I will use my arms to balance my body."
Final Target	Accelerate your pace after you build up to your target time: • Fitness Runners: 30 seconds each leg • Racers: 90 seconds each leg • Total of 10 minutes, continuously, with no break in form.

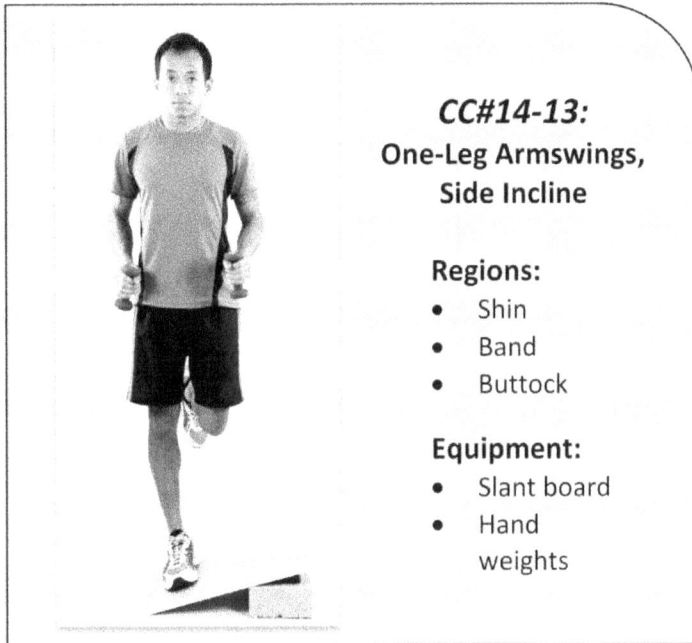

CC#14-13:
One-Leg Armswings,
Side Incline

Regions:
- Shin
- Band
- Buttock

Equipment:
- Slant board
- Hand weights

Starting Position	1. Set up a slant board so that it inclines to one side as you face the mirror. 2. Wearing shoes, stand on the slant board and bend the non-weightbearing knee 90 degrees to the kickback position, keeping a "straight" posture. 3. Holding a hand weight in each hand, bend elbows to 90 degrees.
Action	1. Slowly swing your arms from the shoulder, keeping the elbows bent and close to the body. As one arm moves forward, the other arm moves backward. 2. Repeat on the other leg. 3. Change the slant board to the opposite side and repeat with both legs.
Goals	1. Use your armswings to keep your body straight and balanced over the weightbearing leg on the uneven surface. 2. Create symmetry at glide pace.
Focus Statement	"I will use my arms to balance my body."
Final Target	Accelerate your pace after you build up to your target time: • Fitness Runners: 30 seconds each leg • Racers: 90 seconds each leg • Total of 10 minutes, continuously, with no break in form.

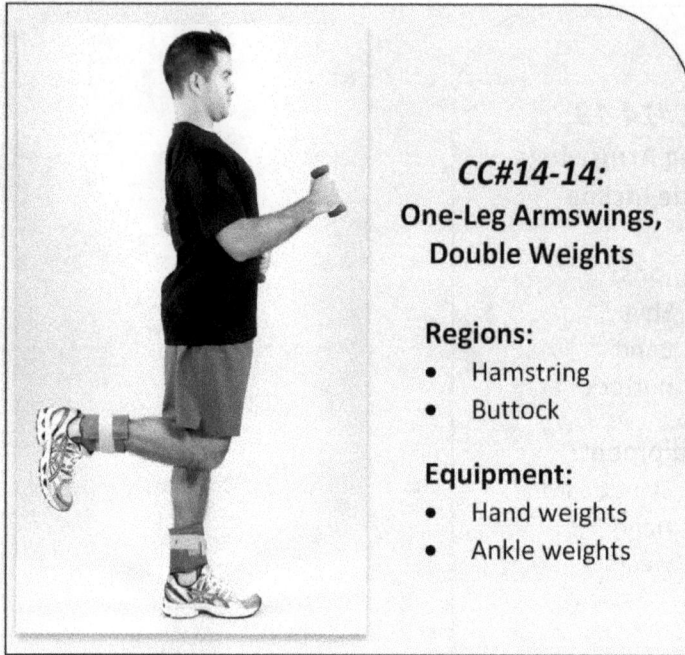

CC#14-14:
One-Leg Armswings, Double Weights

Regions:
- Hamstring
- Buttock

Equipment:
- Hand weights
- Ankle weights

Starting Position	1. Wearing shoes and ankle weights, stand on a level surface with "straight" posture. 2. Bend one knee 90 degrees in the kickback position. 3. Holding a hand weight in each hand, bend elbows to 90 degrees.
Action	1. Slowly swing your arms from the shoulder, keeping the elbows bent and close to the body. As one arm moves forward, the other arm moves backward.
Goals	1. Use your arms to balance your body while keeping the weightbearing leg straight and stationary in the kickback position. 2. Achieve symmetry at glide pace.
Focus Statement	"I will use my arms to balance my body."
Final Target	Accelerate your pace after you build up to your target time: • Fitness Runners: 30 seconds each leg • Racers: 90 seconds each leg • Total of 10 minutes, continuously, with no break in form.

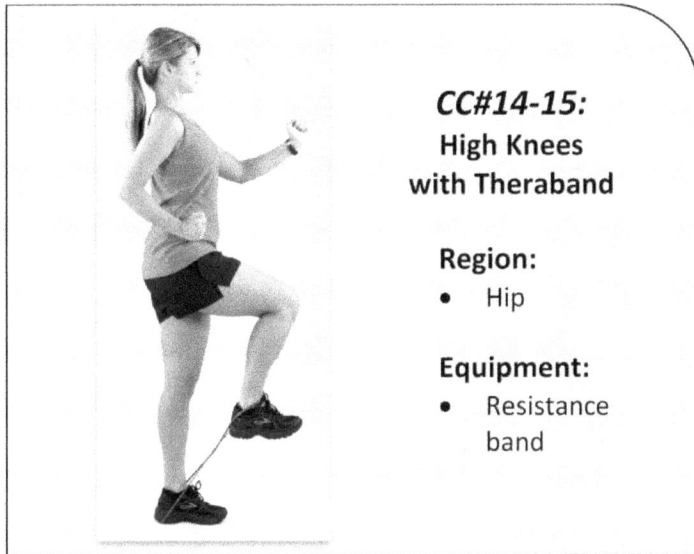

CC#14-15:
**High Knees
with Theraband**

Region:
- Hip

Equipment:
- Resistance band

Starting Position	1. Loop the resistance band under the heel of one shoe so you are standing on the elastic band. This is the weightbearing leg. 2. Make a half-turn in the loop to form a figure "8," and slip the other end of the loop around the other ankle. This is the non-weightbearing leg. 3. Stand in "straight" posture, toes pointed forward, elbows bent 90 degrees.
Action	1. Keeping the weightbearing knee straight, raise the non-weightbearing knee directly forward to the "high knees" position, keeping the foot in neutral position. 2. Coordinate your armswings with your leg motion. 3. Slowly return to the starting position, keeping the foot in neutral position.
Goals	1. Try to maintain a smooth, controlled motion into the high knees position. 2. Tighten your trunk to keep your body straight and balanced over the weight-bearing leg. 3. Create symmetry at glide pace.
Focus Statement	"I will use my arms to balance my body."
Final Target	Build up to your target time at glide pace: • Fitness Runners: 60 seconds each leg • Racers: 2½ minutes each leg • Total of 10 minutes, continuously, with no break in form.

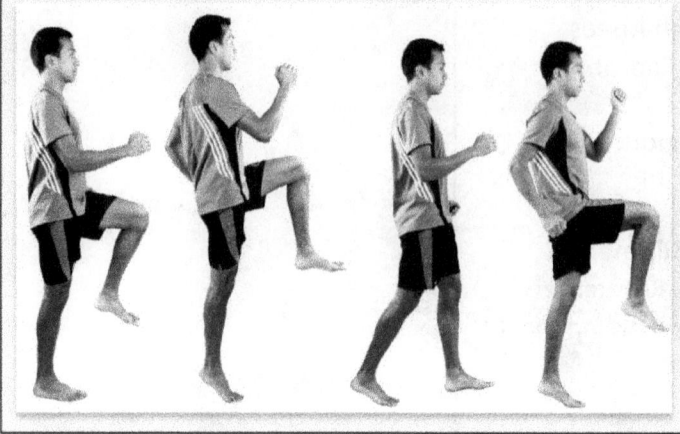

CC#14-16: Barefoot Push-Through

Regions	Toes, arch
Equipment	None
Starting Position	Barefoot, stand in "straight" posture, elbows bent 90 degrees.
Action	1. Walk forward, raising the leading knee to the "high knees" position, keeping your foot aligned under the bent knee. 2. With each step, push up through the big toe of the weightbearing leg, lifting the heel off the ground, keeping the toes flat. 3. Coordinate your armswings with your leg motion.
Goals	1. Use your armswings to maintain a smooth, controlled motion. 2. Tighten your trunk to keep your body straight and balanced as you move forward from the flatfoot strike to the pushoff. 3. Create symmetry at glide pace.
Focus Statement	"I will balance my body to push off through the big toe."
Final Target	Build up to your target time at glide pace: • Fitness Runners: 4½ minute sets with 30 second rest. • Racers: One 10 minute set with no rest. • Total of 10 minutes with no break in form.

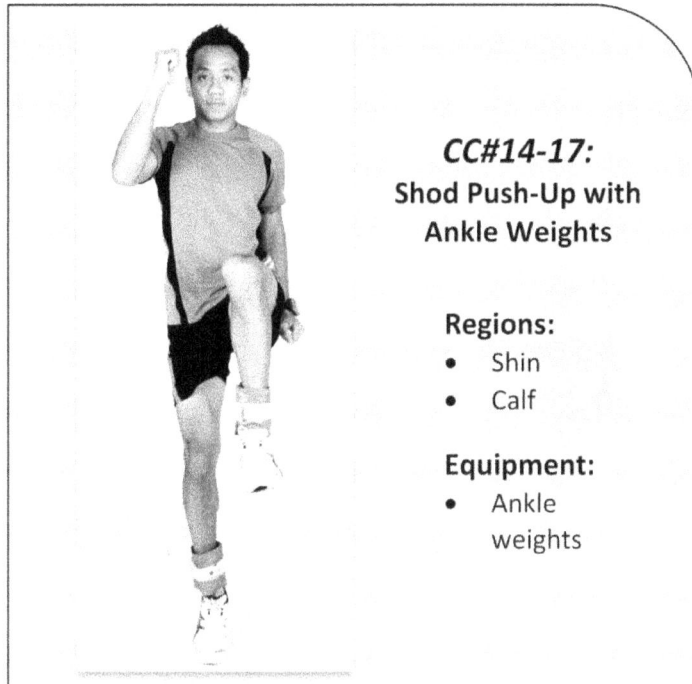

CC#14-17:

Shod Push-Up with Ankle Weights

Regions:
- Shin
- Calf

Equipment:
- Ankle weights

Starting Position	Wearing shoes and ankle weights, stand in "straight" posture, elbows bent 90 degrees.
Action	1. Raise one knee to the "high knees" position, keeping your foot aligned under the bent knee. 2. Simultaneously, push up through the big toe of the weightbearing leg, lifting the heel off the ground. 3. Coordinate your armswings with your leg motion. 4. Return to the starting position and repeat.
Goals	1. Try to maintain a smooth, controlled motion throughout. 2. Tighten your trunk to keep your body straight and balanced over the weight-bearing leg. 3. Create symmetry at glide pace.
Focus Statement	"I will balance my body to push off through the big toe."
Final Target	Accelerate your pace after you build up to your target time: • Fitness Runners: 60 seconds each leg • Racers: 2 ½ minutes each leg • Total of 10 minutes, continuously, with no break in form.

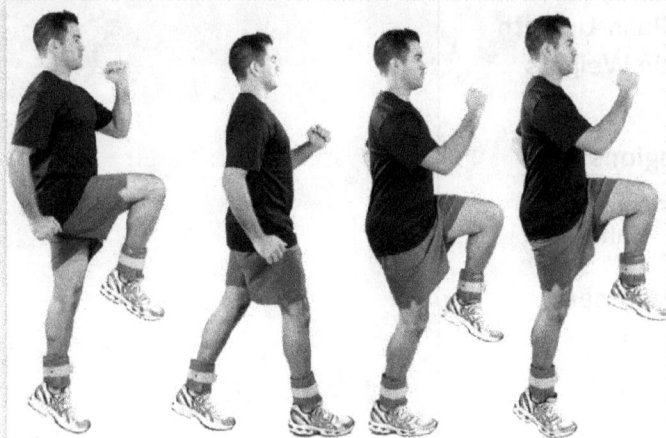

CC#14-18:
Shod Push-Through with Ankle Weights

Regions	Toe, heel, calf, knee, stress fracture
Equipment	Ankle weights
Starting Position	Wearing shoes and ankle weights, stand in "straight" posture, elbows bent 90 degrees.
Action	1. Walk forward, raising the leading knee to the "high knees" position, keeping your foot aligned under the bent knee. 2. With each step, push up through the big toe of the weightbearing leg, lifting the heel off the ground. 3. Coordinate your armswings with your leg motion.
Goals	1. Try to maintain a smooth, controlled motion to keep the weighted foot from slapping on the strike. 2. Tighten your trunk to keep your body straight and balanced as you move forward. 3. Create symmetry at glide pace.
Focus Statement	"I will balance my body to push off through the big toe."
Final Target	Build up to target time at glide pace: • Fitness Runners: 4½ minute sets with 30-second rest • Racers: One 10 minute set with no rest. • Total of 10 minutes with no break in form.

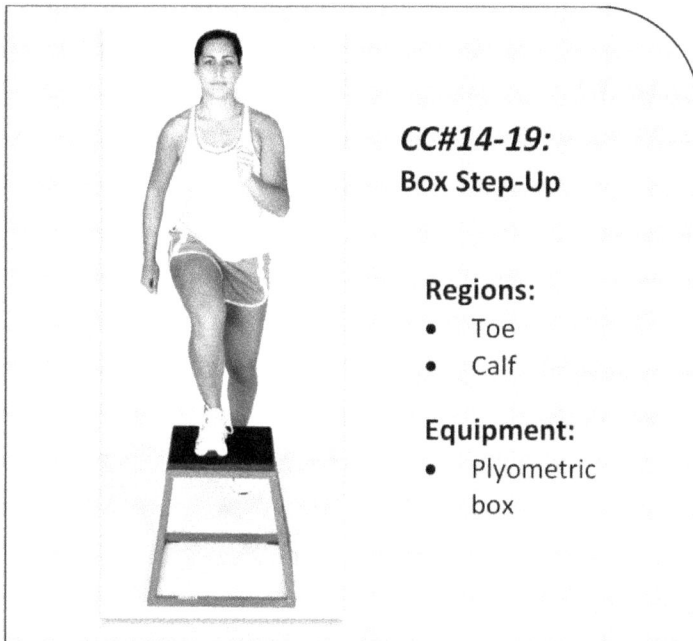

CC#14-19:
Box Step-Up

Regions:
- Toe
- Calf

Equipment:
- Plyometric box

Starting Position	Wearing shoes, stand in "straight" posture with a high box in front of you as you face the mirror; arms bent 90 degrees.
Action	1. Place one foot flat on the box, toes pointed forward. 2. With the lower (second) foot, push up through the big toe. 3. Continuing your motion, step up on the box with both feet. 4. Coordinate your armswings with your leg motion. 5. Leaving the second foot on the box, step backward to the original position with the first foot.
Goals	1. Concentrate on a flatfoot stride and push through with a slow, smooth, controlled motion throughout. 2. Use slow, coordinated armswings to keep your body straight and balanced as you move up and down. 3. Create symmetry at glide pace.
Focus Statement	"I will balance my body to push off through the big toe."
Final Target	1. Gradually raise step height until hip and knee are at high knees position. 2. Build up to target time at glide pace: • Fitness Runners: 2½ minutes each leg • Racers 5: minutes each leg • Total of 10 minutes, continuously, with no break in form.

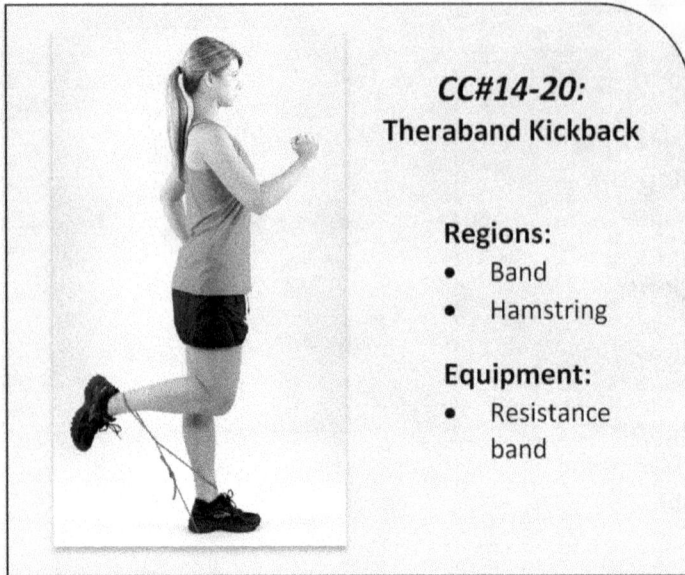

CC#14-20:
Theraband Kickback

Regions:
- Band
- Hamstring

Equipment:
- Resistance band

Starting Position	1. Loop the resistance band under the heel of one shoe so you are standing on the elastic band. This is the weightbearing leg. 2. Make a half-turn in the loop to form a figure "8," and slip the other end of the loop around the other ankle. This is the non-weightbearing leg. 3. Stand in "straight" posture, toes pointed forward, elbows bent 90 degrees. 4. Keeping the knees even, bend the non-weightbearing knee until the toe is just touching down in the "glide" position.
Action	1. Keeping the weightbearing knee straight, slowly bend the non-weightbearing knee to the "kickback" position – raising the heel 90 degrees toward the glutes. 2. Alternately bend and straighten the non-weightbearing knee, coordinating your armswings with your leg motion.
Goals	1. Try to maintain a smooth, controlled motion as you kick back. 2. Tighten your trunk to keep your body straight and balanced over the weight-bearing leg. 3. Create symmetry at glide pace.
Focus Statement	"I will balance my body for a straight kickback."
Final Target	Accelerate your pace after you build up to your target time: • Fitness Runners: 60 seconds each leg • Racers: 2½ minutes each leg • Total of 10 minutes, continuously, with no break in form.

Box 16-2

HOW TO: Hill Closed-Chain

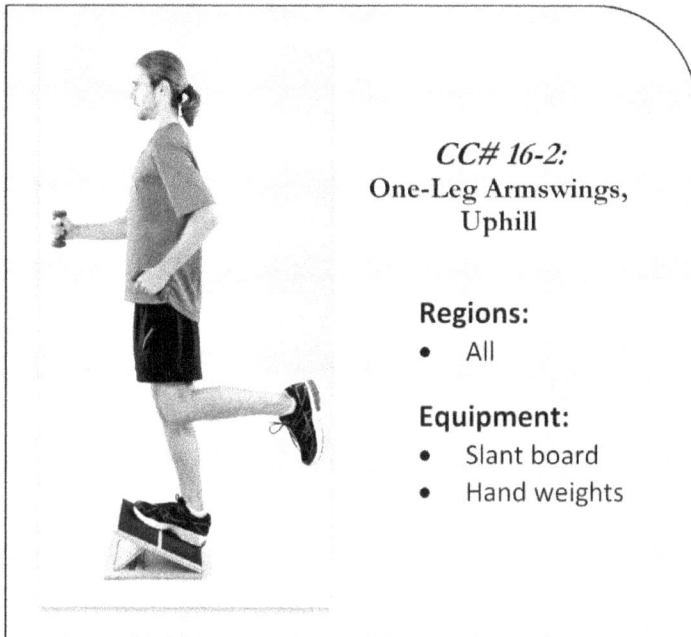

CC# 16-2:
One-Leg Armswings, Uphill

Regions:
- All

Equipment:
- Slant board
- Hand weights

Hill Closed-Chain #1

Starting Position	1. Set up a slant board so that it inclines uphill as you face the mirror. 2. Wearing shoes, stand on the slant board with "straight" posture. 3. Bend one knee 90 degrees to kickback position. 4. Holding a hand weight in each hand, bend elbows to 90 degrees.
Action	1. Swing your arms from the shoulder, keeping the elbows bent and close to the body. 2. Find your uphill balance point by swinging your arms a little farther forward than backward. 3. Build up to your glide rhythm, then accelerate your pace to your target time. 4. Repeat on each leg to create symmetry.
Goal	Use your armswings in a more forward position to keep your body straight and balanced over the weightbearing leg.
Focus Statement	"I will use my armswings to balance my body."
Clearance Target	Create symmetry: • Accelerate to 20 seconds on each leg with no rest in between. • Total of 10 minutes, continuously, with no break in form.
Final Target	Accelerate your pace after you build up to your target time: • Fitness Runners: 30 seconds each leg • Racers: 90 seconds each leg • Total of 10 minutes, continuously, with no break in form.

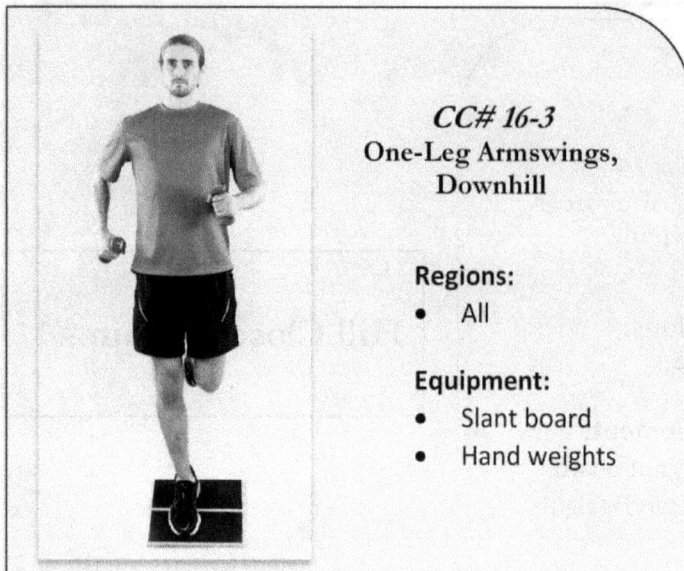

CC# 16-3
One-Leg Armswings, Downhill

Regions:
- All

Equipment:
- Slant board
- Hand weights

Starting Position:	1. Set up a slant board inclining downhill as you face the mirror. 2. Wearing shoes, stand on the slant board with "straight" posture. 3. Bend one knee 90 degrees to kickback position. 4. Slightly bend weightbearing knee. 5. Holding a hand weight in each hand, bend elbows to 90 degrees.
Action	1. Swing your arms from the shoulder, keeping the elbows a little farther from the body to improve balance. 2. Find your downhill balance point by swinging your arms a little farther backward than forward. 3. Build up to your glide rhythm, then accelerate your pace to your target time. 4. Repeat on each leg to create symmetry.
Goal	Hold your elbows farther away from your body and use a more rapid rhythm to keep your body straight and balanced over the weight-bearing leg.
Focus Statement	"I will use my armswings to balance my body."
Clearance Target	Create symmetry: • Accelerate to 20 seconds on each leg with no rest in between. • Total of 10 minutes, continuously, with no break in form.
Final Target	Accelerate your pace after you build up to your target time: • Fitness Runners: 30 seconds each leg • Racers: 90 seconds each leg • Total of 10 minutes, continuously, with no break in form.

Box 15-1	*HOW TO:* Build Your Walk/Glide Program

The formula for a 60-minute training session is **10 minutes fitness walking + [5 minutes (Glide + Walk) x 10 sets] = 60 minutes.** I keep walk/glide sets in units of 5 minutes because it's easy to set your timer.

1. *Warm Up:* Always begin with 10 minutes of **fitness walking** to warm up. If you are not able to fitness walk for 10 minutes without pain or breaking form, do not proceed to walk/glide sets.

2. *Walk/Glide Sets:* After the warm-up, begin your series of 5-minute walk/glide sets. There are five progressive levels of walk/glide sets, each consisting of one or more minutes of **gliding** followed by four or fewer minutes of fitness walking *Table 15-4*]. Follow the instructions for Group 1 (Self-Paced Plan) or Group 2 (Two-Week-Interval Plan).

3. *Glide Drills:* There are five variations of **glide drills [Box 15-4]**.
- For 1-4 sets, insert one 15-second glide drill into each 1-minute glide for a total of 10 glide drills (do each of the five glide drills twice).
- For 2-3 sets and higher, do each of the five glide drills three times for a total of 15 glide drills per training session.

4. *Cool Down:* At the end of each walk/glide session, fitness walk for at least five minutes to cool down.

(Box 15-1 cont.)

Group1: Self-Paced Plan

- Begin at the appropriate level of sets *(Self-Assessment 3E* in the Workbook).
- Progress as your symptoms allow. Symptoms should never go higher than Stage 2 on the Injury Stage Scale.
- If you are starting at Level 1, do ten sets in the 1-4 pattern (alternating one minute of gliding with 4 minutes of fitness walking) for a total 50 minutes.
- When you can complete 50 minutes in the 1-4 pattern without increasing pain or breaking form, progress to Level 2 (2-minute glide, 3-minute walk).
- When you can complete 50 minutes of glides in the 2-3 pattern without increasing pain or breaking form, progress to Level 3. Do the same for Level 4.
- When you can complete 50 minutes of glides in the 4-1 pattern without increasing pain or breaking form, progress to Level 5 (10-minute walk and 50-minute glides).

Group 2: Two-Week-Interval Plan

- Fitness walk your Base Schedule for a *minimum* of two weeks (Log Form S Level 0). You must clear all Basic Closed-Chain Exercises before progressing to walk/glide sets.
- Begin walk/glide sets at Level 1 (1-4 sets) for a total of 10 sets in 50 minutes. Do 1-4 sets for a *minimum* of two weeks, continuing until you can complete the 50 minutes with correct form and no increase in symptoms. Your symptoms should never go above Stage 2 on the Injury Stage Scale.
- When you have cleared the 1-4 sets, you can progress to Level 2 (2-3 sets). Do 2-3 sets for a *minimum* of two weeks, continuing until you can complete 50 minutes with correct form and no increase in symptoms.
- Do the same for Level 3 (3-2 sets) and Level 4 (4-1 sets), for a *minimum* of two weeks each, continuing until you can complete 50 minutes with correct form and no increase in symptoms.
- When you have cleared 4-1 sets with no increase in pain or break in form for two weeks, begin Level 5 (50-minute glides with glide drills).
- Complete at least two weeks at Level 5. Continue until you can complete at least two consecutive workouts with correct form and no increase in pain.

Table 15-4 A

Base Schedule: Level 1

1-4 Sets

- Five 15-second glide drills (2 repetitions each)

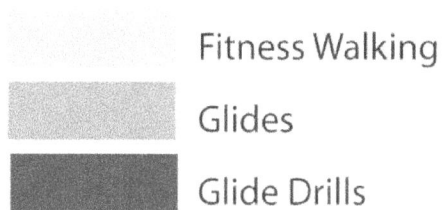

    Fitness Walking

    Glides

    Glide Drills

Minutes & Seconds

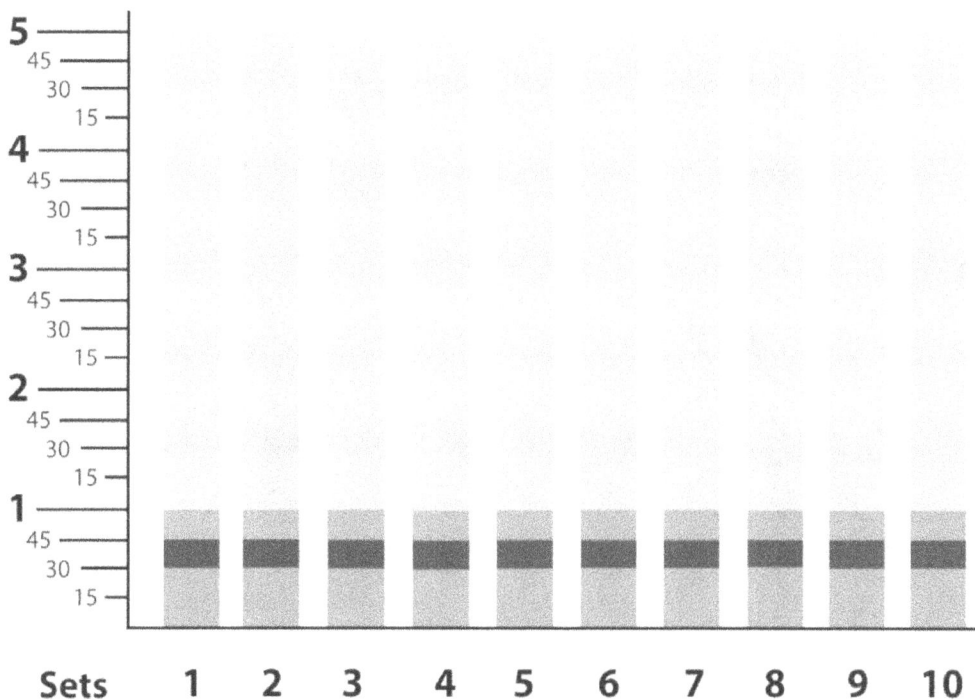

Begin with a 10 minute fitness walk to warm up and finish with a fitness walk to cool down.

Table 15-4 B

Base Schedule: Level 2

2-3 Sets

- Five 15-second glide drills (3 repetitions each)

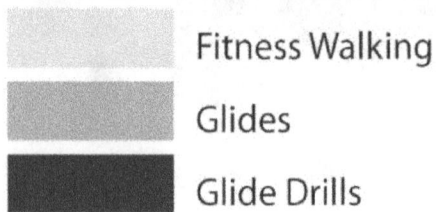

▢	Fitness Walking
▢	Glides
▢	Glide Drills

Minutes & Seconds

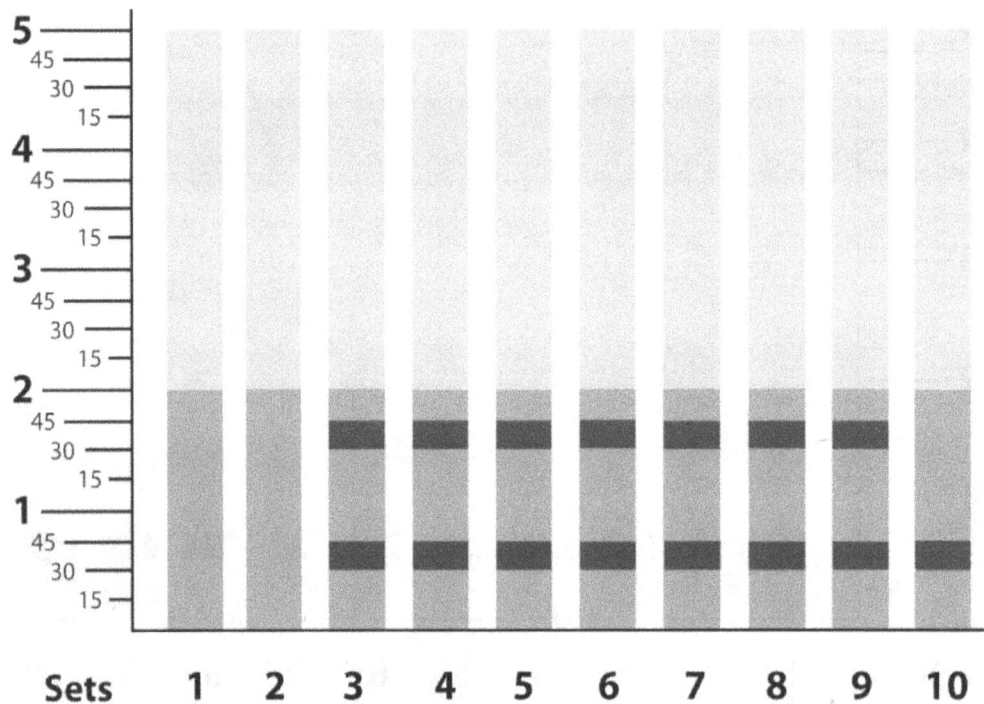

Begin with a 10 minute fitness walk to warm up
and finish with a fitness walk to cool down.

Table 15-4 C

Base Schedule: Level 3

3-2 Sets

- Five 15-second glide drills (3 repetitions each)

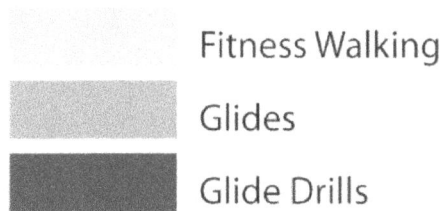

Fitness Walking

Glides

Glide Drills

Minutes & Seconds

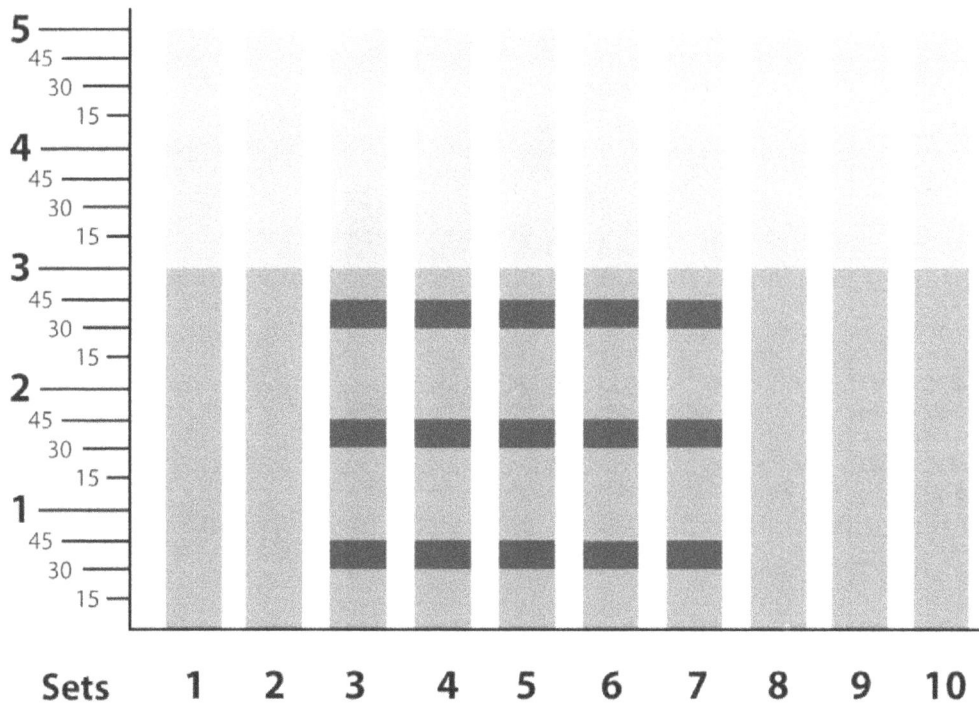

Sets 1 2 3 4 5 6 7 8 9 10

Begin with a 10 minute fitness walk to warm up
and finish with a fitness walk to cool down.

Table 15-4 D

Base Schedule: Level 4

4-1 Sets

- Five 15-second glide drills (3 repetitions each)

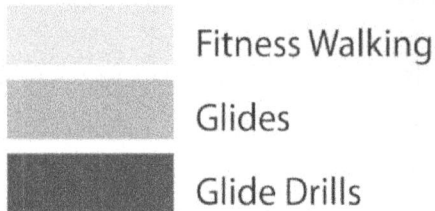

  - Fitness Walking
  - Glides
  - Glide Drills

Minutes & Seconds

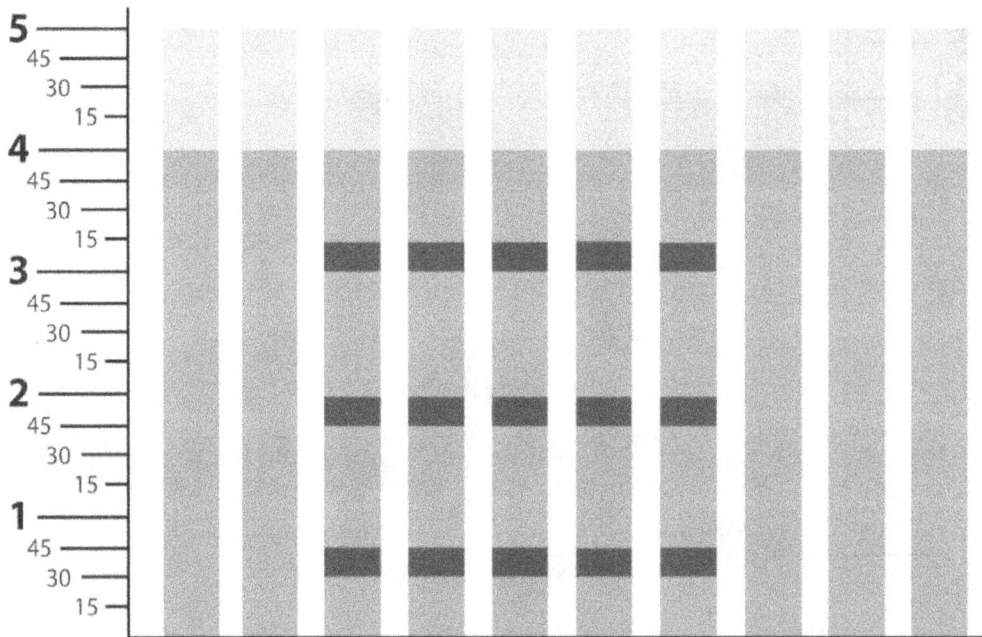

Begin with a 10 minute fitness walk to warm up
and finish with a fitness walk to cool down.

Table 15-4 E
Base Schedule: Level 5

50-Minute Glides

- Five 15-seconds glide drills (3 repetitions each)

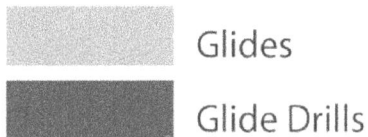

Glides

Glide Drills

Minutes & Seconds

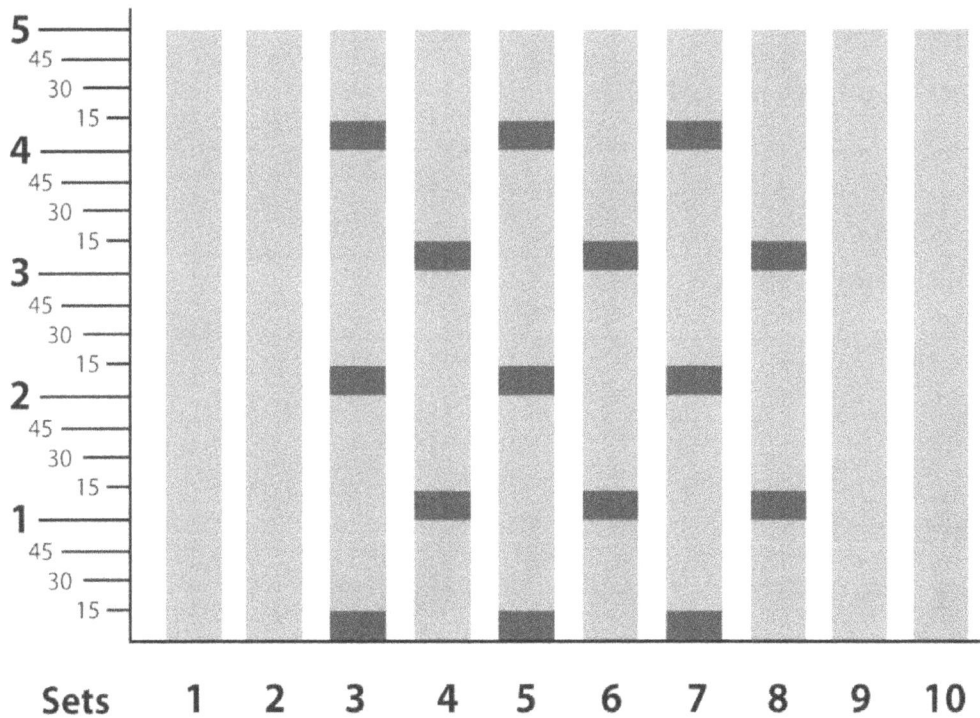

Begin with a 10 minute fitness walk to warm up
and finish with a fitness walk to cool down.

Box 15-2

HOW TO: Fitness Walking

Starting position	1. Stand with "straight" posture. 2. Bend your elbows 90 degrees, keeping your arms close to your body.
Action	1. Walk forward with a **fullfooted stride**, keeping your body balanced and coordinated. 2. Maintain "straight" posture and balance. 3. Coordinate your armswings with your walking motion.
Goal	1. Maintain form, balance, and symmetry. 2. Your effort level should be high enough to raise your heart rate to a moderate exercise level.
Focus Statement	"I will use my arms to balance my body on a straight foot, and push off through my big toe."

Figure 15-1: **Fitness Walking**

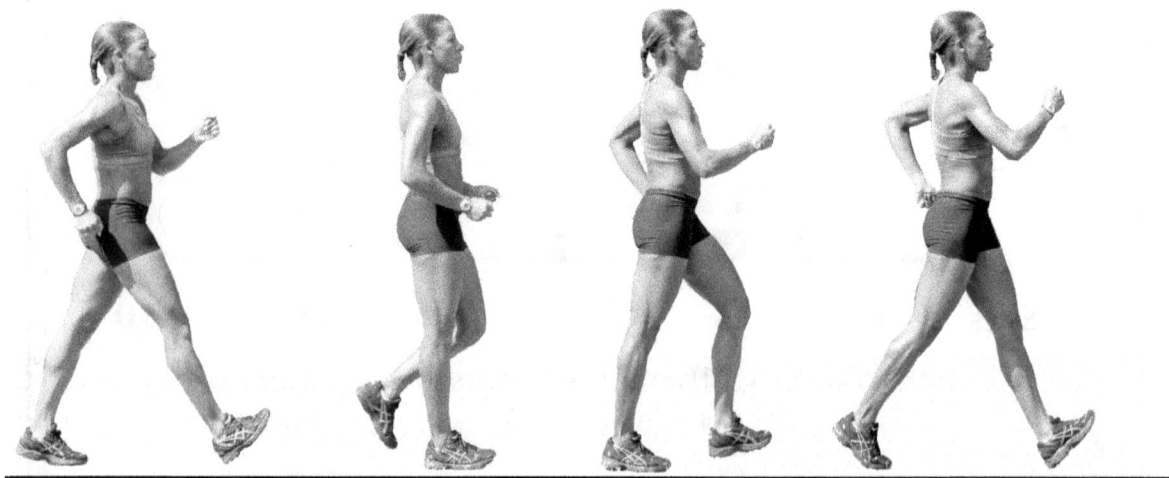

Box 15-3

HOW TO: Glides

Starting position	1. Stand with "straight" posture.
	2. Bend your elbows 90 degrees, keeping your arms close to your body.
Action	1. Using a **flatfooted stride**, run forward slowly and smoothly.
	2. Maintain "straight" posture and balance.
Action (cont.)	3. Keep your kickback straight, in line with your hip.
	4. Coordinate your armswings with your running motion.
Goals	Achieve smooth and efficient forward motion, balance, and symmetry.
Focus Statement	"I will use my arms to balance my body on a straight foot, and push off through my big toe for a straight kickback."

Figure 15-2: Glides

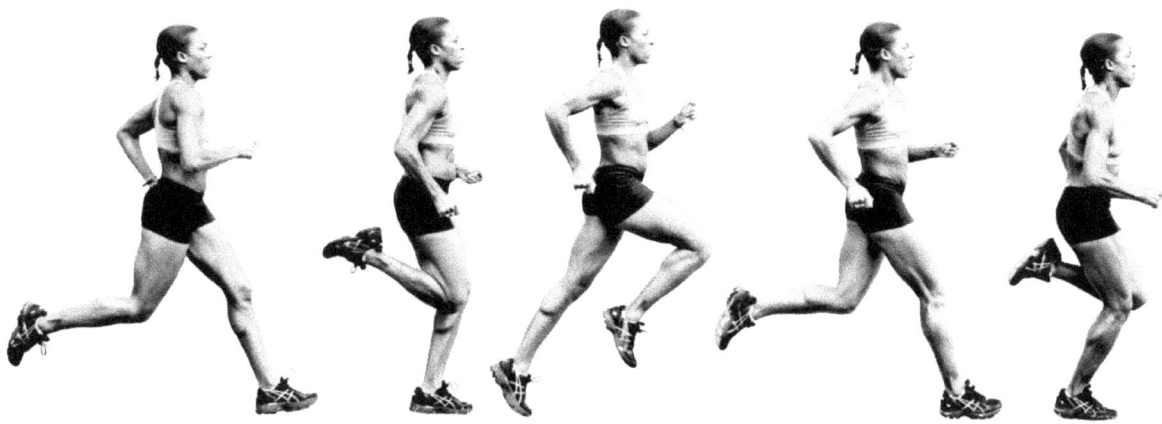

Box 15-4

HOW TO: Glide Drills

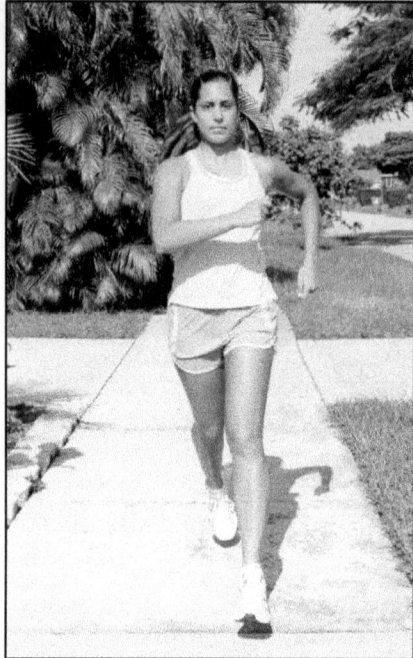

Figure 15-3: Glide Drill #1: Arms In

Action	1. During glides, purposely overswing your arms in front of your body until you begin to feel out of balance.
	2. Bring your arms back into correct armswing position to find your balance.
Goal	Notice how the position and motion of your arms affects your balance.

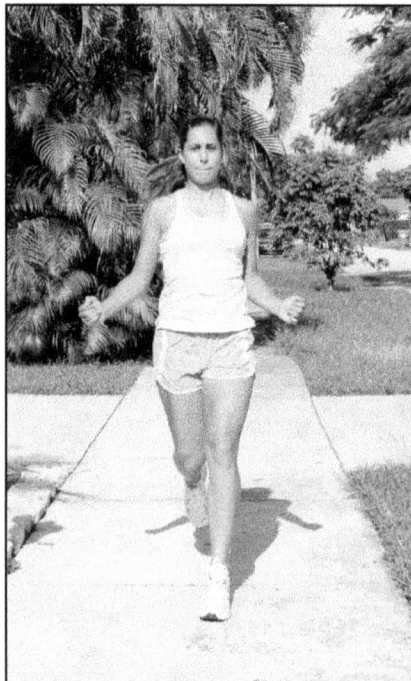

Figure 15-4: Glide Drill #2: Arms Out

Action	1. During glides, purposely rotate your armswings outward, away from your body, until you begin to feel out of balance.
	2. Bring your arms back into correct armswing position to find your balance.
Goal	Notice how the position and motion of your arms affects your balance.

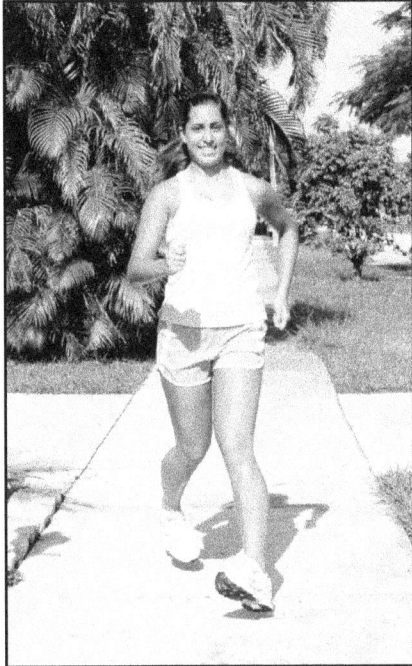

Figure 15-5: Glide Drill #3: Feet In

Action	1. During glides, purposely rotate your leg inwards, toes pointing in, just until you begin to feel out of balance. (Don't rotate so much that it causes you to stumble.) 2. Rotate your legs back into a normal, forward position to find your balance.
Goal	Notice how the alignment of your legs and feet affects your balance.

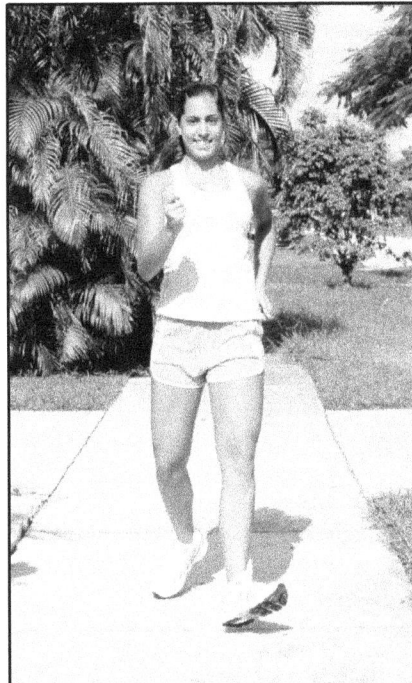

Figure 15-6: Glide Drill #4: Feet Out

Action	1. During glides, purposely rotate your legs outwards, toes pointing out to the sides, just until you begin to feel out of balance. (Don't rotate so much that it causes you to stumble.) 2. Rotate your legs back into a normal, forward position to find your balance.
Goal	Notice how the alignment of your legs and feet affects your balance.

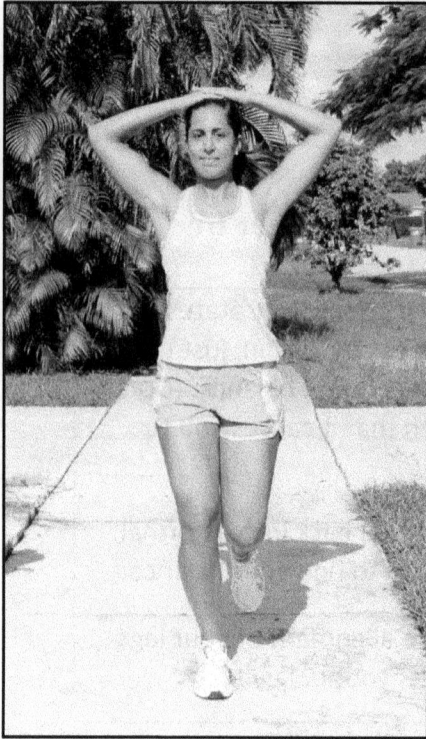

Figure 15-7: Glide Drill #5: Hands on Head

Action	1. During glides, place both hands on top of your head. 2. Keep the elbows pointed straight out to the sides. Do not twist the upper body. 3. Tighten the muscles of the trunk to help control your balance. 4. Run with your body straight, feet straight, and chin tucked. 5. Running motion should be straight forward, not side to side.
Goal	Maintain alignment of the trunk over the pelvis while keeping the arms stationary.

Table 16-2 A (Fitness Runners)
Base Schedule: Level 6, Accelerations

Goals for Fitness Runners

- Three 30-second acceleration drills,
  3 repetitions each (3 minutes in between)

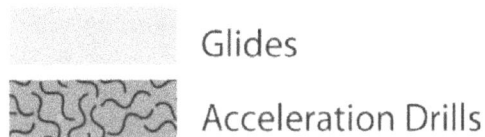

- No glide drills

  Glides

  Acceleration Drills

Minutes & Seconds

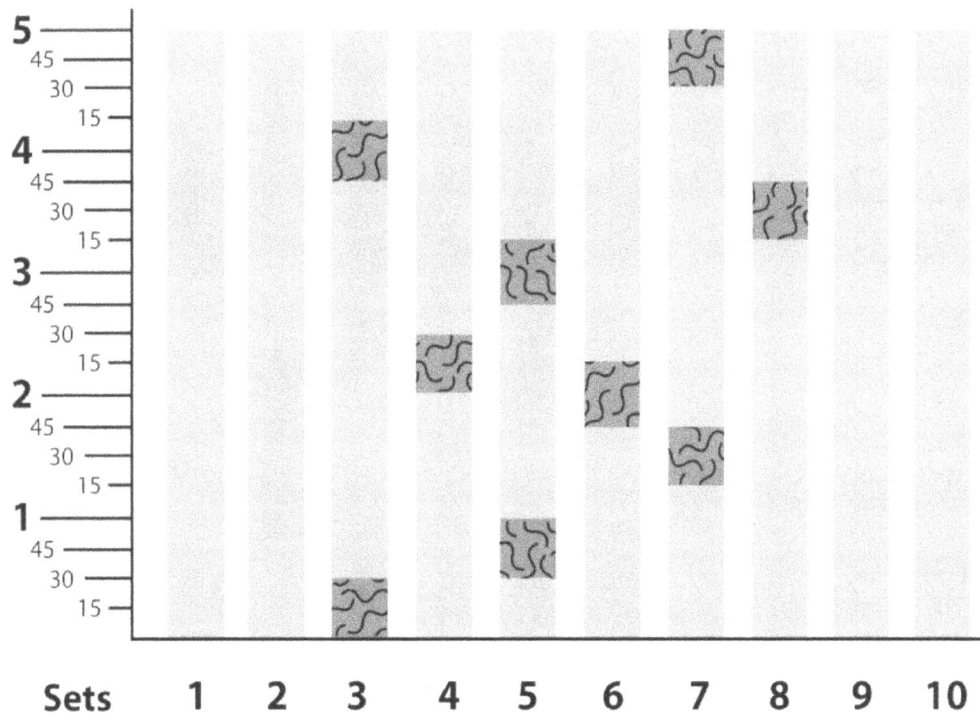

Sets   1   2   3   4   5   6   7   8   9   10

Begin with a 10 minute fitness walk to warm up
and finish with a fitness walk to cool down.

Table 16-2 B (Racers)

Base Schedule: Level 6, Accelerations

Goals for Racers

- Three acceleration drills, 3 repetitions each

- Begin with 30-second accelerations (3 minutes in between)

- Build up to 90-second accelerations (2 minutes in between)

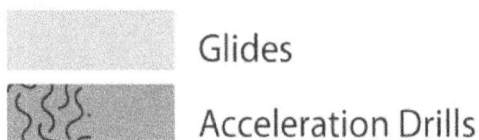

- No glide drills

  Glides

  Acceleration Drills

Minutes & Seconds

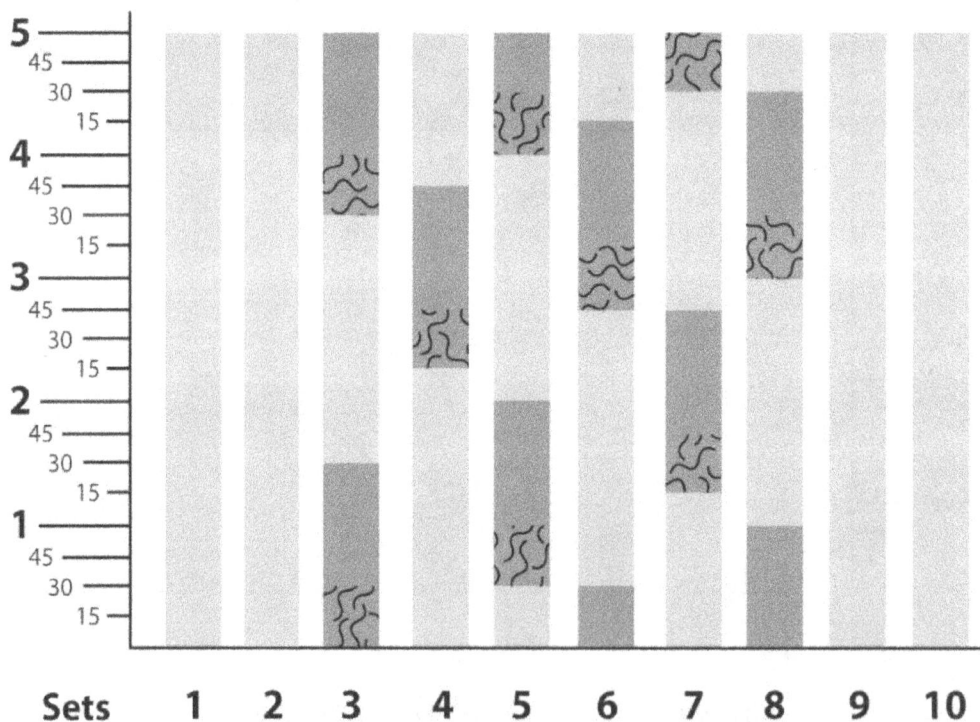

Begin with a 10 minute fitness walk to warm up
and finish with a fitness walk to cool down.

Box 16-1

HOW TO: Acceleratrion Drills

Figure 16-1: Accelerations

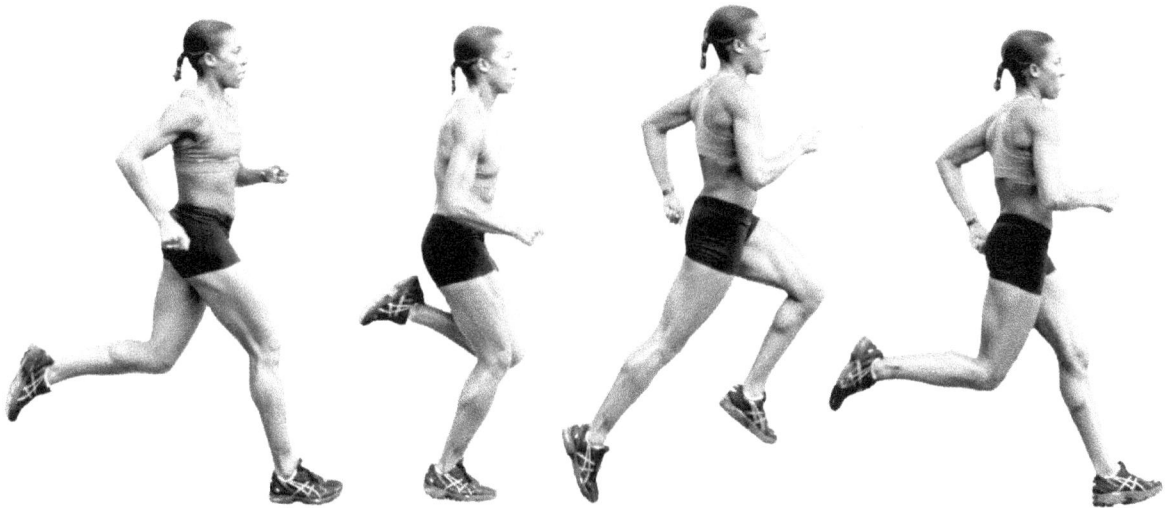

Acceleration Drill #1

Starting position	Gliding with "straight" posture
Action	1. Increase your speed gradually through your Target Time while maintaining glide form and balance. 2. Glide for 2 minutes. 3. Repeat 3 times.
Goal	Try to accelerate without leaning forward.
Focus Statement	Use your specific mental focus statement (*Self-Assessment 3H* in the Workbook)

Acceleration Drill #2

Starting position	Gliding with "straight" posture
Action	1. Accelerate through your Target Time while pumping your arms harder and faster to drive acceleration. 2. Glide for 2 minutes. 3. Repeat 3 times.
Goal	Use your armswings to accelerate and control your balance.
Focus Statement	Use your specific mental focus statement (*Self-Assessment 3H* in the Workbook)

Acceleration Drill #3

Starting position	Gliding with "straight" posture and flatfooted stride
Action	1. Accelerate to a slightly faster **fullfooted stride**, then to a faster **flatfooted stride**, then to an even faster **forefooted stride** [*Table 15-1*]. 2. Glide for 2 minutes. 3. Repeat 3 times.
Goal	Use correct foot position for each of the three strides.
Focus Statement	Use your specific mental focus statement (*Self-Assessment 3H* in the Workbook)

Table 16-3 A (Fitness Runners)
Base Schedule: Level 7, Hills

Goals for Fitness Runners

- 90 seconds uphill and 90 seconds downhill

- 3 repetitions, 7-minute glide in between

- No glide drills

Glides

▲ Uphill Drills

▼ Downhill Drills

Minutes & Seconds

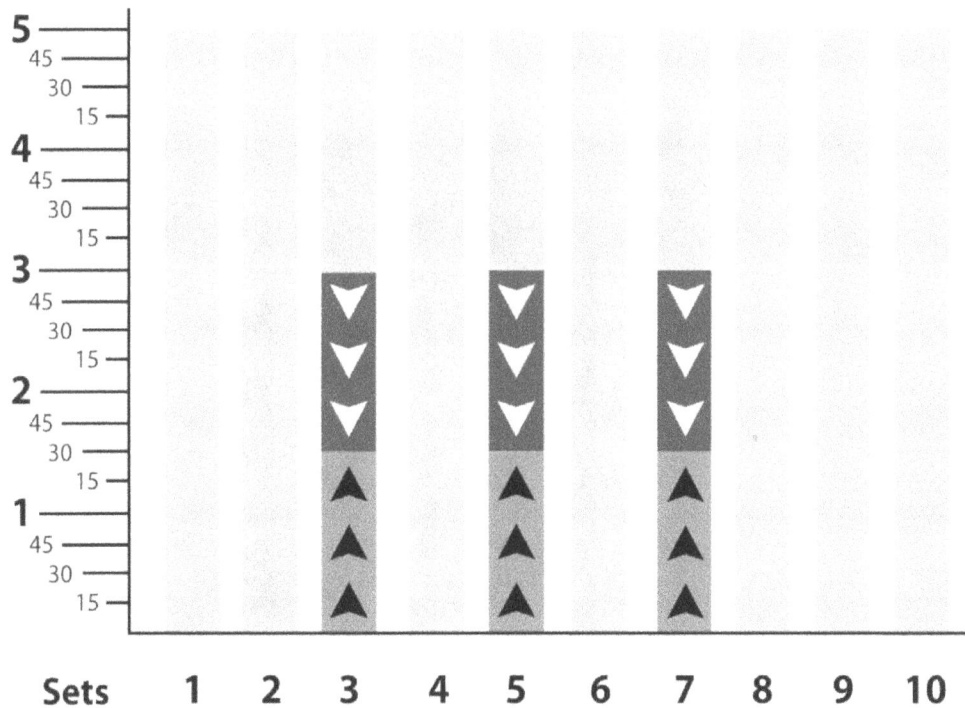

Sets 1 2 3 4 5 6 7 8 9 10

Begin with a 10 minute fitness walk to warm up
and finish with a fitness walk to cool down.

Table 16-3 B (Racers)

Base Schedule: Level 7, Hills

Goals for Racers

- Begin with 90 seconds uphill and 90 seconds downhill

- Build up to 4.5 minutes uphill and 4.5 minutes downhill

- 3 repetitions, 1-minute glide in between

- No glide drills

	Glides
▲	Uphill Drills
▼	Downhill Drills

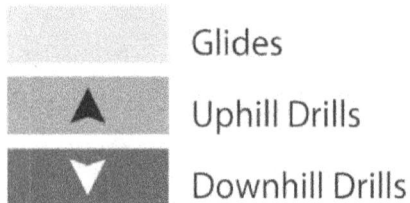

Minutes & Seconds

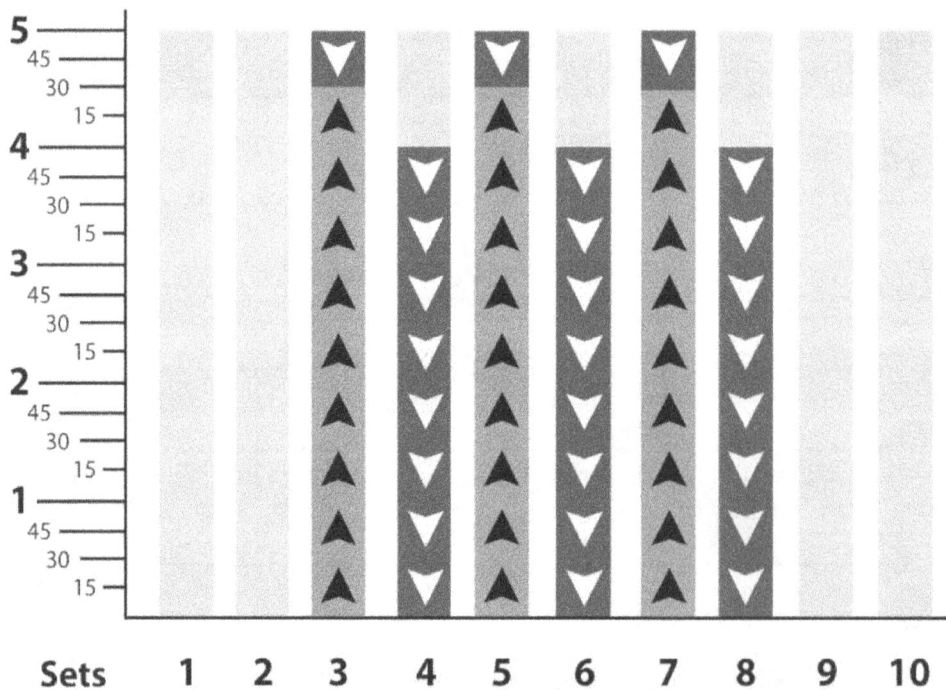

Begin with a 10 minute fitness walk to warm up
and finish with a fitness walk to cool down.

Guidelines for Hill Drills

You may do *Hill Drills* on an adjustable treadmill or street grade with a little more incline than whatever you are normally accustomed to. It should be just a little challenging to work on your balance. Your warmup, glides, and cooldown should always be done on a level surface.

A. Hill Training on the Street

If you are running on the street, you can fit Hill Drills into your 50-minute glides by running uphill, then turning around and running back downhill (or vice versa), with no break in between; then do a short glide interval on a level surface to recover before repeating. Try to avoid *atypical* hills (hills that are different from what you are used to) until you have completed post-injury training.

B. Hill Training on a Treadmill

You can use an adjustable treadmill to simulate running uphill and downhill. When running uphill, increase your incline gradually to maintain upright posture. The treadmill should be at grade 3 to 8, depending upon your ability and what you're accustomed to.

Most treadmills cannot incline downhill. To simulate downhill running on a treadmill that does not decline, keep the treadmill flat, start running at your gliding speed, then add speed to accelerate. While accelerating, practice using your downhill techniques to adjust your balance point.

Uphill Drill

Starting position	Glide with "straight" posture and flatfooted stride on a level surface
Action	1. Run uphill for the specified amount of time. (*See Table 16-3*) 2. Control your balance point by keeping your elbows in, and swinging your arms more to the front than to the back.
Goal	1. Feel how running uphill moves your balance point forward and slows you down. Find your body's specific balance point. 2. Focus on body symmetry and upright posture. Try to avoid moving forward and backward. 3. Build up your speed slowly until you can do hill training at your glide rhythm, without breaking form.
Focus Statement	Use your specific mental focus statement (*Self-Assessment 3H*)

Downhill Drill

Starting position	Glide with "straight" posture and flatfooted stride on a level surface
Action	1. Run downhill for the specified amount of time. (*See Table 16-3*) 2. Lower your center of gravity by bending your knees. Shorten your stride, and increase your step rate. 3. Keep your elbows out, shorten your armswing, and increase your rhythm.
Goal	1. Feel how running downhill moves your balance point back and makes you accelerate faster. Find your body's specific balance point. 2. Focus on body symmetry and upright posture. Try to avoid rocking from side to side as the downhill momentum accelerates you. 3. Build up your speed slowly until you can do hill training at your glide rhythm, without breaking form.
Focus Statement	Use your specific mental focus statement (*Self-Assessment 3H*)

Table 17-1 A (Fitness Runners)
Base Schedule: Level 8, Plyometrics

Goal for Fitness Runners

- Begin with four 15-second plyometric drills (3 reps each)
- Add five 15-second glide drills after plyometrics (2 reps each)

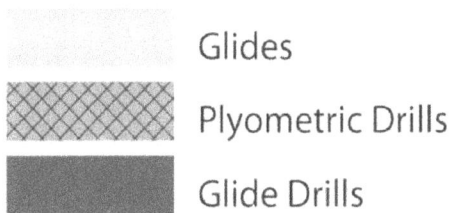

Glides

Plyometric Drills

Glide Drills

Minutes & Seconds

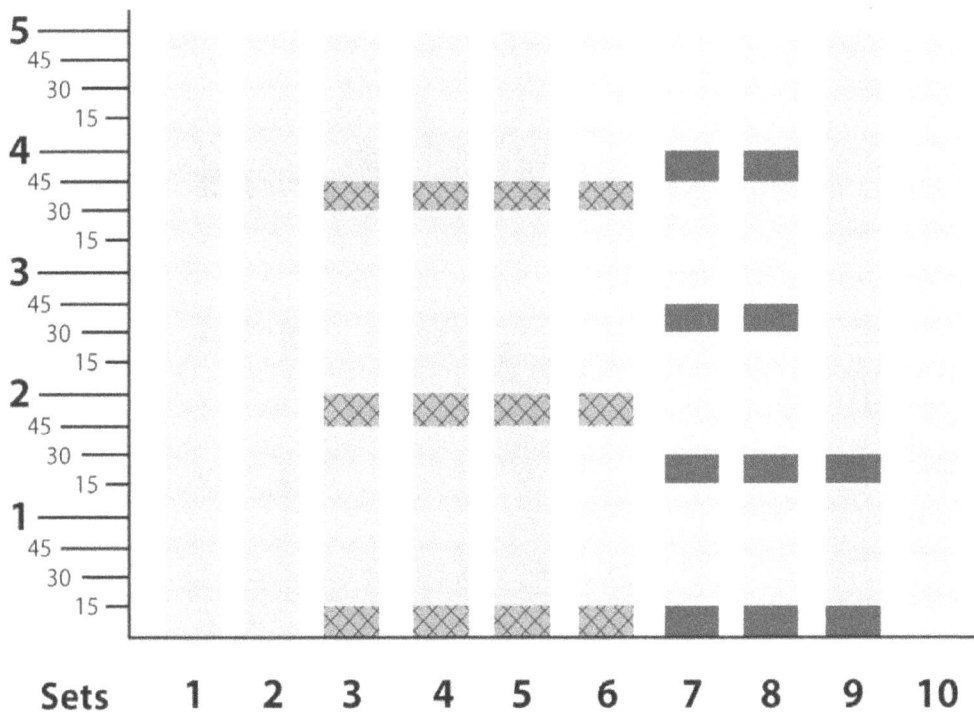

Begin with a 10 minute fitness walk to warm up
and finish with a fitness walk to cool down.

Table 17-1 B (Racers)

Base Schedule: Level 8, Plyometrics

Goal for Racers

- Begin with four 15-second plyometric drills (3 reps each)

- Build up to 45 seconds per exercise (3 reps each)

- Add five 15-second glide drills after plyometrics (2 reps each)

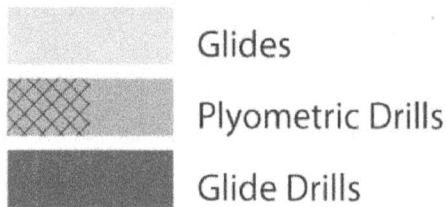

Glides

Plyometric Drills

Glide Drills

Minutes & Seconds

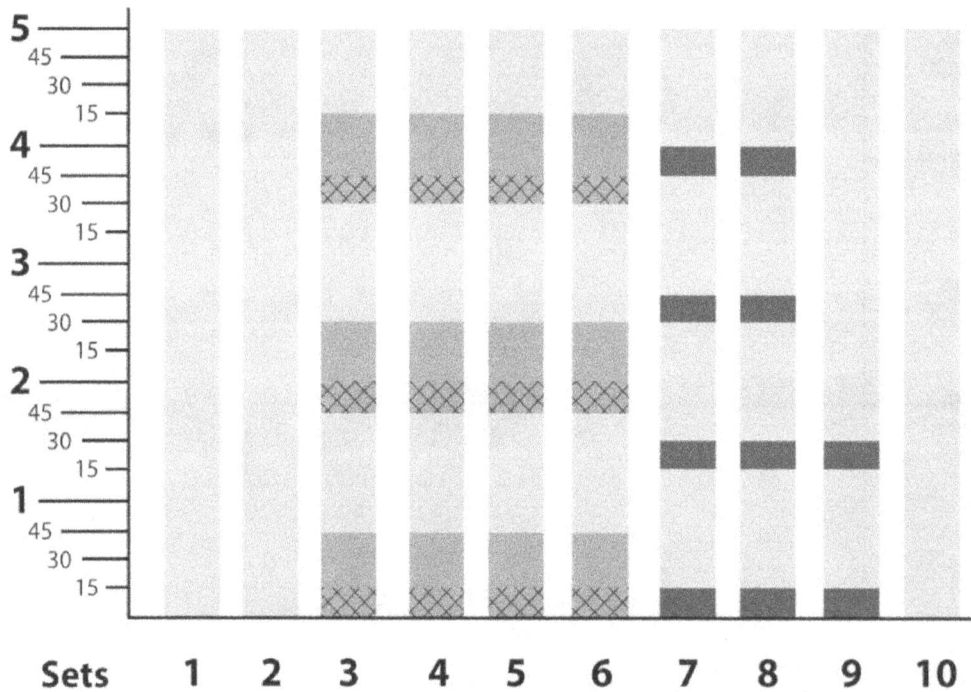

Sets   1   2   3   4   5   6   7   8   9   10

Begin with a 10 minute fitness walk to warm up
and finish with a fitness walk to cool down.

Box 17-1

HOW TO: Plyometric Drills

Plyometric Drill #1: Plyometric High Kickbacks

Starting position	Gliding with "straight" posture and flatfooted stride on a level surface (not a treadmill).
Action	1. Keep your weight on your forefeet throughout the exercise. The balance point is farther back than in *high knees*. 2. Using a fast gliding motion, kick your rear foot up as far as you can toward your butt as you run, keeping the knee pointed down and the foot in straight alignment. 3. When kicking back, coordinate your armswings by snapping the opposite arm back. 4. Flex the weight-bearing foot and ankle downward (plantar flexed) and push up through big toe, keeping your body balanced. 5. When you land, bring the front leg down straight over your foot (forefooted), keeping your weight centered.
Goals	1. Focus on balance, maintaining a straight posture, and having your foot positioned under your knee. 2. Focus on pushing your weight equally through the toes of both feet, and the alignment of the landing. 3. Focus on performing equal kickbacks through both legs.

Figure 17-1: High Kickbacks

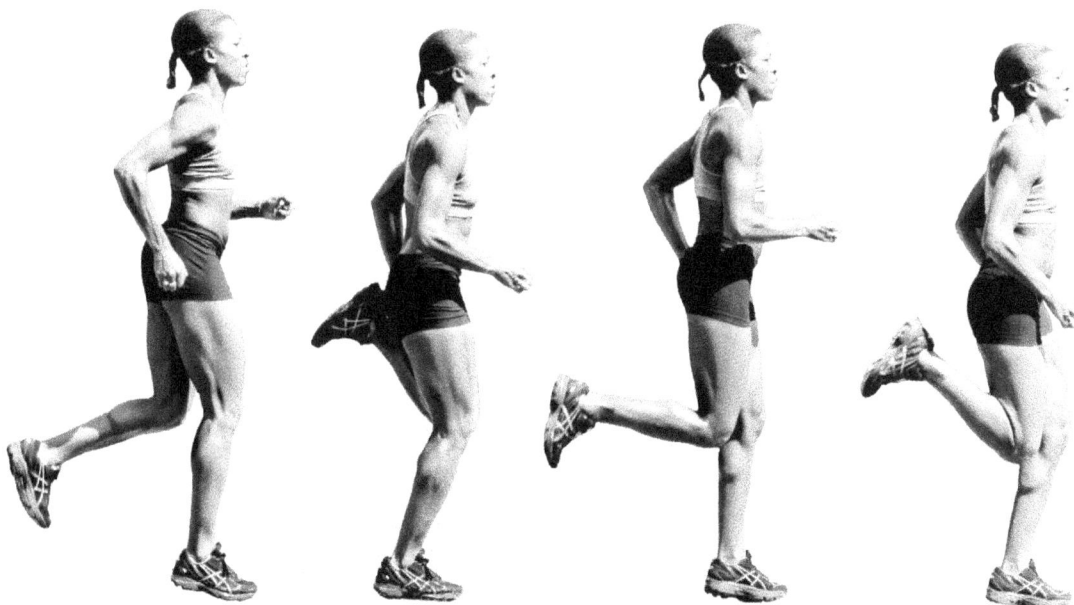

Plyometric Drill #2: Plyometric High Knees

Starting position	Gliding with "straight" posture and flatfooted stride on a level surface (not a treadmill).
Action	1. Keep your weight on your forefeet throughout the exercise. The balance point is farther forward than in *high kickbacks*. 2. Using a fast gliding motion, tighten your trunk muscles and drive each knee upward toward your chest as you run, keeping the foot aligned under the raised knee ("high knees" position). 3. Coordinate your armswings with your leg motion. 4. Flex the weightbearing foot and ankle downward (plantar-flexed) and push up through the big toe. 5. When you land, bring the front leg down straight over your foot (forefooted), keeping your weight centered.
Goals	1. Focus on balance, maintaining a straight posture, and keeping your foot positioned under your knee. 2. Focus on pushing your weight equally through the toes of both feet. 3. Focus on straight alignment of the landing.

Figure 17-2: **High Knees**

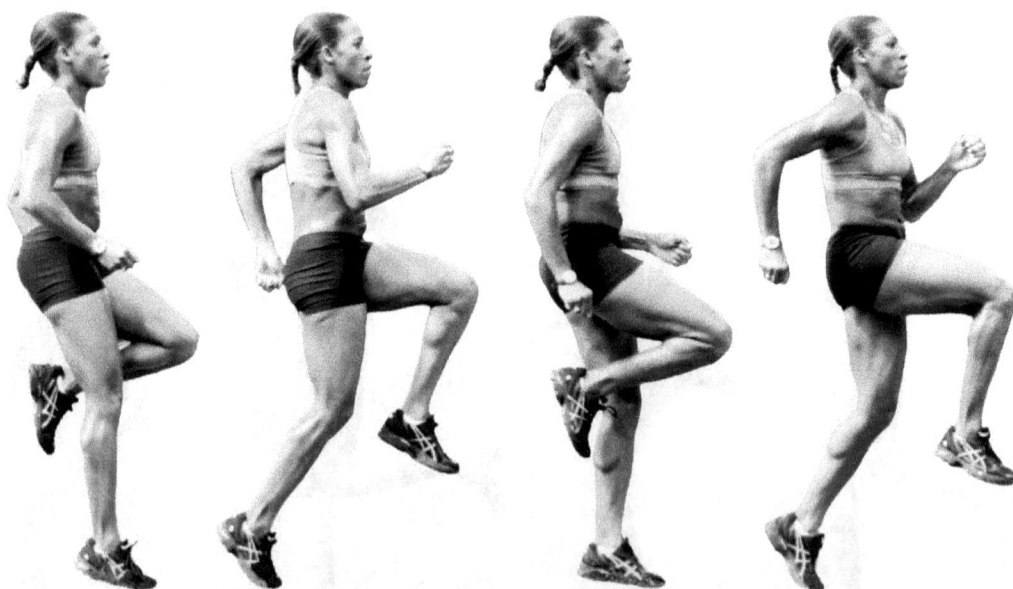

Starting position	Gliding with "straight" posture and flatfooted stride on a level surface (not a treadmill)
Action	1. Keep your weight on your forefeet throughout the exercise. The balance point is farther forward than in *high knees*. 2. Using a fast gliding motion, push off strongly through the big toe and leap forward, leading with the front knee. 3. Extend the leading leg and land on the forefoot with your weight centered, keeping your foot straight and balanced. 4. Coordinate your armswings with your leg motion.
Goals	1. Focus on balance, maintaining a straight posture, and the alignment of the landing. 2. Focus on pushing your weight equally through the toes of both feet. 3. Focus on performing bounds equally through both legs.

Figure 17-3: Bounding

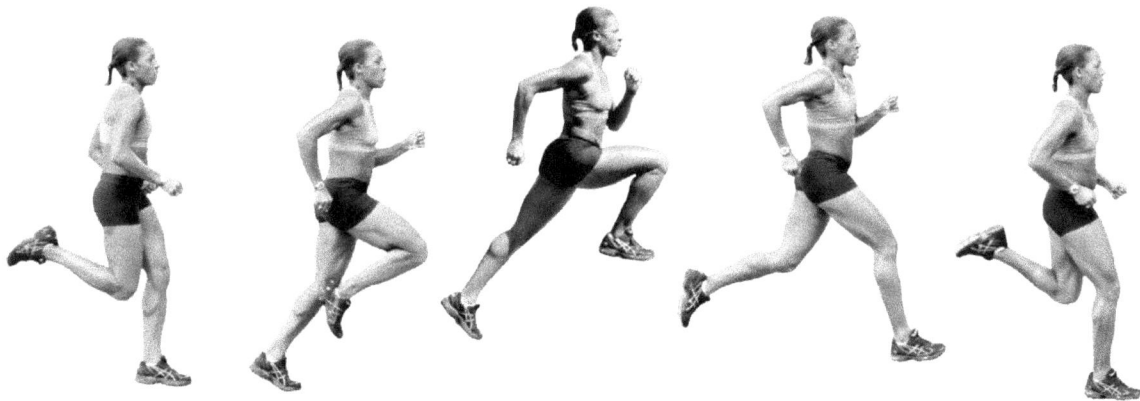

Plyometric Drill #4: Plyometric Skips

Starting position	Gliding with "straight" posture and flatfooted stride on a level surface (not a treadmill).
Action	1. Keep your weight on your forefeet throughout the exercise. The balance point is centered over your pelvis. 2. Using a fast gliding motion, flex the weight-bearing foot and ankle downward (plantar flexed), push off strongly through the big toe, and skip forward, keeping your body upright and balanced. 3. When skipping, coordinate your armswings by snapping the opposite arm back. 4. Land on the same foot, keeping your foot straight and your weight centered. 5. Continue your forward motion onto the opposite foot, and repeat.
Goals	1. Focus on balance, maintaining a straight posture, and the alignment of the landing. 2. Focus on pushing your weight equally through the toes of both feet. 3. Focus on performing skips with equal force through both legs.

Figure 17-4: **Skips**

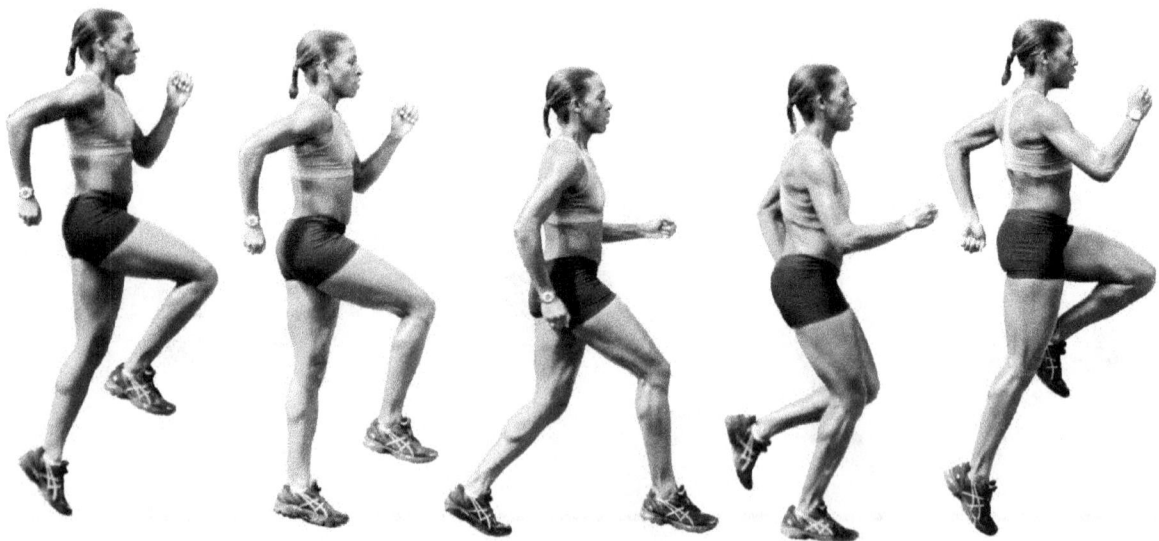

Section 5: References

Appendix A: Index of Affected Regions

Appendix R: Regional Plans

Appendix Z: Regional Closed Chain Tables for Fitness Runners and Racers

This section contains three Appendices that you will use to create your individualized program of Regional Closed-Chain Exercises for P.T. Time.

Appendix A: Index of Affected Regions is used to document the pain pattern and swelling associated with your injury, which will help determine your injury regions and the complexity of your injury.

Appendix R: Regional Plans summarizes the symptoms, treatment program, and goals for each injury region.

Appendix Z: Regional Closed-Chain Tables for Fitness Runners and Racers contains information about specific Regional Closed-Chain Exercises that you will copy to your individualized Log Form R. If you are a Fitness Runner, you will copy the Target Times marked "F" for fitness runners; and if you are a Racer you will copy the Target Times marked "R" for Racers.

Appendix A: Index of Affected Regions

Region 1: Toe (1st Ray)   Secondary Region 1: Outer Toes

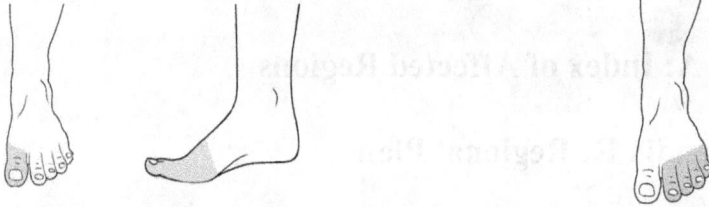

Region 2: Arch

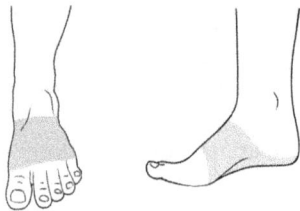

Region 3: Heel

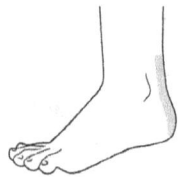

Region 4: Shin   Secondary Region 4: Ankle

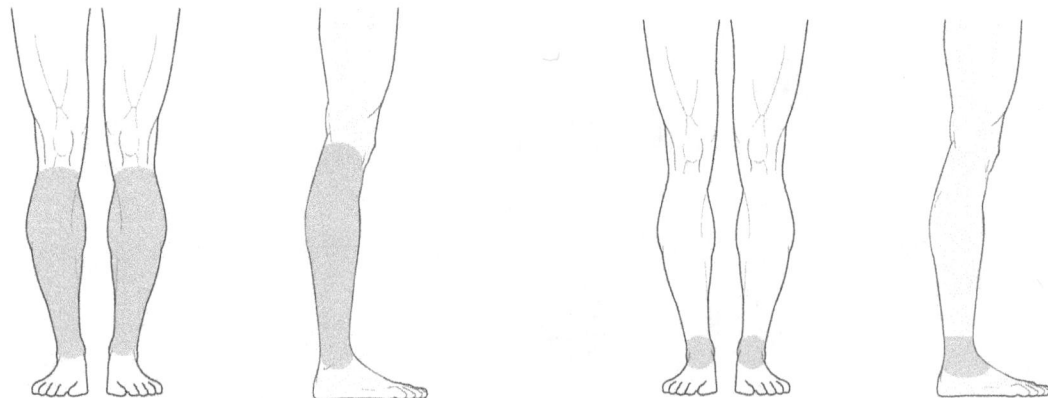

Region 5: Calf

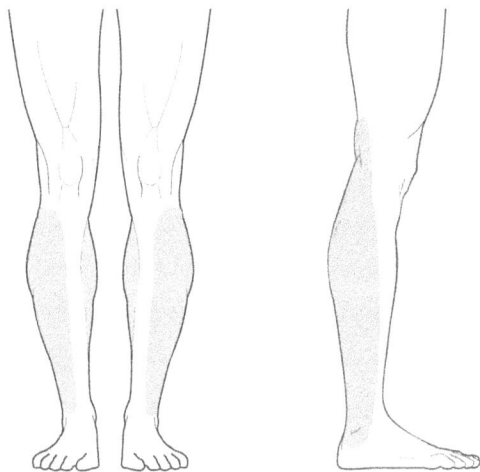

Region 6: Knee

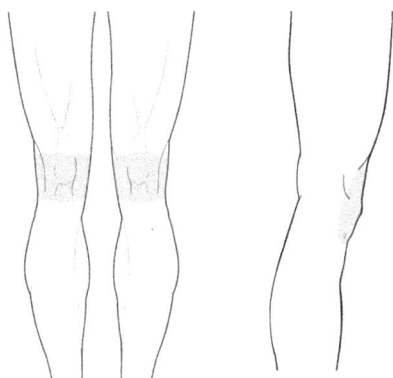

Secondary Region 6: Thigh

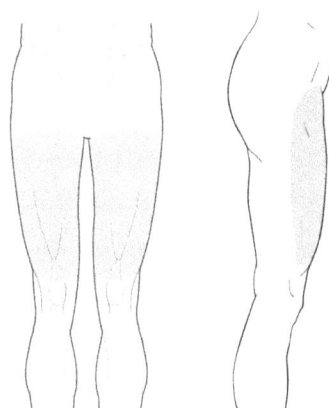

Region 7: Band

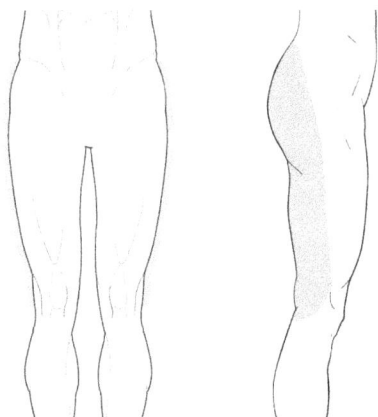

Region 8: Hamstring

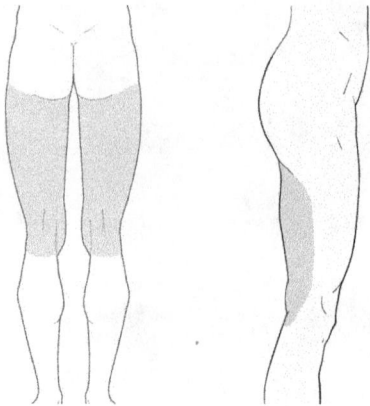

Region 9: Hip

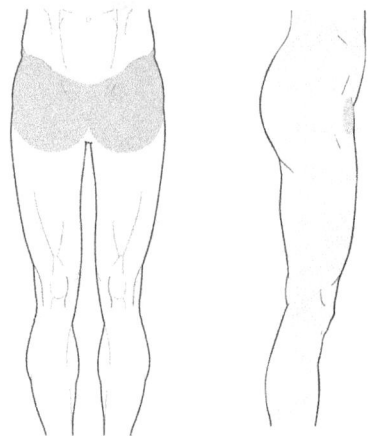

Secondary Region 9: Groin or Inner Thigh

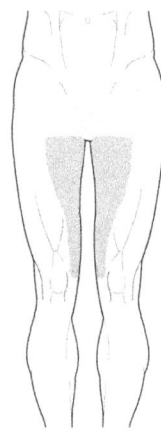

Region 10: Buttocks

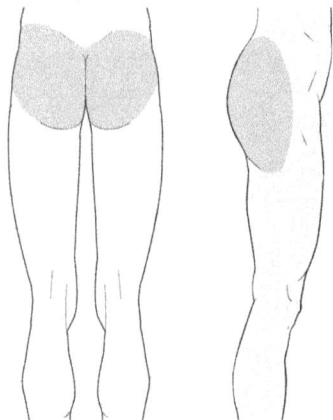

Secondary Region 10: Lateral Hip

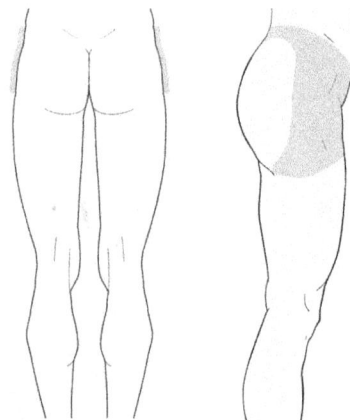

APPENDIX R: REGIONAL PLANS

Recovery Plan, Region 1: Big Toe (1st Ray)
(Secondary Region: Outer Toes)

Region 1: Self-Assessment

Activity	Self-Assessment	
Self-mobilization	I have **tenderness** and/or bruising on the ball of the foot.	
Stretches	I have reduced range of motion **(stiffness)** in the toe region, *resulting in* difficulty flexing the toes up or down.	
Closed-Chain Exercises	I have **weakness** in the toe region, *resulting in*:	A. Difficulty flexing the toes during push off.
		B. Difficulty flexing the toes during step-up.
Pre-Injury Stride Tendency	While running, I have a tendency to:	A. Rotate the leg outward.
		B. Push off from the inner or outer side of the big toe.

Region 1: PT Time

Start Time	Activity	Exercise/Figure Number							
Phase One	ICE position	*5-1*							
Phase Two	Self-Mobs	*10-1*	*10-2*						
	Stretches for Affected Region	*11- 1*	*11-5*						
	Stretches for Unaffected Regions *	*11-2* *11-3*	*11-4* *11-6*	*11-7* *11-8*	*11-9* *11-10*	*11-11* *11-12*	*11-13*		
Phase Three, Part 1	Basic Closed-Chain**	*14-1*	*14-2*	*14-3*	*14-4*	*14-5*	*14-6*	*14-7*	*14-8*
Phase Three, Part 2	Regional Closed-Chain	*14-3*	*14-5*	*14-11*	*14-16*	*14-18*	*14-19*		
Phase Four	Hill Closed-Chain**	*16-2*	*16-3*						

*With self-mobilizations as needed

** Same for all regions

Region 1: Goals

	Regional Focus
Phase Three and Four Stride Changes	1. Smooth, efficient running, keeping the motion straight and centered.
	2. Straight push off and follow-through through the big toe.
Specific Mental Focus Statement	"I will control my body so I can push off through the big toe."

Recovery Plan, Region 2: Arch

Region 2: Self-Assessment

Activity	Self-Assessment	
Self - mobilization	I have **tenderness** in or around the bottom of my foot; or under and/or to the outside of the heel and arch.	
Stretches	I have reduced range of motion **(stiffness)** in the ankle region, *resulting in* difficulty flexing the foot upward.	
Closed-Chain Exercises	I have **weakness** in the toe-flexing muscles, *resulting in* rolling the foot to the inside or outside when standing on one leg.	
Pre-Injury Stride Tendency	While running, I have a tendency to:	A. Turn the leg excessively out or in.
		B. Overstrike and foot-slap into an overpronated foot.

Region 2: PT Time

Start Time	Activity	Exercise/Figure Number							
Phase One	ICE position	*5-1*							
Phase Two	Self-Mobs	*10-3*	*10-4*						
	Stretches for Affected Region	*11-5*	*11-13*						
	Stretches for Unaffected Regions *	*11-1* *11-2*	*11-3* *11-4*	*11-6* *11-7*	*11-8* *11-9*	*11-10* *11-11*	*11-12*		
Phase Three, Part 1	Basic Closed-Chain**	*14-1*	*14-2*	*14-3*	*14-4*	*14-5*	*14-6*	*14-7*	*14-8*
Phase Three, Part 2	Regional Closed-Chain	*14-2*	*14-3*	*14-8*	*14-11*	*14-12*	*14-16*		
Phase Four	Hill Closed-Chain**	*16-2*	*16-3*						

*With self-mobilizations as needed

** Same for all regions

Region 2: Goals

	Regional Focus
Phase Three and Four Stride Changes	1. Initial contact under your center of weight, with your ankle in a neutral position.
	2. Smooth progression into controlled pronation and pushoff through the big toe.
Specific Mental Focus Statement	"I will control my body to land lightly and push off straight through my big toe."

Recovery Plan, Region 3: Heel

Region 3: Self-Assessment

Activity	Self-Assessment	
Self - mobilization	I have **tenderness** at the Achilles tendon, and/or the outer side of the Achilles tendon.	
Stretches	I have reduced range of motion **(stiffness)** in the heel region, *resulting in* tightness in the heel area when standing on an uphill incline.	
Closed-Chain Exercises	I have **weakness** in the heel region, *resulting in*:	A. Difficulty keeping the foot flexed and straight.
		B. Difficulty pushing off.
Pre-Injury Stride Tendency	While running, I have a tendency to:	A. Overstrike, with the lower leg rotated outward.
		B. Slap the foot, with the foot sticking out.
		C. Overstrike on the outer edge of the heel and slap the foot.
		D. Land too hard on the heel.
		E. Overpronate and push off from the inner side of the big toe.
		F. Roll the foot excessively inward.

Region 3: PT Time

Start Time	Activity	Exercise/Figure Number							
Phase One	ICE position	*5-1*							
Phase Two	Self-Mobs	*10-5*	*10-6*						
	Stretches for Affected Region	*11-2*	*11-5*	*11-6*	*11-7*	*11-13*			
	Stretches for Unaffected Regions *	*11-1*	*11-3*	*11-4*	*11-8*	*11-9*	*11-10*	*11-11*	*11-12*
Phase Three, Part 1	Basic Closed-Chain**	*14-1*	*14-2*	*14-3*	*14-4*	*14-5*	*14-6*	*14-7*	*14-8*
Phase Three, Part 2	Regional Closed-Chain	*14-5*	*14-6*	*14-8*	*14-11*	*14-12*	*14-18*		
Phase Four	Hill Closed-Chain**	*16-2*	*16-3*						

*With self-mobilizations as needed
** Same for all regions

Region 3: Goals

	Regional Focus
Phase Three and Four Stride Changes	1. Initial contact under your center of weight with your ankle in a neutral position.
	2. Run balanced with your foot straight.
	3. Smooth progression into controlled transition and pushoff through the big toe.
	4. Control your balance from foot strike through push off.
Specific Mental Focus Statement	"I will control my body to land lightly and push off through my big toe."

Recovery Plan, Region 4: Shin
(Secondary Region: Ankle)

Region 4: Self-Assessment

Activity	Self-Assessment	
Self-mobilization	I have **tenderness** on either side of the shin, extending down to the tendons near the foot.	
Stretches	I have reduced range of motion **(stiffness)** in the leg, *resulting in* reduced range of motion in the ankle.	
Closed-Chain Exercises	I have **weakness** in the shin region, *resulting in* twisting and leaning that causes excessive exertion in my shin.	
Pre-Injury Stride Tendency	While running, I have a tendency to:	A. A running stride that puts excessive stress on the shin.
		B. Over-lean in any plane.
		C. Overstrike on the heel.
		D. Twist the knee and turn the foot outward.
		E. Wobble at the hip.

Region 4: PT Time

Start Time	Activity	Exercise/Figure Number							
Phase One	ICE position	5-1							
Phase Two	Self-Mobs	10-7	10-8						
	Stretches for Affected Region	11-2	11-5	11-6	11-7	11-13			
	Stretches for Unaffected Regions *	11-1 11-3	11-4 11-8	11-9 11-10	11-11 11-12				
Phase Three, Part 1	Basic Closed-Chain**	14-1	14-2	14-3	14-4	14-5	14-6	14-7	14-8
Phase Three, Part 2	Regional Closed-Chain	14-1	14-2	14-11	14-12	14-13	14-17		
Phase Four	Hill Closed-Chain**	16-2	16-3						

*With self-mobilizations as needed

** Same for all regions

Region 4: Goals

	Regional Focus
Phase Three and Four Stride Changes	1. Maintain correct posture and balance while placing my weight through the shin.
	2. Progressively increase the weight load on the shin, increasing the frequency, speed, and duration of training.
Specific Mental Focus Statement	"I will control my body while running to maintain a balanced force on my shin."

Recovery Plan, Region 5: Calf

Region 5: Self-Assessment

Activity	Self-Assessment	
Self - mobilization	I have **tenderness** in the thick part of the calf muscle.	
Stretches	I have reduced range of motion **(stiffness)** in the calf region, *resulting in* difficulty flexing the foot upward.	
Closed-Chain Exercises	I have **weakness** in the calf region, *resulting in* difficulty flexing the foot downward.	
Pre-Injury Stride Tendency	While running, I have a tendency to:	A. Not be able to kick back straight and/or fully after pushoff.
		B. Rotate the leg outward.
		C. Have a circular movement of the lower leg.
		D. Push off from the inner side of the big toe.

Region 5: PT Time

Start Time	Activity	Exercise/Figure Number							
Phase One	ICE position	*5-1*							
Phase Two	Self-Mobs	*10-9*	*10-10*						
	Stretches for Affected Region	*11-2*	*11-5*	*11-6*	*11-7*	*11-13*			
	Stretches for Unaffected Regions	*11-1* *11-3*	*11-4* *11-8*	*11-9* *11-10*	*11-11* *11-12*				
Phase Three, Part 1	Basic Closed-Chain**	*14-1*	*14-2*	*14-3*	*14-4*	*14-5*	*14-6*	*14-7*	*14-8*
Phase Three, Part 2	Regional Closed-Chain	***14-2***	***14-6***	***14-12***	***14-17***	***14-18***	***14-19***		
Phase Four	Hill Closed-Chain**	*16-2*	*16-3*						

*With self-mobilizations as needed
** Same for all regions

Region 5: Goals

	Regional Focus
Phase Three and Four Stride Changes	1. Initial contact under my center of mass.
	2. Smooth pushoff through the big toe.
	3. Straight kickback.
Specific Mental Focus Statement	"I will control my body to land lightly and push off through my big toe."

Recovery Plan, Region 6: Knee
(Secondary Region: Thigh)

Region 6: Self-Assessment

Activity	Self-Assessment	
Self-mobilization	I have **tenderness** anywhere around the whole knee cap (usually to the outside of the knee cap), with or without generalized knee swelling.	
Stretches	I have reduced range of motion **(stiffness)** in the knee region, *resulting in* tightness and inability to bend the knee, and generalized stiffness.	
Closed-Chain Exercises	I have **weakness** in the knee region, *resulting in*:	A. Leg twisting inward during exercise.
		B. Difficulty bearing weight while stepping down.
		C. Difficulty kicking back straight.
		D. Difficulty balancing on one leg.
		E. Inability to maintain knee control when stepping down (descending stairs).
Pre-Injury Stride Tendency	While running, I have a tendency to:	A. Twist at the knee.
		B. Run with the foot pointed outward.

Region 6: PT Time

Start Time	Activity	Exercise/Figure Number							
Phase One	ICE position	*5-1*							
Phase Two	Self-Mobs	*10-11*							
	Stretches for Affected Region	*11-5*	*11-10*						
	Stretches for Unaffected Regions *	*11-1* *11-2*	*11-3* *11-4*	*11-6* *11-7*	*11-8* *11-9*	*11-11* *11-12*	*11-13* *11-14*		
Phase Three, Part 1	Basic Closed-Chain**	*14-1*	*14-2*	*14-3*	*14-4*	*14-5*	*14-6*	*14-7*	*14-8*
Phase Three, Part 2	Regional Closed-Chain	*14-2*	*14-7*	*14-8*	*14-11*	*14-12*	*4-18*		
Phase Four	Hill Closed-Chain**	*16-2*	*16-3*						

*with self-mobilizations as needed

** same for all regions

Region 6: Goals

	Regional Focus
Phase Three and Four Stride Changes	1. Maintain hip, knee, and ankle in neutral alignment.
	2. Avoid twisting the knee.
Specific Mental Focus Statement	"I will control my body to avoid twisting my knee while running."

Recovery Plan, Region 7: Band

Region 7: Self-Assessment

Activity	Self-Assessment	
Self - mobilization	I have **tenderness** on the outside of the knee, with or without visible swelling.	
Stretches	I have reduced range of motion **(stiffness)** from the hip and buttock down to the upper leg.	
Closed-Chain Exercises	I have **weakness** in the band region, *resulting in*:	A. Difficulty staying balanced on one leg.
		B. Difficulty kicking out to the side.
Pre-Injury Stride Tendency	While running, I have a tendency to:	A. Wobble side-to-side at the hip.
		B. Lean to the outside with my foot sticking out, causing my knee to go to the inside.

Region 7: PT Time

Start Time	Activity	Exercise/Figure Number							
Phase One	ICE position	*5-2*							
Phase Two	Self-Mobs	*10-12*	*10-13*	*10-14*					
	Stretches for Affected Region	*11-7*	*11-8*	*11-9*					
	Stretches for Unaffected Regions *	*11-1* *11-2*	*11-3* *11-4*	*11-5* *11-6*	*11-10* *11-11*	*11-12* *11-13*			
Phase Three, Part 1	Basic Closed-Chain**	*14-1*	*14-2*	*14-3*	*14-4*	*14-5*	*14-6*	*14-7*	*14-8*
Phase Three, Part 2	Regional Closed-Chain	*14-2*	*14-8*	*14-9*	*14-12*	*14-13*	*14-20*		
Phase Four	Hill Closed-Chain**	*16-2*	*16-3*						

*With self-mobilizations as needed
** Same for all regions

Region 7: Goals

	Regional Focus
Phase Three and Four Stride Changes	1. Maintain pelvic stability and hip stability.
	2. Minimize excessive side-to-side movements.
Specific Mental Focus Statement	"I will control my body to run while keeping my feet, hip, and pelvis straight."

Recovery Plan, Region 8: Hamstring

Region 8: Self-Assessment

Activity	Self-Assessment	
Self-mobilization	1. I have **tenderness** in the back of the leg between the knee and buttock.	
Stretches	I have reduced range of motion **(stiffness)** in the Straight Leg Raise.	
Closed-Chain Exercises	I have **weakness** in the hamstring region, *resulting in* asymmetrical weakness and inflexibility in the hamstring area during kickback.	
Pre-Injury Stride Tendency	While running, I have a tendency to:	A. Push off from the inner side of the big toe.
		B. Have a kickback that is short, asymmetrical, or twists.

Region 8: PT Time

Start Time	Activity	Exercise/Figure Number							
Phase One	ICE position	5-1							
Phase Two	Self-Mobs	10-15	10-16						
	Stretches for Affected Region	11-3	11-4	11-5	11-6	11-7			
	Stretches for Unaffected Regions *	11-1 11-2	11-8 11-9	11-10 11-11	11-12 11-13				
Phase Three, Part 1	Basic Closed-Chain**	14-1	14-2	14-3	14-4	14-5	14-6	14-7	14-8
Phase Three, Part 2	Regional Closed-Chain	14-2	14-7	14-8	14-12	14-14	14-20		
Phase Four	Hill Closed-Chain**	16-2	16-3						

*With self-mobilizations as needed

** Same for all regions

Region 8: Goals

	Regional Focus
Phase Three and Four Stride Changes	1. Push off straight through the big toe.
	2. Straight, smooth forward progression.
	3. Symmetrical kickback.
Specific Mental Focus Statement	"I will control my body to run with a straight and strong kickback."

Recovery Plan, Region 9: Hip
(Secondary Regions: Groin or Inner Thigh)

Region 9: Self-Assessment

Activity	Self-Assessment
Self - mobilization	I have **tenderness** and/or swelling in the front of the hip.
Stretches	I have reduced range of motion **(stiffness)** in the hip region, *resulting in* inability to bring the ankle and/or knee all the way up, down, or back on the injured side when doing stretches.
Closed-Chain Exercises	I have **weakness** in the hip region, *resulting in* difficulty kicking up to "high knees" position.
Pre-Injury Stride Tendency	While running, I have a tendency to lean too far forward and toward the side of the injured hip.

Region 9: PT Time

Start Time	Activity	Exercise/Figure Number							
Phase One	ICE position	*5-3*							
Phase Two	Self-Mobs	*10-17*							
	Stretches for Affected Region	*11-4*	*11-10*	*11-11*	*11-12*				
	Stretches for Unaffected Regions *	*11-1* *11-2*	*11-3* *11-5*	*11-6* *11-7*	*11-8* *11-9*	*11-13*			
Phase Three, Part 1	Basic Closed-Chain**	*14-1*	*14-2*	*14-3*	*14-4*	*14-5*	*14-6*	*14-7*	*14-8*
Phase Three, Part 2	Regional Closed-Chain	*14-2*	*14-8*	*14-10*	*14-11*	*14-12*	*14-15*		
Phase Four	Hill Closed-Chain**	*16-2*	*16-3*						

*With self-mobilizations as needed

** Same for all regions

Region 9: Goals

	Regional Focus
Phase Three and Four Stride Changes	1. Running with upright posture (not leaning forward).
	2. Minimize lean toward the injured side.
Specific Mental Focus Statement	"I will control my body to run balanced, straight, and smooth."

Recovery Plan, Region 10: Buttock
(Secondary Region: Lateral hip)

Region 10: Self Assessment

Activity	Self-Assessment	
Self - mobilization	I have **tenderness** and swelling to the rear and side of the hip.	
Stretches	I have reduced range of motion **(stiffness)** in any hip stretching exercise.	
Closed-Chain Exercises:	I have **weakness** in the hip and buttock region that affects symmetrical kickback and overall balance.	
Pre-Injury Stride Tendency	While running, I have a tendency to:	A. Wobble side-to-side at the hip.
		B. Not be able to kick back straight and/or fully.
		C. Have asymmetrical rotation of the pelvis.

Region 10: PT Time

Start Time	Activity	Exercise/Figure Number							
Phase One	ICE position	5-4							
Phase Two	Self-Mobs	10-18	10-19						
	Stretches for Affected Region	11-4	11-8	11-9	11-11				
	Stretches for Unaffected Regions *	11-1 11-2	11-3 11-5	11-6 11-7	11-12 11-13				
Phase Three, Part 1	Basic Closed-Chain**	14-1	14-2	14-3	14-4	14-5	14-6	14-7	14-8
Phase Three, Part 2	Regional Closed-Chain	14-6	14-7	14-8	14-9	14-13	14-14		
Phase Four	Hill Closed-Chain**	16-2	16-3						

*With self-mobilizations as needed
** Same for all regions

Region 10: Goals

	Regional Focus
Phase Three and Four Stride Changes	1. Eliminate any side-to-side wobble.
	2. Keep your pelvis centered and stable, with symmetrical gliding motion in the hips and pelvis.
	3. Make the length of your stride equal on both sides.
Specific Mental Focus Statement	"I will control my body to run straight and evenly."

Recovery Plan 11: Regional Injury with Stress Fracture

Region 11 (Stress Fracture) Self Assessment

Activity	Self-Assessment
Self - mobilization	I have **tenderness** in any weight-bearing bone in my injury region (anywhere from the foot to the pelvis).
Stretches	I have reduced range of motion **(stiffness)** in the region where I have bone tenderness.
Closed-Chain Exercises:	After icing *and* not running for at least 3 weeks, I can still **reproduce my injury pain** when I hop on the injured leg (Square Hops).
	After icing *and* not running for at least 3 weeks, I may still **reproduce my injury pain** when I try to place equal amounts of weight or impact on both legs during any closed-chain exercise.
Pre-Injury Stride Tendency	While running, I feel pain in the region where I have bone tenderness.

If you are *unable* to clear Square Hops, follow your Regional Plan(s) with the following additions:

PT Time Phase Three, Part 2	All regional closed-chain exercises for your injury region(s)				
	Add Stress Fracture Closed-Chain	*14-1*	*14-2*	*14-8*	*14-18*
Goals	**Phase Three and Four Stride Changes**	Progressively increase ability to put weight on the injured region, without going back to pain that alters your stride.			
	Specific Mental Focus Statement	"I will train consistently and thoughtfully on a balanced body."			

APPENDIX Z: Regional Closed-Chain Tables for Fitness Runners and Racers

Notes for Appendix Z:

(1) Symmetry Target: Calculate this number in your Regional Closed-Chain Initial Assessment (see **Instructions for Log Form R, Line 8**).

(2) Rest Between Sets: Based on instructions for individual Closed-Chain Exercises in Box 14-2. For CC#16 and CC#18, copy only the rest time that applies to your group (Fitness Runner or Racer) to **Log Form R**.

(3) Final Target for Fitness Runners or Racers: Based on instructions for individual Closed-Chain Exercises in Box 14-2. Copy only the target time that applies to your group (Fitness Runner or Racer) to **Log Form R**.

(4) Build pace as: Based on instructions for individual Closed-Chain Exercises in Box 14-2. After achieving symmetry, build toward your *Final Target* time at glide rhythm, or as an acceleration.

(5) Symmetry Goal: Based on **Table R1: Symmetry Goals for Closed-Chain** in **Instructions for Log Form R**. Enter the time that represents 5% of your *Symmetry Target* (in Stage 1) or *Final Target* (in Stage 2).

Note for CC#4: This exercise is used in Basic Closed-Chain only, not in Regional Closed-Chain.

Special Instructions for CC#6 (Quick Steps), CC#16 (Barefoot Push-Through), and CC#18 (Shod Push-Through): Modify your **Log Form R** to look like the examples in *Appendix Z*. Cross out *Left* and *Right* on the line for *Set Times*, and write in "Both." Cross out *one* of each pair of boxes numbered 1 through 5. Also cross out the boxes for *Left/Right Difference* and *Symmetry Goal* (see sample **Log Forms R** in *Case Studies*).

Regional Closed-Chain Exercise	CC#1 Square Hops		CC#2 Side Step-Down		CC#3 One-Leg Armswings, Barefoot		CC#4	
Symmetry Target [1]								
Rest Between Sets [2]	10 sec		0		0			
Final Target for Fitness or Racing [3]	F: 30sec	R: 90sec	F: 30sec	R: 90sec	F: 30sec	R: 90sec		
Build pace as: [4]	acceleration		glide [A]		glide			
Set Times	Left	Right	Left	Right	Left	Right	Left	Right
1								
2								
3								
4								
5								
Total								
Avg Set Time								
L/R Difference								
Symmetry Goal [5]		sec		sec		sec		sec
Maximum Pain (0-10)	Left	Right	Left	Right	Left	Right	Left	Right

Footnotes: [A] See instructions to build box height in Box 14-2: Closed-Chain Exercises.

Regional Closed-Chain Exercise	CC#5 Barefoot Push-Up		CC#6 Quick Steps [B]		CC#7 Weighted Kickback		CC#8 Box Step Up and Over	
Symmetry Target [1]								
Rest Between Sets [2]	0		10 sec		0		0	
Final Target for Fitness or Racing [3]	F: 30 sec	R: 90 sec	F: 50 sec	R: 1m 50s	F: 2.5 min	R: 5 min	F: 2.5 min	R: 5 min
Build pace as: [4]	glide		acceleration [A]		glide		glide [A]	
Set Times	Left	Right	Both Legs		Left	Right	Left	Right
1								
2								
3								
4								
5								
Total								
Avg Set Time								
L/R Difference								
Symmetry Goal [2]		sec				sec		sec
Maximum Pain (0-10)	Left	Right	Left	Right	Left	Right	Left	Right

Footnotes:
[A] See instructions to build box height in Box 14-2: Closed-Chain Exercises.
[B] CC#6: See Special Instructions for Quick Steps.

~ 333 ~

Regional Closed-Chain Exercise	CC#9 Hip Abduction w/ Theraband		CC#10 Lateral Straight-Leg Raise w/ Theraband		CC#11 Straight-Leg Raise w/ Theraband		CC#12 One-Leg Armswings, Double Pillows	
Symmetry Target [1]								
Rest Between Sets [2]	0		0		0		0	
Final Target for Fitness or Racing [3]	F: 60 sec	R: 2.5 min	F: 60 sec	R: 2.5 min	F: 60 sec	R: 2.5 min	F: 30 sec	R: 90 sec
Build pace as: [4]	glide		glide		glide		acceleration	
Set Times	Left	Right	Left	Right	Left	Right	Left	Right
1								
2								
3								
4								
5								
Total								
Avg Set Time								
L/R Difference								
Symmetry Goal [5]	sec		sec		sec		sec	
Maximum Pain (0-10)	Left	Right	Left	Right	Left	Right	Left	Right

Regional Closed-Chain Exercise	CC#13 One-Leg Armswings, Side Incline		CC#14 One-Leg Armswings, Double Weights		CC#15 High Knees w/ Theraband		CC#16 Barefoot Push-Through [B]	
Symmetry Target [1]								
Rest Between Sets [2]	0		0		0		30 sec	0
Final Target for Fitness or Racing [3]	F: 30 sec	R: 90 sec	F: 30 sec	R: 90 sec	F: 60 sec	R: 2.5 min	F: 4.5 min	R: 10 min
Build pace as: [4]	acceleration		acceleration		glide		glide	
Set Times	Left	Right	Left	Right	Left	Right	Both Legs	
1								
2								
3								
4								
5								
Total								
Avg Set Time								
L/R Difference								
Symmetry Goal [5]	sec		sec		sec			
Maximum Pain (0-10)	Left	Right	Left	Right	Left	Right	Left	Right

Footnotes: [B] CC#16: See Special Instructions for Push-Throughs.

Regional Closed-Chain Exercise	CC#17 Shod Push-Up w/ Ankle Weights		CC#18 Shod Push-Through w/ Ankle Weights [B]		CC#19 Box Step-Up		CC#20 Theraband Kickback	
Symmetry Target [1]								
Rest Between Sets [2]	0		F:30sec	R: 0	0		0	
Final Target for Fitness or Racing [3]	F: 60 sec	R: 2.5 min	F: 4.5 min	R: 10 min	F: 2.5 min	R: 5 min	F: 60 sec	R: 2.5 min
Build pace as: [4]	acceleration		glide		glide [A]		acceleration	
Set Times	Left	Right	Both Legs		Left	Right	Left	Right
1								
2								
3								
4								
5								
Total								
Avg Set Time								
L/R Difference								
Symmetry Goal [4]		sec				sec		sec
Maximum Pain (0-10)	Left	Right	Left	Right	Left	Right	Left	Right

Footnotes:
[A] See instructions to build box height in Box 14-2: Closed-Chain Exercises.
[B] CC#18: See Special Instructions for Push-Throughs.

Hill Closed-Chain Exercises	Hill CC#1 Uphill Incline		Hill CC#2 Downhill Incline	
Symmetry Target	20 sec [C]		20 sec [C]	
Rest Between Sets	0		0	
Final Target for Fitness or Racing	F: 30 sec	R: 90 sec	F: 30 sec	R: 90 sec
Build pace as:	acceleration		acceleration	
Set Times	Left	Right	Left	Right
1				
2				
3				
4				
5				
Total				
Avg Set Time				
L/R Difference				
Symmetry Goal	1 sec		1 sec	
Maximum Pain (0-10)	Left	Right	Left	Right

Footnotes: [C] Achieve symmetry in Hill Closed-Chain before starting Hill Drills.

Section 6: Blank Worksheets and Log Forms

In this section you will find blank copies of all Worksheets and Log Forms. You may download additional Worksheets and Log Forms at www.postinjuryrunning.com.

Worksheets
1A1: Identifying a Running Injury
1B1: Running History
1C1: Medical History
1D1: Pain Pattern
1D2: Swelling Within Past 2 Weeks
1D3: Injury Stage
1D4: Summary of Original Injury
1D5: Phase One Treatment Group
1E1: Phase One Clearance

2A1: Mobility Self-Assessment
2A2: Ranking Affected Regions
2B1: Phase Two Treatment Group and Subgroup
2D1: Regional Tenderness

3A1: Evaluation of Basic Closed-Chain Exercises
3B1: Regional Self-Assessment Tables
3B2: Injury Regions in Order of Severity
3C1: Regional Closed-Chain Exercises in Order of Severity
Table 3D1: Balance Problems and Impairment Statements
3D1: Treatment Groups for Phase Three Part Two
Worksheet T: Training Plan for Phase Three Part Two
3G1: Evaluate Log Form S for Self-Paced Plan
3G2: Evaluate Log Form S for Two-Week-Interval Plan
3H1: Phase Three Clearance

4A1: Level 6 Clearance
4B1: Level 7 Clearance
4C1: Level 8 Clearance
4D1: Habits for Post-Recovery Running

Log Forms
Log Form I: Group 2 ICE Log
Log Form C: Stretch/Mobilization Cycles
Log Form M: Maintain Mobility
Log Form B: Basic Closed-Chain
Log Form R: Regional Closed-Chain
Log Form S: Base Schedule, Levels 0-8

Worksheet 1A1: Identifying a Running Injury		
1. Do you think you might have a running injury?	No	Yes
2. Do you have pain that only appears or gets worse *while* you are running OR that only appears in a regular pattern some time *after* you run?	No	Yes
3. Do your symptoms always lessen when you *stop* running (either immediately or after not running for up to two weeks)?	No	Yes

Worksheet 1B1: Running History

1. Write the exact day and date of the **last day you ran** (your last regular training session):
   _____.

2. How many years have you been running on a regular basis?
   - a. Less than 1 year
   - b. 1 to 3 years
   - c. More than 3 years

3. Which type of runner are you?
   - a. My primary goal is to improve my fitness (**Fitness Runner**).
   - b. My primary goal is to run faster in competitions (**Racer**).

4. Before your injury, how many *days* per week were you running on a regular basis?
   - a. 2 days or less per week
   - b. 3 to 5 days per week
   - c. More than 5 days per week

5. Before your injury, how many *miles* per week were you running on a regular basis?
   - a. Less than 10 miles per week
   - b. 10 to 25 miles per week
   - c. More than 25 miles per week

6. With this injury, how long could you run before the pain started?
   - a. Less than 10 minutes or 1 mile
   - b. 10 to 20 minutes, or 1 to 2 miles
   - c. 20 to 30 minutes, or 2 to 3 miles
   - d. 30 to 40 minutes, or 3 to 4 miles
   - e. 40 to 50 minutes, or 4 to 5 miles
   - f. More than 50 minutes or 5 miles

7. Based on the examples in Chapter 1 of *The Running Injury Recovery Program*, list any *intrinsic* or *extrinsic* factors that you need to work on:

Worksheet 1C1: Medical History

1. Have you had any previous running injuries that are not completely resolved and may still affect your running?	Yes	No
2. Have you had any traumatic injuries such as a fall, twist, sprain, or other accident within the past 12 months that affect your running?	Yes	No
3. Have you ever had surgery on any body part that might affect your running?	Yes	No
4. Do you have any pre-existing medical condition that affects your ability to run, such as osteoarthritis?	Yes	No
5. Do you take any medication for a medical condition which affects your ability to feel pain, such as a steroid or anti-inflammatory medication?	Yes	No

If you answered "Yes" to any question, list your conditions and/or medications here:

Worksheet 1D:
Document Your Injury and Phase One Treatment Group

Last day you ran: _____   Today's date: _____

Worksheet 1D1: Pain Pattern

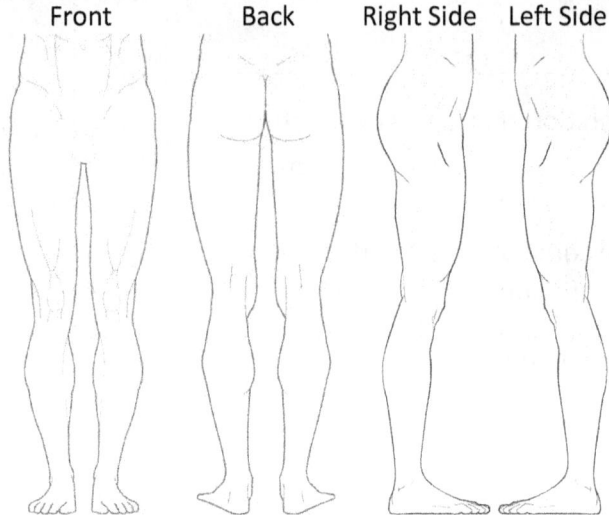

Front   Back   Right Side   Left Side

Compare to *Appendix A* and list your *possible affected regions* and side here:

_____

_____

_____

_____

_____

_____

Worksheet 1D2: Swelling Within Past 2 Weeks

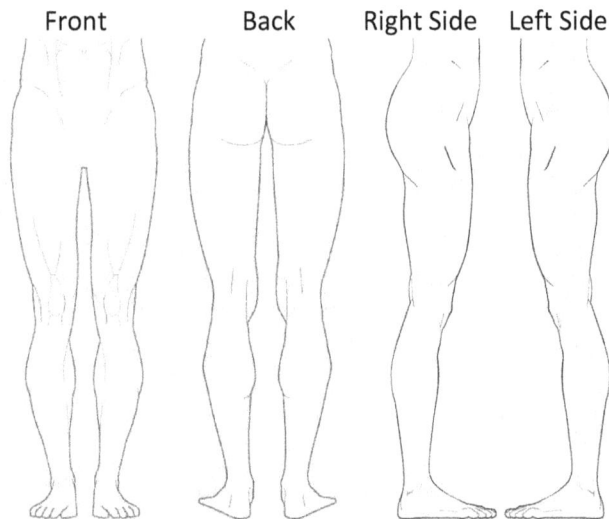

Front   Back   Right Side   Left Side

Compare to *Appendix A* and list your *possible affected regions* and side here:

_____

_____

_____

_____

_____

_____

Worksheet 1D3: Injury Stage

Injury Side and *possible affected region(s)*: _____

Table A: Maximum Symptoms *within the past 2 weeks*

Injury Stages	Emerging Symptoms	*Red Flags*	Which region(s)?
Stage 1	Pain while running	Pain that alters your stride	
Stage 2	Pain at rest (after running)	Pain that disturbs your rest	
Stage 3	Pain during your normal daily activities	Pain that interferes with or makes you avoid ADLs	
Stage 4	Running injury pain that you take medication for	Being in Stage 4	
Stage 5	Pain that cripples you	Being in Stage 5	

Table B: Maximum Symptoms *from more than 2 weeks ago*

Injury Stages	Emerging Symptoms	*Red Flags*	Which region(s)?
Stage 1	Pain while running	Pain that alters your stride	
Stage 2	Pain at rest (after running)	Pain that disturbs your rest	
Stage 3	Pain during your normal daily activities	Pain that interferes with or makes you avoid ADLs	
Stage 4	Running injury pain that you take medication for	Being in Stage 4	
Stage 5	Pain that cripples you	Being in Stage 5	

Worksheet 1D4: Summary of Original Injury

Refer to →	Worksheet 1D1: Pain Pattern	Worksheet 1D2: Swelling	Worksheet 1D3: Table A Injury Stage in Past 2 Weeks	
Left Leg Circle *Possible Affected Regions*	**Pain Severity (1-10)**	**Swelling in past 2 weeks (yes/no)**	**Injury Stage Scale (1-5)**	**Red Flag (yes/no)**
1 Toe				
2 Arch				
3 Heel				
4 Shin				
5 Calf				
6 Knee				
7 Band				
8 Hamstring				
9 Hip				
10 Buttock				

Refer to →	Worksheet 1D1: Pain Pattern	Worksheet 1D2: Swelling	Worksheet 1D3: Table A Injury Stage in Past 2 Weeks	
Right Leg Circle *Possible Affected Regions*	**Pain Severity (1-10)**	**Swelling in past 2 weeks (yes/no)**	**Injury Stage Scale (1-5)**	**Red Flag (yes/no)**
1 Toe				
2 Arch				
3 Heel				
4 Shin				
5 Calf				
6 Knee				
7 Band				
8 Hamstring				
9 Hip				
10 Buttock				

Worksheet 1D5: Phase One Treatment Group	
Circle ONE of the two statements below:	
I will enter Phase One injury management in treatment Group 1, and I do not have to ICE.	I will enter Phase One injury management in treatment Group 2, and I will now begin to ICE (**Log Form I**).

Worksheet 1E1: Phase One Clearance		
I have *no* Red Flag symptoms or visible swelling.	No	Yes
All of the emerging symptoms I recorded in Worksheets 1D1 through 1D4 have improved.	No	Yes
My sleep is not disturbed by pain due to this injury.	No	Yes
I can perform my activities of daily living (ADLs) normally, with less pain.	No	Yes
I do not need to take medication for pain and inflammation due to my running injury.	No	Yes
I have checked lines 5.1 through 9.4 on my Course Map.	No	Yes
I have followed all of the instructions in chapters 5 through 9 to implement protection and recovery for my running injury.	No	Yes
Group 2 ONLY: I have Iced 3 times a day, and the symptoms I have recorded on **Log Form I** have improved.	No	Yes

Worksheet 2A1: Mobility Self-Assessment

Circle *Possible Affected Region* and Side →		1: Toe	2: Arch	3: Heel	4: Shin	5: Calf	6: Knee	7: Band	8: Hams	9: Hip	10:Butt
		Left	Left	Left	Left	Left	Left	Left	Left	Left	Left
Stretch	**SIDE / Rank #**	Right	Right	Right	Right	Right	Right	Right	Right	Right	Right
11-1	Left:										
	Right:										
Notes:											
11-2	Left:										
	Right:										
Notes:											
11-3	Left:										
	Right:										
Notes:											
11-4	Left:										
	Right:										
Notes:											
11-5	Left:										
	Right:										
Notes:											
11-6	Left:										
	Right:										
Notes:											
11-7	Left:										
	Right:										
Notes:											
11-8	Left:										
	Right:										
Notes:											
11-9	Left:										
	Right:										
Notes:											
11-10	Left:										
	Right:										
Notes:											
11-11	Left:										
	Right:										
Notes:											
11-12	Left:										
	Right:										
Notes:											
11-13	Left:										
	Right:										
Notes:											

Worksheet 2A2: Ranking Affected Regions

SIDE:		From Worksheet 2A1			From Worksheet 1D4			Summary	
Possible Affected Regions		Maximum Stiffness		Maximum Asymmetry (left/right)	Pain (0-10)	Swelling yes/no	Injury Stage (1-5)	Assessment	Rank #
		Left	Right						
1	Toe								
2	Arch								
3	Heel								
4	Shin								
5	Calf								
6	Knee								
7	Band								
8	Hams								
9	Hip								
10	Butt								

Worksheet 2B1: Phase Two Treatment Group and Subgroup

1. Did you begin Phase One in Group 2 (with *Red Flags* or swelling)?

    A. No

    B. Yes

2. Do you *now* have any *Red Flags* or visible swelling in the injured region?

    A. No

    B. Yes

3. Based on your answers to questions 1 and 2, find your Phase Two treatment group:

Question 1:	Question 2:	Treatment Group
A. No	*and* A. No	*Group 1*
A. No	*and* B. Yes	*Group 2*
B. Yes	*and* A. No	*Group 2*
B. Yes	*and* B. Yes	*Group 2*

4. Go to your completed **Worksheet 2A2: Ranking Affected Regions**. How many regions did you assess as *possibly affected regions*?

   A. If you have only one *possible affected region* on one side (no regions on the other side), then count your injury as **one region**.

   B. If you have two or three *possible affected regions* on one side (and no regions on the other side), AND your *possible affected regions* are in closely associated areas (such as 1, 2, 3 or 6, 7, 8), AND you have decided, based on the guidelines in this book, that your symptoms are due to one simple injury, then count your injury as **one region**.

   C. If you circled one or more *possible affected region* on the left side AND one or more *possible affected region* on the right side, count your injury as **two or more regions**.

   D. If you circled two or more *possible affected regions* on one side, and they are NOT all closely associated with each other (such as 2, 3 and 7), count your injury as **two or more regions**.

5. Go to your **Self-Assessment 1C: Medical History**.

   A. If you answered NO to *all* questions in **Self-Assessment 1C**, you have **NO pre-existing condition** that might affect your running.

   B. If you answered YES to *any* question in **Self-Assessment 1C**, you have a **pre-existing condition** that might affect your running.

6. Based on your answers to questions 4 and 5 above, find your complexity subgroup below:

Question 4:	Question 5:	Subgroup
A or B (One region)	*and* A. NO pre-existing condition	*Simple Injury*
A or B (One region)	*and* B. Pre-existing condition	*Complex Injury*
C or D (Two or more regions)	*and* A.NO pre-existing condition	*Complex Injury*
C or D (Two or more regions)	*and* B. Pre-existing condition	*Complex Injury*

7. Fill in your Phase Two Recovery Group and Complexity Subgroup here:

   Entering Phase Two, I am in recovery group (*1 or 2*) _____, and I will follow

   the guidelines for (*simple or complex*) _____ injuries.

Worksheet 2D1: Regional Tenderness

List *possible affected regions* from **Log Form C**	Max tenderness on *more affected* side:	Max tenderness on *less affected* side:	Left/Right Difference	Assessment (affected or not)

Worksheet 3A1: Evaluation of Basic Closed-Chain Exercises

1. Based on your daily assessments, list all eight Basic Closed-Chain Exercises **in order of difficulty**:

    1. CC#_____

    2. CC#_____

    3. CC#_____

    4. CC#_____

    5. CC#_____

    6. CC#_____

    7. CC#_____

    8. CC#_____

2. Count the number of days since you started your Basic Closed-Chain exercises, and **circle** the statement below that applies to you:

I was *able* to clear all Basic Closed-Chain Exercises in 7 days or less, and I am progressing to Regional Closed-Chain Exercises.	I was *unable* to clear all Basic Closed-Chain Exercises in 7 days or less, and I am continuing with Basic Closed-Chain Exercises.

Worksheet 3B1: Regional Self-Assessment Tables

Region 1: Big Toe (1st Ray)
(Secondary Region: Outer Toes)

Activity	Self-Assessment		Left	Right
Self - mobilization	I have **tenderness** and/or bruising on the ball of the foot.			
Stretches	I have reduced range of motion **(stiffness)** in the toe region, *resulting in* difficulty flexing the toes up or down.			
Closed-Chain Exercises	I have **weakness** in the toe region, *resulting in*:	A. Difficulty flexing the toes during push off.		
		B. Difficulty flexing the toes during step-up.		
Pre-Injury Stride Tendency	While running, I have a tendency to:	A. Rotate the leg outward.		
		B. Push off from the inner or outer side of the big toe.		

Region 2: Arch

Activity	Self-Assessment		Left	Right
Self - mobilization	I have **tenderness** in or around the bottom of my foot; or under and/or to the outside of the heel and arch.			
Stretches	I have reduced range of motion **(stiffness)** in the ankle region, *resulting in* difficulty flexing the foot upward.			
Closed-Chain Exercises	I have **weakness** in the toe-flexing muscles, *resulting in* rolling the foot to the inside or outside when standing on one leg.			
Pre-Injury Stride Tendency	While running, I have a tendency to:	A. Turn the leg excessively out or in.		
		B. Overstrike and foot-slap into an overpronated foot.		

Region 3: Heel

Activity	Self-Assessment		Left	Right
Self - mobilization	I have **tenderness** at the Achilles tendon, and/or the outer side of the Achilles tendon.			
Stretches	I have reduced range of motion **(stiffness)** in the heel region**,** *resulting in* tightness in the heel area when standing on an uphill incline.			
Closed-Chain Exercises	I have **weakness** in the heel region, *resulting in*:	A. Difficulty keeping the foot flexed and straight.		
		B. Difficulty pushing off.		
Pre-Injury Stride Tendency	While running, I have a tendency to:	A. Overstrike, with the lower leg rotated outward.		
		B. Slap the foot, with the foot sticking out.		
		C. Overstrike on the outer edge of the heel and slap the foot.		
		D. Land too hard on the heel.		
		E. Overpronate and push off from the inner side of the big toe.		
		F. Roll the foot excessively inward.		

Region 4: Shin
(Secondary Region: Ankle)

Activity	Self-Assessment		Left	Right
Self - mobilization	I have **tenderness** on either side of the shin, extending down to the tendons near the foot.			
Stretches	I have reduced range of motion **(stiffness)** in the leg**,** *resulting in* reduced range of motion in the ankle.			
Closed-Chain Exercises	I have **weakness** in the shin region, *resulting in* twisting and leaning that causes excessive exertion in my shin.			
Pre-Injury Stride Tendency	While running, I have a tendency to:	A. A running stride that puts excessive stress on the shin.		
		B. Over-lean in any plane.		
		C. Overstrike on the heel.		
		D. Twist the knee and turn the foot outward.		
		E. Wobble at the hip.		

Region 5: Calf

Activity	Self-Assessment		Left	Right
Self - mobilization	I have **tenderness** in the thick part of the calf muscle			
Stretches	I have reduced range of motion **(stiffness)** in the calf region, *resulting in* difficulty flexing the foot upward.			
Closed-Chain Exercises	I have **weakness** in the calf region, *resulting in* difficulty flexing the foot downward.			
Pre-Injury Stride Tendency	While running, I have a tendency to:	A. Not be able to kick back straight and/or fully after pushoff.		
		B. Rotate the leg outward.		
		C. Have a circular movement of the lower leg.		
		D. Push off from the inner side of the big toe.		

Region 6: Knee
(Secondary Region: Thigh)

Activity	Self-Assessment		Left	Right
Self - mobilization	I have **tenderness** anywhere around the whole knee cap (usually to the outside of the knee cap), with or without generalized knee swelling.			
Stretches	I have reduced range of motion **(stiffness)** in the knee region, *resulting in* tightness and inability to bend the knee, and generalized stiffness.			
Closed-Chain Exercises	I have **weakness** in the knee region, *resulting in*:	A. Leg twisting inward during exercise.		
		B. difficulty bearing weight while stepping down.		
		C. Difficulty kicking back straight.		
		D. Difficulty balancing on one leg.		
		E. Inability to maintain knee control when stepping down stairs.		
Pre-Injury Stride Tendency	While running, I have a tendency to:	A. Twist at the knee.		
		B. Run with the foot pointed outward.		

Region 7: Band

Activity	Self-Assessment		Left	Right
Self - mobilization	I have **tenderness** on the outside of the knee, with or without visible swelling.			
Stretches	I have reduced range of motion **(stiffness)** from the hip and buttock down to the upper leg.			
Closed-Chain Exercises	I have **weakness** in the band region, *resulting in*:	A. Difficulty staying balanced on one leg.		
		B. Difficulty kicking out to the side.		
Pre-Injury Stride Tendency	While running, I have a tendency to:	A. Wobble side-to-side at the hip.		
		B. Lean to the outside with my foot sticking out, causing my knee to go to the inside.		

Region 8: Hamstring

Activity	Self-Assessment		Left	Right
Self - mobilization	I have **tenderness** in the back of the leg between the knee and buttock.			
Stretches	I have reduced range of motion **(stiffness)** in the Straight Leg Raise.			
Closed-Chain Exercises	I have **weakness** in the hamstring region, *resulting in* asymmetrical weakness and inflexibility in the hamstring area during kickback.			
Pre-Injury Stride Tendency	While running, I have a tendency to:	A. Push off from the inner side of the big toe.		
		B. Have a kickback that is short, asymmetrical, or twists.		

Region 9: Hip

Activity	Self-Assessment	Left	Right
Self - mobilization	I have **tenderness** and/or swelling in the front of the hip.		
Stretches	I have reduced range of motion **(stiffness)** in the hip region, *resulting in* inability to bring the ankle and/or knee all the way up, down, or back on the injured side when doing stretches.		
Closed-Chain Exercises	I have **weakness** in the hip region, *resulting in* difficulty kicking up to "high knees" position.		
Pre-Injury Stride Tendency	While running, I have a tendency to lean too far forward and toward the side of the injured hip.		

Region 10: Buttock
(Secondary Region: Lateral hip)

Activity	Self-Assessment		Left	Right
Self - mobilization	I have **tenderness** and swelling to the rear and side of the hip.			
Stretches	I have reduced range of motion **(stiffness)** in any hip stretching exercise.			
Closed-Chain Exercises:	I have **weakness** in the hip and buttock region that affects symmetrical kickback and overall balance.			
Pre-Injury Stride Tendency	While running, I have a tendency to:	A. Wobble side-to-side at the hip.		
		B. Be unable to kick back straight and/or fully.		
		C. Have asymmetrical rotation of the pelvis.		

Region 11: Regional Injury with Stress Fracture

Activity	Self-Assessment	Left	Right
Self - mobilization	I have **tenderness** in any weight-bearing bone in my injury region (anywhere from the foot to the pelvis), with or without pain in the associated soft tissues.		
Stretches	I have reduced range of motion **(stiffness)** in the region where I have bone tenderness.		
Closed-Chain Exercises:	After icing *and* not running for at least 3 weeks, I can *still* **reproduce my injury pain** when I hop on the injured leg (unable to clear CC#1 Square Hop Exercise).		
Pre-Injury Stride Tendency	While running, I feel pain in the region where I have bone tenderness.		

Worksheet 3B2: Injury Regions in Order of Severity		
Rank #	**Side (left/right)**	**Injury Region**
1.		Region #
2.		Region #
3.		Region #
4.		Region #

Worksheet 3C1: Regional Closed-Chain Exercises in Order of Severity

1st Injury Region and Side:	
Box 1: Regional Closed-Chain Exercises	
CC#	
CC#	
CC#	
CC#	
CC#	
CC#	

2nd Injury Region and Side:	
Box 2: Regional Closed-Chain Exercises	
CC#	
CC#	
CC#	
CC#	
CC#	
CC#	

3rd Injury Region and Side:	
Box 3: Regional Closed-Chain Exercises	
CC#	
CC#	
CC#	
CC#	
CC#	
CC#	

Stress Fracture, Side:	
Box 4: Regional Closed-Chain Exercises	
CC# 1	
CC# 2	
CC# 8	

Table 3D1: Basic Closed-Chain Balance Problems	
Basic Closed-Chain Exercise	Basic Balance Problem
CC# 1 or 2	Difficulty maintaining balance over a straight foot.
CC# 3 or 4	Difficulty using armswings to maintain balance while standing on one leg.
CC# 5 or 6	Difficulty maintaining balance while pushing off straight through the big toe.
CC# 7 or 8	Difficulty maintaining balance while kicking straight back.

Impairment Statement 1:

Impairment Statement 2:

Impairment Statement 3 (for injuries in the second leg only):

Worksheet 3D1: Treatment Groups for Phase Three Part Two

1. Which of the following statements applies to you?

    A. I have cleared all eight Basic Closed-Chain Exercises in 7 Days or less.

    B. I have completed Day 7 of Basic Closed-Chain Exercises, and I still have *not* cleared one or more of the eight Basic Closed-Chain Exercises.

2. Based on your **Self-Assessment 2B**, which complexity subgroup are you in?

    A. *Simple Injuries.*

    B. *Complex Injuries.*

3. How many Injury Regions did you list in **Worksheet 3B2: Injury Regions in Order of Severity**?

    A. One

    B. More than one

4. Look at the top section of today's **Log Form B: Basic Closed-Chain**, and find the box for "Days since *last day you ran*." Which of the following statements applies to you?

    A. Today is 42 days or less (6 weeks or less) since the last day I ran.

    B. Today is 43 days or more (more than 6 weeks) since the last day I ran.

---

5. Based on questions 1 through 4, find your Treatment Group for Phase Three Part Two:

You are in:	If your answers to questions 1 though 4 are:
GROUP 1A	"A" to ALL FOUR questions
GROUP 1B	"B" to question 1 AND "A" to ALL of questions 2, 3 and 4
GROUP 2A	"A" to question 1 AND "B" to ONE OR MORE of questions 2, 3, and 4
GROUP 2B	"B" to question 1 AND "B" to ONE OR MORE of questions 2, 3, and 4

Worksheet T: Training Plan for Phase Three Part Two

1. I am a (Fitness Runner or Racer): _____.

2. I plan to do my P.T. Time (**Log Form M** and **Log Form B** or **Log Form R**) 60 minutes per day, two days per week, on these days: _____ and _____.
(*Note:* P.T. Time may be done on the same days as your Base Schedule, or on different days).

3. I plan to do my Base Schedule (**Log Form S**) 60 minutes per day, _____ days per week, on these days:

_____

4. I am in Treatment Group Number (1A, 1B, 2A, or 2B) _____.

5. I am following the (*Self-Paced Plan* or *Two-Week-Interval Plan*):

_____

6. I will start my Base Schedule at Level _____.

7. My weekly mileage *goal* is _____ miles per week.

8. My daily mileage *maximum* is _____ miles per day (divide line 7 by line 3).

Write your personalized *Impairment Statements* from *Self-Assessment 3D* here:

Worksheet 3G1: Evaluate Log Form S for Self-Paced Plan (Level 0)

1. Evaluate your ability to fitness-walk your *Base Schedule* according to the instructions in Chapter 15:	Did you have any increase in pain or break in form during your 60-minute fitness walk?	Yes	No
2. Evaluate your notes:	A. Did you note any weakness, asymmetry, or problem with your stride?	Yes	No
	B. Are you aware of any other problem that you need to work on before progressing to Walk/Glide sets?	Yes	No

Worksheet 3G1: Evaluate Log Form S for Self-Paced Plan (Levels 1 through 5)

1. Evaluate your ability to perform each part of your *Base Schedule* according to the instructions in Chapter 15:	A. *Warmup:* Did you have any increase in pain or break in form during your 10-minute fitness walk?	Yes	No
	B. *Walk/glide sets:* Did you have any increase in pain or break in form during walk/glide sets?	Yes	No
	C. *Glide drills:* Did you have any difficulty performing any of the drills with correct form (as described in the instructions for that drill)?	Yes	No
	D. *Cooldown:* Did you have any increase in pain or break in form during your 5-minute fitness walk?	Yes	No
2. Evaluate completion of all drills:	A. Were you *unable* to complete the required time (*duration*) for any drill?	Yes	No
	B. Were you *unable* to complete the required number of sets (*repetitions*) for any drill?	Yes	No
3. Evaluate your notes:	A. Did you note any weakness, asymmetry, or problem with your stride?	Yes	No
	B. Are you aware of any other problem that you need to work on before progressing to the next level?	Yes	No
4. Level 5 only: Continue until the two numbers on the right match:	Write your number of *Target Days per Week* (3, 4, or 5).		
	Write the number of consecutive days you have cleared your Base Schedule at Level 5 with no break in form and no increase in symptoms.		

Worksheet 3G2: Evaluate Log Form S for Two-Week-Interval Plan (Level 0)

1. Evaluate your ability to fitness-walk your Base Schedule according to the instructions in Chapter 15:	Did you have any increase in pain or break in form during your 60-minute fitness walk?	Yes	No
2. Evaluate your notes:	A. Did you note any weakness, asymmetry, or problem with your stride?	Yes	No
	B. Are you aware of any other problem that you need to work on before progressing to Walk/Glide sets?	Yes	No
3. Level 0: Continue until the two numbers on the right match:	Multiply your number of *Target Days per Week* (3, 4, or 5) times two.		
	Write the number of consecutive days you have cleared your Base Schedule at Level 0 with no break in form and no increase in symptoms.		

Worksheet 3G2: Evaluate Log Form S for Two-Week-Interval Plan (Levels 1 through 5)

1. Evaluate your ability to perform each part of your Base Schedule according to the instructions in Chapter 15:	A. *Warmup:* Did you have any increase in pain or break in form during your 10-minute fitness walk?	Yes	No
	B. *Walk/glide sets:* Did you have any increase in pain or break in form during walk/glide sets?	Yes	No
	C. *Glide drills:* Did you have any difficulty performing any of the drills with correct form (as described in the instructions for that drill)?	Yes	No
	D. *Cooldown:* Did you have any increase in pain or break in form during your 5-minute fitness walk?	Yes	No
2. Evaluate completion of all drills:	A. Were you *unable* to complete the required time (*duration*) for any drill?	Yes	No
	B. Were you *unable* to complete the required number of sets (*repetitions*) for any drill?	Yes	No
3. Evaluate your notes:	A. Did you note any weakness, asymmetry, or problem with your stride?	Yes	No
	B. Are you aware of any other problem that you need to work on before progressing to the next level?	Yes	No
4. Levels 1 through 5: Continue until the two numbers on the right match.	Multiply your number of *Target Days per Week* (3, 4, or 5) times two.		
	Write the number of consecutive days you have cleared your Base Schedule at this level with no break in form and no increase in symptoms?		

Worksheet 3H1: Phase Three Clearance		
1. Have you cleared all of your Regional Closed-Chain Exercises through Stage 1 (*Self-Assessment 3F*)?	No	Yes
2. Have you cleared your Base Schedule through Level 5 (*Self-Assessment 3G1 or 3G2*)?	No	Yes

Specific Mental Focus Statement:

Worksheet 4A1: Level 6 Clearance			
Log Form S Level 6:	1. Are you able to perform all nine of your acceleration drills for the time required for your group (Fitness Runner or Racer), with no break in form and no increase in pain?	No	Yes
	2. Are you able to complete your Base Schedule (glides and acceleration drills) continuously for 50 minutes, with no break in form or significant increase in pain?	No	Yes
Log Form R (Stage 2)	3. Are you maintaining symmetry in all of your Regional Closed-Chain Exercises, with no significant increase in pain?	No	Yes
	4. Have you reached your *Symmetry Target* for Hill Closed-Chain Exercises 1 and 2?	No	Yes

Worksheet 4B1: Level 7 Clearance			
Log Form S Level 7:	1. Are you able to perform all six of your Hill Training drills for the time required for your group (Fitness Runner or Racer), with no break in form and no increase in pain?	No	Yes
	2. Are you able to complete your Base Schedule (glides and Hill-Training drills) continuously for 50 minutes, with no break in form or significant increase in pain?	No	Yes

Worksheet 4C1: Level 8 Clearance			
Log Form S Level 8:	1. Are you able to perform all twelve of your Plyometric Drills for the time required for your group (Fitness Runner or Racer), with no break in form and no increase in pain?	No	Yes
	2. Are you able to complete your Base Schedule (glides and Plyometric Drills and Glide Drills) continuously for 50 minutes, with no break in form or significant increase in pain?	No	Yes

Worksheet 4D1: Habits for Post-Recovery Running		
Post-Recovery Running Habits Checklist:	1. I will make a plan, and train consistently.	
	2. I will set realistic running goals.	
	3. I will start each run with a proper warmup.	
	4. I will pay close attention to my equipment, particularly my footwear.	
	5. I will focus on functional running.	
	6. I will manage my running injuries early, before they become severe.	

The most important lessons I have learned from my *Running Injury Recovery Program* that I will use when I return to regular training are:

Log Form I: Group 2 ICE Log

Phase #		Starting DAY/DATE:		Number of ICE Days:	

Week 1 (Day/Date/Phase)	ICE#	Symptoms (0 to 10)	Week 2 (Day/Date/Phase)	ICE#	Symptoms (0 to 10)
Day:	1		Day:	1	
Date:	2		Date:	2	
Phase:	3		Phase:	3	
Day:	1		Day:	1	
Date:	2		Date:	2	
Phase:	3		Phase:	3	
Day:	1		Day:	1	
Date:	2		Date:	2	
Phase:	3		Phase:	3	
Day:	1		Day:	1	
Date:	2		Date:	2	
Phase:	3		Phase:	3	
Day:	1		Day:	1	
Date:	2		Date:	2	
Phase:	3		Phase:	3	
Day:	1		Day:	1	
Date:	2		Date:	2	
Phase:	3		Phase:	3	
Day:	1		Day:	1	
Date:	2		Date:	2	
Phase:	3		Phase:	3	

Week 3	ICE#	Symptoms	Week 4	ICE#	Symptoms
Day:	1		Day:	1	
Date:	2		Date:	2	
Phase:	3		Phase:	3	
Day:	1		Day:	1	
Date:	2		Date:	2	
Phase:	3		Phase:	3	
Day:	1		Day:	1	
Date:	2		Date:	2	
Phase:	3		Phase:	3	
Day:	1		Day:	1	
Date:	2		Date:	2	
Phase:	3		Phase:	3	
Day:	1		Day:	1	
Date:	2		Date:	2	
Phase:	3		Phase:	3	
Day:	1		Day:	1	
Date:	2		Date:	2	
Phase:	3		Phase:	3	
Day:	1		Day:	1	
Date:	2		Date:	2	
Phase:	3		Phase:	3	

Log Form C: Stretch/Mobilization Cycles

DAY/DATE:	Days since *last day you ran*:
PHASE #	Days in this Phase:
AFFECTED SIDE:	AFFECTED REGION(S):

Circle affected side →		Left		Right	Symmetry	
Enter your exercise list from *Worksheets 2A1* and *2A2*	Rank #	**Stretches: Stiffness (0-5)** **Self Mobs: Tenderness (0-5)**	Rank#	**Stretches: Stiffness (0-5)** **Self Mobs: Tenderness (0-5)**	No	Yes
Stretch # 11-						
Self-Mob:						
Stretch # 11-						
Self-Mob:						
Stretch # 11-						
Self-Mob:						
Stretch # 11-						
Self-Mob:						
Stretch # 11-						
Self-Mob:						
Stretch # 11-						
Self-Mob:						
Stretch # 11-						
Self-Mob:						
Stretch # 11-						
Self-Mob:						
Stretch # 11-						
Self-Mob:						
Stretch # 11-						
Self-Mob:						
Stretch # 11-						
Self-Mob:						
Stretch # 11-						
Self-Mob:						
Stretch # 11-						
Self-Mob:						
Stretch # 11-						
Self-Mob:						

Log Form C: Stretch/Mobilization Cycles

DAY/DATE:	Days since *last day you ran*:
PHASE #	Days in this Phase:
AFFECTED SIDE:	AFFECTED REGION(S):

Circle affected side →		Left		Right		Symmetry	
Enter your exercise list from *Worksheets 2A1* and *2A2*	Rank #	**Stretches: Stiffness (0-5)** **Self Mobs: Tenderness (0-5)**	Rank#	**Stretches: Stiffness (0-5)** **Self Mobs: Tenderness (0-5)**		No	Yes
Stretch # 11-							
Self-Mob:							
Stretch # 11-							
Self-Mob:							
Stretch # 11-							
Self-Mob:							
Stretch # 11-							
Self-Mob:							
Stretch # 11-							
Self-Mob:							
Stretch # 11-							
Self-Mob:							
Stretch # 11-							
Self-Mob:							
Stretch # 11-							
Self-Mob:							
Stretch # 11-							
Self-Mob:							
Stretch # 11-							
Self-Mob:							
Stretch # 11-							
Self-Mob:							
Stretch # 11-							
Self-Mob:							
Stretch # 11-							
Self-Mob:							

Log Form C: Stretch/Mobilization Cycles

DAY/DATE:	Days since *last day you ran*:
PHASE #	Days in this Phase:
AFFECTED SIDE:	AFFECTED REGION(S):

Circle affected side →		Left		Right		Symmetry	
Enter your exercise list from *Worksheets 2A1* and *2A2*	Rank #	**Stretches: Stiffness (0-5)** **Self Mobs: Tenderness (0-5)**	Rank#	**Stretches: Stiffness (0-5)** **Self Mobs: Tenderness (0-5)**	No	Yes	
Stretch # 11-							
Self-Mob:							
Stretch # 11-							
Self-Mob:							
Stretch # 11-							
Self-Mob:							
Stretch # 11-							
Self-Mob:							
Stretch # 11-							
Self-Mob:							
Stretch # 11-							
Self-Mob:							
Stretch # 11-							
Self-Mob:							
Stretch # 11-							
Self-Mob:							
Stretch # 11-							
Self-Mob:							
Stretch # 11-							
Self-Mob:							
Stretch # 11-							
Self-Mob:							
Stretch # 11-							
Self-Mob:							
Stretch # 11-							
Self-Mob:							

Log Form C: Stretch/Mobilization Cycles

DAY/DATE:	Days since *last day you ran*:
PHASE #	Days in this Phase:
AFFECTED SIDE:	AFFECTED REGION(S):

Circle affected side →		Left		Right		Symmetry	
Enter your exercise list from *Worksheets 2A1* and *2A2*	Rank #	**Stretches: Stiffness (0-5)** **Self Mobs: Tenderness (0-5)**		Rank#	**Stretches: Stiffness (0-5)** **Self Mobs: Tenderness (0-5)**	No	Yes
Stretch # 11-							
Self-Mob:							
Stretch # 11-							
Self-Mob:							
Stretch # 11-							
Self-Mob:							
Stretch # 11-							
Self-Mob:							
Stretch # 11-							
Self-Mob:							
Stretch # 11-							
Self-Mob:							
Stretch # 11-							
Self-Mob:							
Stretch # 11-							
Self-Mob:							
Stretch # 11-							
Self-Mob:							
Stretch # 11-							
Self-Mob:							
Stretch # 11-							
Self-Mob:							
Stretch # 11-							
Self-Mob:							
Stretch # 11-							
Self-Mob:							

Log Form C: Stretch/Mobilization Cycles

DAY/DATE:	Days since *last day you ran*:
PHASE #	Days in this Phase:
AFFECTED SIDE:	AFFECTED REGION(S):

Circle affected side →		Left		Right	Symmetry	
Enter your exercise list from *Worksheets 2A1* and *2A2*	Rank #	**Stretches: Stiffness (0-5)** **Self Mobs: Tenderness (0-5)**	Rank#	**Stretches: Stiffness (0-5)** **Self Mobs: Tenderness (0-5)**	No	Yes
Stretch # 11-						
Self-Mob:						
Stretch # 11-						
Self-Mob:						
Stretch # 11-						
Self-Mob:						
Stretch # 11-						
Self-Mob:						
Stretch # 11-						
Self-Mob:						
Stretch # 11-						
Self-Mob:						
Stretch # 11-						
Self-Mob:						
Stretch # 11-						
Self-Mob:						
Stretch # 11-						
Self-Mob:						
Stretch # 11-						
Self-Mob:						
Stretch # 11-						
Self-Mob:						
Stretch # 11-						
Self-Mob:						
Stretch # 11-						
Self-Mob:						

Log Form C: Stretch/Mobilization Cycles

DAY/DATE:	Days since *last day you ran*:
PHASE #	Days in this Phase:
AFFECTED SIDE:	AFFECTED REGION(S):

Circle affected side →		Left		Right		Symmetry	
Enter your exercise list from *Worksheets 2A1* and *2A2*	**Rank #**	**Stretches:** **Stiffness (0-5)** / **Self Mobs:** **Tenderness (0-5)**		**Rank#**	**Stretches:** **Stiffness (0-5)** / **Self Mobs:** **Tenderness (0-5)**		No	Yes
Stretch # 11-							
Self-Mob:							
Stretch # 11-							
Self-Mob:							
Stretch # 11-							
Self-Mob:							
Stretch # 11-							
Self-Mob:							
Stretch # 11-							
Self-Mob:							
Stretch # 11-							
Self-Mob:							
Stretch # 11-							
Self-Mob:							
Stretch # 11-							
Self-Mob:							
Stretch # 11-							
Self-Mob:							
Stretch # 11-							
Self-Mob:							
Stretch # 11-							
Self-Mob:							
Stretch # 11-							
Self-Mob:							
Stretch # 11-							
Self-Mob:							

Log Form M: Maintain Mobility

DAY/DATE		Days since *last day you ran*:
PHASE #		Days in this Phase:

	Stretch/Mobilization Cycles	Left		Right		Symmetry	
Enter your exercise list from *Self-Assessment*		**Pain** (0-10)	**Stiffness / Tenderness** (0-5)	**Pain** (0-10)	**Stiffness / Tenderness** (0-5)	No	Yes
Set 1	Stretch #						
	Self-Mobs						
Set 2	Stretch #						
	Self-Mobs						
Set 3	Stretch #						
	Self-Mobs						
Set 4	Stretch #						
	Self-Mobs						
Set 5	Stretch #						
	Self-Mobs						
Set 6	Stretch #						
	Self-Mobs						
Set 7	Stretch #						
	Self-Mobs						
Set 8	Stretch #						
	Self-Mobs						
Set 9	Stretch #						
	Self-Mobs						
Set 10	Stretch #						
	Self-Mobs						
Set 11	Stretch #						
	Self-Mobs						
Set 12	Stretch #						
	Self-Mobs						
Set 13	Stretch #						
	Self-Mobs						

Log Form M: Maintain Mobility

DAY/DATE	Days since *last day you ran*:
PHASE #	Days in this Phase:

Stretch/Mobilization Cycles		Left		Right		Symmetry	
Enter your exercise list from *Self-Assessment*		Pain (0-10)	Stiffness / Tenderness (0-5)	Pain (0-10)	Stiffness / Tenderness (0-5)	No	Yes
Set 1	Stretch #						
	Self-Mobs						
Set 2	Stretch #						
	Self-Mobs						
Set 3	Stretch #						
	Self-Mobs						
Set 4	Stretch #						
	Self-Mobs						
Set 5	Stretch #						
	Self-Mobs						
Set 6	Stretch #						
	Self-Mobs						
Set 7	Stretch #						
	Self-Mobs						
Set 8	Stretch #						
	Self-Mobs						
Set 9	Stretch #						
	Self-Mobs						
Set 10	Stretch #						
	Self-Mobs						
Set 11	Stretch #						
	Self-Mobs						
Set 12	Stretch #						
	Self-Mobs						
Set 13	Stretch #						
	Self-Mobs						

Log Form M: Maintain Mobility

DAY/DATE	Days since *last day you ran*:
PHASE #	Days in this Phase:

	Stretch/Mobilization Cycles	Left		Right		Symmetry	
Enter your exercise list from *Self-Assessment*		**Pain** (0-10)	**Stiffness / Tenderness** (0-5)	**Pain** (0-10)	**Stiffness / Tenderness** (0-5)	No	Yes
Set 1	Stretch #						
	Self-Mobs						
Set 2	Stretch #						
	Self-Mobs						
Set 3	Stretch #						
	Self-Mobs						
Set 4	Stretch #						
	Self-Mobs						
Set 5	Stretch #						
	Self-Mobs						
Set 6	Stretch #						
	Self-Mobs						
Set 7	Stretch #						
	Self-Mobs						
Set 8	Stretch #						
	Self-Mobs						
Set 9	Stretch #						
	Self-Mobs						
Set 10	Stretch #						
	Self-Mobs						
Set 11	Stretch #						
	Self-Mobs						
Set 12	Stretch #						
	Self-Mobs						
Set 13	Stretch #						
	Self-Mobs						

Log Form M: Maintain Mobility

DAY/DATE		Days since *last day you ran*:
PHASE #		Days in this Phase:

	Stretch/Mobilization Cycles	Left		Right		Symmetry	
Enter your exercise list from *Self-Assessment*		**Pain** (0-10)	**Stiffness / Tenderness** (0-5)	**Pain** (0-10)	**Stiffness / Tenderness** (0-5)	No	Yes
Set 1	Stretch #						
	Self-Mobs						
Set 2	Stretch #						
	Self-Mobs						
Set 3	Stretch #						
	Self-Mobs						
Set 4	Stretch #						
	Self-Mobs						
Set 5	Stretch #						
	Self-Mobs						
Set 6	Stretch #						
	Self-Mobs						
Set 7	Stretch #						
	Self-Mobs						
Set 8	Stretch #						
	Self-Mobs						
Set 9	Stretch #						
	Self-Mobs						
Set 10	Stretch #						
	Self-Mobs						
Set 11	Stretch #						
	Self-Mobs						
Set 12	Stretch #						
	Self-Mobs						
Set 13	Stretch #						
	Self-Mobs						

Log Form M: Maintain Mobility

DAY/DATE	Days since *last day you ran*:
PHASE #	Days in this Phase:

	Stretch/Mobilization Cycles	Left		Right		Symmetry	
Enter your exercise list from *Self-Assessment*		Pain (0-10)	Stiffness / Tenderness (0-5)	Pain (0-10)	Stiffness / Tenderness (0-5)	No	Yes
Set 1	Stretch #						
	Self-Mobs						
Set 2	Stretch #						
	Self-Mobs						
Set 3	Stretch #						
	Self-Mobs						
Set 4	Stretch #						
	Self-Mobs						
Set 5	Stretch #						
	Self-Mobs						
Set 6	Stretch #						
	Self-Mobs						
Set 7	Stretch #						
	Self-Mobs						
Set 8	Stretch #						
	Self-Mobs						
Set 9	Stretch #						
	Self-Mobs						
Set 10	Stretch #						
	Self-Mobs						
Set 11	Stretch #						
	Self-Mobs						
Set 12	Stretch #						
	Self-Mobs						
Set 13	Stretch #						
	Self-Mobs						

Log Form M: Maintain Mobility

DAY/DATE	Days since *last day you ran*:
PHASE #	Days in this Phase:

Stretch/Mobilization Cycles		Left		Right		Symmetry	
Enter your exercise list from *Self-Assessment*		**Pain** (0-10)	**Stiffness / Tenderness** (0-5)	**Pain** (0-10)	**Stiffness / Tenderness** (0-5)	No	Yes
Set 1	Stretch #						
	Self-Mobs						
Set 2	Stretch #						
	Self-Mobs						
Set 3	Stretch #						
	Self-Mobs						
Set 4	Stretch #						
	Self-Mobs						
Set 5	Stretch #						
	Self-Mobs						
Set 6	Stretch #						
	Self-Mobs						
Set 7	Stretch #						
	Self-Mobs						
Set 8	Stretch #						
	Self-Mobs						
Set 9	Stretch #						
	Self-Mobs						
Set 10	Stretch #						
	Self-Mobs						
Set 11	Stretch #						
	Self-Mobs						
Set 12	Stretch #						
	Self-Mobs						
Set 13	Stretch #						
	Self-Mobs						

Log Form M: Maintain Mobility

DAY/DATE	Days since *last day you ran*:
PHASE #	Days in this Phase:

	Stretch/Mobilization Cycles	Left		Right		Symmetry	
Enter your exercise list from *Self-Assessment*		**Pain** (0-10)	**Stiffness / Tenderness** (0-5)	**Pain** (0-10)	**Stiffness / Tenderness** (0-5)	No	Yes
Set 1	Stretch #						
	Self-Mobs						
Set 2	Stretch #						
	Self-Mobs						
Set 3	Stretch #						
	Self-Mobs						
Set 4	Stretch #						
	Self-Mobs						
Set 5	Stretch #						
	Self-Mobs						
Set 6	Stretch #						
	Self-Mobs						
Set 7	Stretch #						
	Self-Mobs						
Set 8	Stretch #						
	Self-Mobs						
Set 9	Stretch #						
	Self-Mobs						
Set 10	Stretch #						
	Self-Mobs						
Set 11	Stretch #						
	Self-Mobs						
Set 12	Stretch #						
	Self-Mobs						
Set 13	Stretch #						
	Self-Mobs						

Log Form M: Maintain Mobility

DAY/DATE		Days since *last day you ran*:
PHASE #		Days in this Phase:

	Stretch/Mobilization Cycles	Left		Right		Symmetry	
Enter your exercise list from *Self-Assessment*		**Pain** (0-10)	**Stiffness / Tenderness** (0-5)	**Pain** (0-10)	**Stiffness / Tenderness** (0-5)	No	Yes
Set 1	Stretch #						
	Self-Mobs						
Set 2	Stretch #						
	Self-Mobs						
Set 3	Stretch #						
	Self-Mobs						
Set 4	Stretch #						
	Self-Mobs						
Set 5	Stretch #						
	Self-Mobs						
Set 6	Stretch #						
	Self-Mobs						
Set 7	Stretch #						
	Self-Mobs						
Set 8	Stretch #						
	Self-Mobs						
Set 9	Stretch #						
	Self-Mobs						
Set 10	Stretch #						
	Self-Mobs						
Set 11	Stretch #						
	Self-Mobs						
Set 12	Stretch #						
	Self-Mobs						
Set 13	Stretch #						
	Self-Mobs						

Log Form M: Maintain Mobility

DAY/DATE		Days since *last day you ran*:
PHASE #		Days in this Phase:

	Stretch/Mobilization Cycles	Left		Right		Symmetry	
Enter your exercise list from *Self-Assessment*		**Pain** (0-10)	**Stiffness / Tenderness** (0-5)	**Pain** (0-10)	**Stiffness / Tenderness** (0-5)	No	Yes
Set 1	Stretch #						
	Self-Mobs						
Set 2	Stretch #						
	Self-Mobs						
Set 3	Stretch #						
	Self-Mobs						
Set 4	Stretch #						
	Self-Mobs						
Set 5	Stretch #						
	Self-Mobs						
Set 6	Stretch #						
	Self-Mobs						
Set 7	Stretch #						
	Self-Mobs						
Set 8	Stretch #						
	Self-Mobs						
Set 9	Stretch #						
	Self-Mobs						
Set 10	Stretch #						
	Self-Mobs						
Set 11	Stretch #						
	Self-Mobs						
Set 12	Stretch #						
	Self-Mobs						
Set 13	Stretch #						
	Self-Mobs						

Log Form M: Maintain Mobility

DAY/DATE	Days since *last day you ran*:
PHASE #	Days in this Phase:

	Stretch/Mobilization Cycles	Left		Right		Symmetry	
	Enter your exercise list from *Self-Assessment*	**Pain (0-10)**	**Stiffness / Tenderness (0-5)**	**Pain (0-10)**	**Stiffness / Tenderness (0-5)**	No	Yes
Set 1	Stretch #						
	Self-Mobs						
Set 2	Stretch #						
	Self-Mobs						
Set 3	Stretch #						
	Self-Mobs						
Set 4	Stretch #						
	Self-Mobs						
Set 5	Stretch #						
	Self-Mobs						
Set 6	Stretch #						
	Self-Mobs						
Set 7	Stretch #						
	Self-Mobs						
Set 8	Stretch #						
	Self-Mobs						
Set 9	Stretch #						
	Self-Mobs						
Set 10	Stretch #						
	Self-Mobs						
Set 11	Stretch #						
	Self-Mobs						
Set 12	Stretch #						
	Self-Mobs						
Set 13	Stretch #						
	Self-Mobs						

Log Form B: Basic Closed-Chain

DAY/DATE		Days since *last day you ran:*
PHASE 3, Part#		Days in this Phase
AFFECTED SIDE and REGION(S)		

Basic Closed-Chain Exercise	CC#1 Square Hops		CC#2 Side Step-Down		CC#3 One-Leg Armswings, Barefoot		CC#4 One-Leg Armswings, 1 Pillow	
Target Time	20 sec		20 sec		15 sec		30 sec	
Rest Between Sets	10 sec		0		0		0	
Set Times	Left	Right	Left	Right	Left	Right	Left	Right
1								
2								
3								
4								
5								
Total								
Avg Set Time								
L/R Difference								
Symmetry Goal	1 sec		1 sec		1 sec		2 sec	
Max Pain (0-10)	L:	R:	L:	R:	L:	R:	L:	R:
NOTES:								

DAY/DATE		Days since *last day you ran:*		Days in this Phase:

Basic Closed-Chain Exercise	CC#5 Barefoot Push-Up		CC#6 Quick Steps		CC#7 Weighted Kickback		CC#8 Box Step Up and Over	
Target Time	15 sec		20 sec		60 sec		60 sec	
Rest Between Sets	0		10 sec		0		0	
Set Times	Left	Right	Both Legs [A]		Left	Right	Left	Right
1								
2								
3								
4								
5								
Total								
Avg Set Time								
L/R Difference								
Symmetry Goal	1 sec				3 sec		3 sec	
Max Pain (0-10)	L:	R:	L:	R:	L:	R:	L:	R:
NOTES:								

[A] See Instructions line 9: *Special Instructions for Quick Steps*

Log Form B: Basic Closed-Chain

DAY/DATE		Days since *last day you ran:*
PHASE 3, Part#		Days in this Phase
AFFECTED SIDE and REGION(S)		

Basic Closed-Chain Exercise	CC#1 Square Hops		CC#2 Side Step-Down		CC#3 One-Leg Armswings, Barefoot		CC#4 One-Leg Armswings, 1 Pillow	
Target Time	20 sec		20 sec		15 sec		30 sec	
Rest Between Sets	10 sec		0		0		0	
Set Times	Left	Right	Left	Right	Left	Right	Left	Right
1								
2								
3								
4								
5								
Total								
Avg Set Time								
L/R Difference								
Symmetry Goal	1 sec		1 sec		1 sec		2 sec	
Max Pain (0-10)	L:	R:	L:	R:	L:	R:	L:	R:
NOTES:								

DAY/DATE		Days since *last day you ran:*	Days in this Phase:

Basic Closed-Chain Exercise	CC#5 Barefoot Push-Up		CC#6 Quick Steps		CC#7 Weighted Kickback		CC#8 Box Step Up and Over	
Target Time	15 sec		20 sec		60 sec		60 sec	
Rest Between Sets	0		10 sec		0		0	
Set Times	Left	Right	Both Legs [(A)]		Left	Right	Left	Right
1								
2								
3								
4								
5								
Total								
Avg Set Time								
L/R Difference								
Symmetry Goal	1 sec				3 sec		3 sec	
Max Pain (0-10)	L:	R:	L:	R:	L:	R:	L:	R:
NOTES:								

[(A)] See Instructions line 9: *Special Instructions for Quick Steps*

Log Form B: Basic Closed-Chain

DAY/DATE		Days since *last day you ran:*	
PHASE 3, Part#		Days in this Phase	
AFFECTED SIDE and REGION(S)			

Basic Closed-Chain Exercise	CC#1 Square Hops		CC#2 Side Step-Down		CC#3 One-Leg Armswings, Barefoot		CC#4 One-Leg Armswings, 1 Pillow	
Target Time	20 sec		20 sec		15 sec		30 sec	
Rest Between Sets	10 sec		0		0		0	
Set Times	Left	Right	Left	Right	Left	Right	Left	Right
1								
2								
3								
4								
5								
Total								
Avg Set Time								
L/R Difference								
Symmetry Goal	1 sec		1 sec		1 sec		2 sec	
Max Pain (0-10)	L:	R:	L:	R:	L:	R:	L:	R:
NOTES:								

DAY/DATE		Days since *last day you ran:*		Days in this Phase:

Basic Closed-Chain Exercise	CC#5 Barefoot Push-Up		CC#6 Quick Steps		CC#7 Weighted Kickback		CC#8 Box Step Up and Over	
Target Time	15 sec		20 sec		60 sec		60 sec	
Rest Between Sets	0		10 sec		0		0	
Set Times	Left	Right	Both Legs [A]		Left	Right	Left	Right
1								
2								
3								
4								
5								
Total								
Avg Set Time								
L/R Difference								
Symmetry Goal	1 sec				3 sec		3 sec	
Max Pain (0-10)	L:	R:	L:	R:	L:	R:	L:	R:
NOTES:								

[A] See Instructions line 9: *Special Instructions for Quick Steps*

Log Form B: Basic Closed-Chain

DAY/DATE	Days since *last day you ran:*
PHASE 3, Part#	Days in this Phase
AFFECTED SIDE and REGION(S)	

Basic Closed-Chain Exercise	CC#1 Square Hops		CC#2 Side Step-Down		CC#3 One-Leg Armswings, Barefoot		CC#4 One-Leg Armswings, 1 Pillow	
Target Time	20 sec		20 sec		15 sec		30 sec	
Rest Between Sets	10 sec		0		0		0	
Set Times	Left	Right	Left	Right	Left	Right	Left	Right
1								
2								
3								
4								
5								
Total								
Avg Set Time								
L/R Difference								
Symmetry Goal	1 sec		1 sec		1 sec		2 sec	
Max Pain (0-10)	L:	R:	L:	R:	L:	R:	L:	R:
NOTES:								

DAY/DATE	Days since *last day you ran:*	Days in this Phase:

Basic Closed-Chain Exercise	CC#5 Barefoot Push-Up		CC#6 Quick Steps		CC#7 Weighted Kickback		CC#8 Box Step Up and Over	
Target Time	15 sec		20 sec		60 sec		60 sec	
Rest Between Sets	0		10 sec		0		0	
Set Times	Left	Right	Both Legs [A]		Left	Right	Left	Right
1								
2								
3								
4								
5								
Total								
Avg Set Time								
L/R Difference								
Symmetry Goal	1 sec				3 sec		3 sec	
Max Pain (0-10)	L:	R:	L:	R:	L:	R:	L:	R:
NOTES:								

[A] See Instructions line 9: *Special Instructions for Quick Steps*

Log Form R: Regional Closed-Chain

DAY/DATE:		Days since *last day you ran:*
PHASE (3 or 4):		Days in this Phase:
Injury Region(s) and Side:		

Regional Closed-Chain Exercise (number and name)	CC#		CC#		CC#		CC#	
Symmetry Target								
Rest Between Sets								
Final Target								
Build pace as:								
Set Times	Left	Right	Left	Right	Left	Right	Left	Right
1								
2								
3								
4								
5								
Total								
Avg Set Time								
L/R Difference								
Symmetry Goal	sec		sec		sec		sec	
Max Pain (0-10)	L:	R:	L:	R:	L:	R:	L:	R:
NOTES:								
FOOTNOTES:								

DAY/DATE:		Days since *last day you ran:*	Days in this Phase:

Regional Closed-Chain Exercise (number and name)	CC#		CC#		CC#		CC#	
Symmetry Target								
Rest Between Sets								
Final Target								
Build pace as:								
Set Times	Left	Right	Left	Right	Left	Right	Left	Right
1								
2								
3								
4								
5								
Total								
Avg Set Time								
L/R Difference								
Symmetry Goal	sec		sec		sec		sec	
Max Pain (0-10)	L:	R:	L:	R:	L:	R:	L:	R:
NOTES:								
FOOTNOTES:								

Log Form R: Regional Closed-Chain

DAY/DATE:		Days since *last day you ran:*
PHASE (3 or 4):		Days in this Phase:
Injury Region(s) and Side:		

Regional Closed-Chain Exercise (number and name)	CC#		CC#		CC#		CC#	
Symmetry Target								
Rest Between Sets								
Final Target								
Build pace as:								
Set Times	Left	Right	Left	Right	Left	Right	Left	Right
1								
2								
3								
4								
5								
Total								
Avg Set Time								
L/R Difference								
Symmetry Goal		sec		sec		sec		sec
Max Pain (0-10)	L:	R:	L:	R:	L:	R:	L:	R:
NOTES:								
FOOTNOTES:								

DAY/DATE:		Days since *last day you ran:*	Days in this Phase:

Regional Closed-Chain Exercise (number and name)	CC#		CC#		CC#		CC#	
Symmetry Target								
Rest Between Sets								
Final Target								
Build pace as:								
Set Times	Left	Right	Left	Right	Left	Right	Left	Right
1								
2								
3								
4								
5								
Total								
Avg Set Time								
L/R Difference								
Symmetry Goal		sec		sec		sec		sec
Max Pain (0-10)	L:	R:	L:	R:	L:	R:	L:	R:
NOTES:								
FOOTNOTES:								

Log Form R: Regional Closed-Chain

DAY/DATE:				Days since *last day you ran:*			
PHASE (3 or 4):				Days in this Phase:			
Injury Region(s) and Side:							

Regional Closed-Chain Exercise (number and name)	CC#		CC#		CC#		CC#	
Symmetry Target								
Rest Between Sets								
Final Target								
Build pace as:								
Set Times	Left	Right	Left	Right	Left	Right	Left	Right
1								
2								
3								
4								
5								
Total								
Avg Set Time								
L/R Difference								
Symmetry Goal		sec		sec		sec		sec
Max Pain (0-10)	L:	R:	L:	R:	L:	R:	L:	R:
NOTES:								
FOOTNOTES:								

DAY/DATE:				Days since *last day you ran:*		Days in this Phase:	

Regional Closed-Chain Exercise (number and name)	CC#		CC#		CC#		CC#	
Symmetry Target								
Rest Between Sets								
Final Target								
Build pace as:								
Set Times	Left	Right	Left	Right	Left	Right	Left	Right
1								
2								
3								
4								
5								
Total								
Avg Set Time								
L/R Difference								
Symmetry Goal		sec		sec		sec		sec
Max Pain (0-10)	L:	R:	L:	R:	L:	R:	L:	R:
NOTES:								
FOOTNOTES:								

Log Form R: Regional Closed-Chain

DAY/DATE:				Days since *last day you ran:*			
PHASE (3 or 4):				Days in this Phase:			
Injury Region(s) and Side:							

Regional Closed-Chain Exercise (number and name)	CC#		CC#		CC#		CC#	
Symmetry Target								
Rest Between Sets								
Final Target								
Build pace as:								
Set Times	Left	Right	Left	Right	Left	Right	Left	Right
1								
2								
3								
4								
5								
Total								
Avg Set Time								
L/R Difference								
Symmetry Goal		sec		sec		sec		sec
Max Pain (0-10)	L:	R:	L:	R:	L:	R:	L:	R:
NOTES:								
FOOTNOTES:								

DAY/DATE:				Days since *last day you ran:*		Days in this Phase:	

Regional Closed-Chain Exercise (number and name)	CC#		CC#		CC#		CC#	
Symmetry Target								
Rest Between Sets								
Final Target								
Build pace as:								
Set Times	Left	Right	Left	Right	Left	Right	Left	Right
1								
2								
3								
4								
5								
Total								
Avg Set Time								
L/R Difference								
Symmetry Goal		sec		sec		sec		sec
Max Pain (0-10)	L:	R:	L:	R:	L:	R:	L:	R:
NOTES:								
FOOTNOTES:								

Log Form R: Regional Closed-Chain

DAY/DATE:			Days since *last day you ran:*				
PHASE (3 or 4):			Days in this Phase:				
Injury Region(s) and Side:							

Regional Closed-Chain Exercise (number and name)	CC#		CC#		CC#		CC#	
Symmetry Target								
Rest Between Sets								
Final Target								
Build pace as:								
Set Times	Left	Right	Left	Right	Left	Right	Left	Right
1								
2								
3								
4								
5								
Total								
Avg Set Time								
L/R Difference								
Symmetry Goal		sec		sec		sec		sec
Max Pain (0-10)	L:	R:	L:	R:	L:	R:	L:	R:
NOTES:								
FOOTNOTES:								

DAY/DATE:			Days since *last day you ran:*			Days in this Phase:	

Regional Closed-Chain Exercise (number and name)	CC#		CC#		CC#		CC#	
Symmetry Target								
Rest Between Sets								
Final Target								
Build pace as:								
Set Times	Left	Right	Left	Right	Left	Right	Left	Right
1								
2								
3								
4								
5								
Total								
Avg Set Time								
L/R Difference								
Symmetry Goal		sec		sec		sec		sec
Max Pain (0-10)	L:	R:	L:	R:	L:	R:	L:	R:
NOTES:								
FOOTNOTES:								

Log Form R: Regional Closed-Chain

DAY/DATE:			Days since *last day you ran:*					
PHASE (3 or 4):			Days in this Phase:					
Injury Region(s) and Side:								

Regional Closed-Chain Exercise (number and name)	CC#		CC#		CC#		CC#	
Symmetry Target								
Rest Between Sets								
Final Target								
Build pace as:								
Set Times	Left	Right	Left	Right	Left	Right	Left	Right
1								
2								
3								
4								
5								
Total								
Avg Set Time								
L/R Difference								
Symmetry Goal		sec		sec		sec		sec
Max Pain (0-10)	L:	R:	L:	R:	L:	R:	L:	R:
NOTES:								
FOOTNOTES:								

DAY/DATE:		Days since *last day you ran:*		Days in this Phase:	

Regional Closed-Chain Exercise (number and name)	CC#		CC#		CC#		CC#	
Symmetry Target								
Rest Between Sets								
Final Target								
Build pace as:								
Set Times	Left	Right	Left	Right	Left	Right	Left	Right
1								
2								
3								
4								
5								
Total								
Avg Set Time								
L/R Difference								
Symmetry Goal		sec		sec		sec		sec
Max Pain (0-10)	L:	R:	L:	R:	L:	R:	L:	R:
NOTES:								
FOOTNOTES:								

Log Form R: Regional Closed-Chain

DAY/DATE:	Days since *last day you ran:*
PHASE (3 or 4):	Days in this Phase:
Injury Region(s) and Side:	

Regional Closed-Chain Exercise (number and name)	CC#		CC#		CC#		CC#	
Symmetry Target								
Rest Between Sets								
Final Target								
Build pace as:								
Set Times	Left	Right	Left	Right	Left	Right	Left	Right
1								
2								
3								
4								
5								
Total								
Avg Set Time								
L/R Difference								
Symmetry Goal		sec		sec		sec		sec
Max Pain (0-10)	L:	R:	L:	R:	L:	R:	L:	R:
NOTES:								
FOOTNOTES:								

DAY/DATE:	Days since *last day you ran:*	Days in this Phase:

Regional Closed-Chain Exercise (number and name)	CC#		CC#		CC#		CC#	
Symmetry Target								
Rest Between Sets								
Final Target								
Build pace as:								
Set Times	Left	Right	Left	Right	Left	Right	Left	Right
1								
2								
3								
4								
5								
Total								
Avg Set Time								
L/R Difference								
Symmetry Goal		sec		sec		sec		sec
Max Pain (0-10)	L:	R:	L:	R:	L:	R:	L:	R:
NOTES:								
FOOTNOTES:								

Log Form R: Regional Closed-Chain

DAY/DATE:					Days since *last day you ran:*			
PHASE (3 or 4):					Days in this Phase:			
Injury Region(s) and Side:								

Regional Closed-Chain Exercise (number and name)	CC#		CC#		CC#		CC#	
Symmetry Target								
Rest Between Sets								
Final Target								
Build pace as:								
Set Times	Left	Right	Left	Right	Left	Right	Left	Right
1								
2								
3								
4								
5								
Total								
Avg Set Time								
L/R Difference								
Symmetry Goal	sec		sec		sec		sec	
Max Pain (0-10)	L:	R:	L:	R:	L:	R:	L:	R:
NOTES:								
FOOTNOTES:								

DAY/DATE:			Days since *last day you ran:*		Days in this Phase:	

Regional Closed-Chain Exercise (number and name)	CC#		CC#		CC#		CC#	
Symmetry Target								
Rest Between Sets								
Final Target								
Build pace as:								
Set Times	Left	Right	Left	Right	Left	Right	Left	Right
1								
2								
3								
4								
5								
Total								
Avg Set Time								
L/R Difference								
Symmetry Goal	sec		sec		sec		sec	
Max Pain (0-10)	L:	R:	L:	R:	L:	R:	L:	R:
NOTES:								
FOOTNOTES:								

Log Form R: Regional Closed-Chain

DAY/DATE:			Days since *last day you ran:*		
PHASE (3 or 4):			Days in this Phase:		
Injury Region(s) and Side:					

Regional Closed-Chain Exercise (number and name)	CC#		CC#		CC#		CC#	
Symmetry Target								
Rest Between Sets								
Final Target								
Build pace as:								
Set Times	Left	Right	Left	Right	Left	Right	Left	Right
1								
2								
3								
4								
5								
Total								
Avg Set Time								
L/R Difference								
Symmetry Goal		sec		sec		sec		sec
Max Pain (0-10)	L:	R:	L:	R:	L:	R:	L:	R:
NOTES:								
FOOTNOTES:								

DAY/DATE:			Days since *last day you ran:*		Days in this Phase:	

Regional Closed-Chain Exercise (number and name)	CC#		CC#		CC#		CC#	
Symmetry Target								
Rest Between Sets								
Final Target								
Build pace as:								
Set Times	Left	Right	Left	Right	Left	Right	Left	Right
1								
2								
3								
4								
5								
Total								
Avg Set Time								
L/R Difference								
Symmetry Goal		sec		sec		sec		sec
Max Pain (0-10)	L:	R:	L:	R:	L:	R:	L:	R:
NOTES:								
FOOTNOTES:								

Log Form R: Regional Closed-Chain

DAY/DATE:			Days since *last day you ran*:			
PHASE (3 or 4):			Days in this Phase:			
Injury Region(s) and Side:						

Regional Closed-Chain Exercise (number and name)	CC#		CC#		CC#		CC#	
Symmetry Target								
Rest Between Sets								
Final Target								
Build pace as:								
Set Times	Left	Right	Left	Right	Left	Right	Left	Right
1								
2								
3								
4								
5								
Total								
Avg Set Time								
L/R Difference								
Symmetry Goal		sec		sec		sec		sec
Max Pain (0-10)	L:	R:	L:	R:	L:	R:	L:	R:
NOTES:								
FOOTNOTES:								

DAY/DATE:		Days since *last day you ran*:	Days in this Phase:

Regional Closed-Chain Exercise (number and name)	CC#		CC#		CC#		CC#	
Symmetry Target								
Rest Between Sets								
Final Target								
Build pace as:								
Set Times	Left	Right	Left	Right	Left	Right	Left	Right
1								
2								
3								
4								
5								
Total								
Avg Set Time								
L/R Difference								
Symmetry Goal		sec		sec		sec		sec
Max Pain (0-10)	L:	R:	L:	R:	L:	R:	L:	R:
NOTES:								
FOOTNOTES:								

Log Form S: Base Schedule
Level 0 (Groups 1B, 2A and 2B Only)

	Starting Day/Date:			Days since *last day you ran* (on starting day):		
	Target Days per week (3, 4, 5)			Clearance date:		
	Activity	**Type**	**Repetitions**	**Duration**		**Total Time**
Warmup	Fitness walk					10 min
Base Schedule	Fitness walk					50 min
Cooldown	Fitness walk					5 min

	Day/Date	Day/Date	Day/Date	Day/Date	Day/Date
Week 1	/	/	/	/	/
Pain (0-10)					
Notes:					
Week 2	/	/	/	/	/
Pain (0-10)					
Notes:					
Week 3	/	/	/	/	/
Pain (0-10)					
Notes:					
Week 4	/	/	/	/	/
Pain (0-10)					
Notes:					

Log Form S: Base Schedule
Level 1

Starting Day/Date:			Days since *last day you ran* (on starting day):		
Target Days per week (3, 4, 5)			Clearance date:		
	Activity	**Type**	**Repetitions**	**Duration**	**Total Time**
Warmup	Fitness Walk				10 min
Base Schedule (*Table 15-4A*)	Walk/glide sets	Glide 1min/walk 4 min	10		
	10 Glide Drills:	Drill #1	2	15 sec	50 min
		Drill #2	2	15 sec	
		Drill #3	2	15 sec	
		Drill #4	2	15 sec	
		Drill #5	2	15 sec	
Cooldown	Fitness Walk				5 min

	Day/Date	Day/Date	Day/Date	Day/Date	Day/Date
Week 1	/	/	/	/	/
Pain (0-10)					
Drills/Form					
Notes:					
Week 2	/	/	/	/	/
Pain (0-10)					
Drills/Form					
Notes:					
Week 3	/	/	/	/	/
Pain (0-10)					
Drills/Form					
Notes:					
Week 4	/	/	/	/	/
Pain (0-10)					
Drills/Form					
Notes:					

Log Form S: Base Schedule
Level 2

Starting Day/Date:			Days since *last day you ran* (on starting day):		
Target Days per week (3, 4, 5)			Clearance date:		
	Activity	**Type**	**Repetitions**	**Duration**	**Total Time**
Warmup	Fitness Walk				10 min
Base Schedule (*Table 15-4B*)	Walk/glide sets	Glide 2 min/walk 3 min	10		50 min
	15 Glide Drills:	Drill #1	3	15 sec	
		Drill #2	3	15 sec	
		Drill #3	3	15 sec	
		Drill #4	3	15 sec	
		Drill #5	3	15 sec	
Cooldown	Fitness Walk				5 min

	Day/Date	Day/Date	Day/Date	Day/Date	Day/Date
Week 1	/	/	/	/	/
Pain (0-10)					
Drills/Form					
Notes:					
Week 2	/	/	/	/	/
Pain (0-10)					
Drills/Form					
Notes:					
Week 3	/	/	/	/	/
Pain (0-10)					
Drills/Form					
Notes:					
Week 4	/	/	/	/	/
Pain (0-10)					
Drills/Form					
Notes:					

Log Form S: Base Schedule
Level 3

Starting Day/Date:			Days since *last day you ran* (on starting day):		
Target Days per week (3, 4, 5)			**Clearance date:**		
	Activity	**Type**	**Repetitions**	**Duration**	**Total Time**
Warmup	Fitness Walk				10 min
Base Schedule *(Table 15-4C)*	Walk/glide sets	Glide 3 min/walk 2 min	10		50 min
	15 Glide Drills:	Drill #1	3	15 sec	
		Drill #2	3	15 sec	
		Drill #3	3	15 sec	
		Drill #4	3	15 sec	
		Drill #5	3	15 sec	
Cooldown	Fitness Walk				5 min

	Day/Date	Day/Date	Day/Date	Day/Date	Day/Date
Week 1	/	/	/	/	/
Pain (0-10)					
Drills/Form					
Notes:					
Week 2	/	/	/	/	/
Pain (0-10)					
Drills/Form					
Notes:					
Week 3	/	/	/	/	/
Pain (0-10)					
Drills/Form					
Notes:					
Week 4	/	/	/	/	/
Pain (0-10)					
Drills/Form					
Notes:					

Log Form S: Base Schedule
Level 4

Starting Day/Date:			Days since *last day you ran* (on starting day):		
Target Days per week (3, 4, 5)			Clearance date:		
	Activity	Type	Repetitions	Duration	Total Time
Warmup	Fitness Walk				10 min
Base Schedule (*Table 15-4D*)	Walk/glide sets	Glide 4 min/walk 1 min	10		50 min
	15 Glide Drills:	Drill #1	3	15 sec	
		Drill #2	3	15 sec	
		Drill #3	3	15 sec	
		Drill #4	3	15 sec	
		Drill #5	3	15 sec	
Cooldown	Fitness Walk				5 min

	Day/Date	Day/Date	Day/Date	Day/Date	Day/Date
Week 1	/	/	/	/	/
Pain (0-10)					
Drills/Form					
Notes:					
Week 2	/	/	/	/	/
Pain (0-10)					
Drills/Form					
Notes:					
Week 3	/	/	/	/	/
Pain (0-10)					
Drills/Form					
Notes:					
Week 4	/	/	/	/	/
Pain (0-10)					
Drills/Form					
Notes:					

Log Form S: Base Schedule
Level 5

Starting Day/Date:			Days since *last day you ran* (on starting day):			
Target Days per week (3, 4, 5)			Clearance date:			
	Activity	**Type**	**Repetitions**	**Duration**	**Total Time**	
Warmup	Fitness Walk				10 min	
Base Schedule (*Table 15-4E*)	Glides	50-minute glides				
	15 Glide Drills:	Drill #1	3	15 sec ea		
		Drill #2	3	15 sec ea	50 min	
		Drill #3	3	15 sec ea		
		Drill #4	3	15 sec ea		
		Drill #5	3	15 sec ea		
Cooldown	Fitness Walk				5 min	

	Day/Date	Day/Date	Day/Date	Day/Date	Day/Date
Week 1	/	/	/	/	/
Pain (0-10)					
Drills/Form					
Notes:					
Week 2	/	/	/	/	/
Pain (0-10)					
Drills/Form					
Notes:					
Week 3	/	/	/	/	/
Pain (0-10)					
Drills/Form					
Notes:					
Week 4	/	/	/	/	/
Pain (0-10)					
Drills/Form					
Notes:					

Log Form S: Base Schedule
Level 6

Starting Day/Date:			Days since *last day you ran* (on starting day):			
Target Days per week (3, 4, 5)			Clearance date:			
	Activity	Type	Reps	A. Fitness Runners	B. Racers	Total Time
Warmup	Fitness Walk					10 min
Base Schedule (*Table 16-2*)	Glides	50-min. glides				
	9 Acceleration Drills:	Drill #1	3	30 sec each	Build to 90 sec each	50 min
		Drill #2	3			
		Drill #3	3			
Cooldown	Fitness Walk					5 min
Mental Focus Statement:						

	Day/Date	Day/Date	Day/Date	Day/Date	Day/Date
Week 1	/	/	/	/	/
Pain (0-10)					
Drills/Form					
Notes:					
Week 2	/	/	/	/	/
Pain (0-10)					
Drills/Form					
Notes:					
Week 3	/	/	/	/	/
Pain (0-10)					
Drills/Form					
Notes:					
Week 4	/	/	/	/	/
Pain (0-10)					
Drills/Form					
Notes:					

Log Form S: Base Schedule
Level 7

Starting Day/Date:			**Days since *last day you ran* (on starting day):**			
Target Days per week (3, 4, 5)			**Clearance date:**			
	Activity	**Type**	**Reps**	**A. Fitness Runners**	**B. Racers**	**Total Time**
Warmup	Fitness Walk					10 min
Base Schedule (*Table 16-3*)	Glides	50-min. glides				50 min
	6 Hill Drills:	Uphill Drill	3	90 sec each	Build to 4.5 min each	
		Downhill Drill	3	90 sec each	Build to 4.5 min each	
Cooldown	Fitness Walk					5 min
Mental Focus Statement:						

	Day/Date	Day/Date	Day/Date	Day/Date	Day/Date
Week 1	/	/	/	/	/
Pain (0-10)					
Drills/Form					
Notes:					
Week 2	/	/	/	/	/
Pain (0-10)					
Drills/Form					
Notes:					
Week 3	/	/	/	/	/
Pain (0-10)					
Drills/Form					
Notes:					
Week 4	/	/	/	/	/
Pain (0-10)					
Drills/Form					
Notes:					

Log Form S: Base Schedule
Level 8

Starting Day/Date:			Days since *last day you ran* (on starting day):			
Target Days per week (3, 4, 5)			Clearance date:			
	Activity	Type	Reps	A. Fitness Runners	B. Racers	Total Time
Warmup	Fitness Walk					10 min
Base Schedule (*Table 17-1*)	Glides	50-min. glides				50 min
	12 Plyometric Drills:	Drill #1	3	15 sec each	Build to 45 sec each	
		Drill #2	3			
		Drill #3	3			
		Drill #4	3			
	10 Glide Drills	5 glide drills	2 each	15 sec each	15 sec each	
Cooldown	Fitness Walk					5 min
Mental Focus Statement:						

	Day/Date	Day/Date	Day/Date	Day/Date	Day/Date
Week 1	/	/	/	/	/
Pain (0-10)					
Drills/Form					
Notes:					
Week 2	/	/	/	/	/
Pain (0-10)					
Drills/Form					
Notes:					
Week 3	/	/	/	/	/
Pain (0-10)					
Drills/Form					
Notes:					
Week 4	/	/	/	/	/
Pain (0-10)					
Drills/Form					
Notes:					

Frequently Asked Questions (FAQ's)

Q1: What is the _Running Injury Recovery Program WORKBOOK_?

- The _Running Injury Recovery Program WORKBOOK_ contains all the step-by-step instructions for the _Running Injury Recovery Program_, including the _Course Map_, _Guidelines_, _Self-Assessments_, _Log Forms_, examples in _Case Studies_, and important references in _Appendices_.

Q2: Why is the _WORKBOOK_ so long and complicated?

- This _Running Injury Recovery Program_ covers nearly every possible combination of scenarios for every type of running injury that I have encountered in my P.T. practice over the past 30 years. Your individual journey will not be that complicated.

- Once you have read through _The Running Injury Recovery Program_ and learned the "education" part, the _WORKBOOK_ will guide you step-by-step through the recovery process.

- The first time you use this program, take the time to understand the goals and follow the instructions carefully. The next time you have an injury, it will go much quicker.

Q3: What are all these confusing numbers?

- All the exercises you will use in your _WORKBOOK_ are numbered, starting with the chapter number where they are introduced in _The Running Injury Recovery Program_. For example, you'll find the instructions for stretch number 11-4 in Chapter 11 of the _Program_ book, and the instructions for exercise 14-8 in Chapter 14.

- Except for the Checkpoints between phases, all lines in the _Course Map_ are numbered for a chapter number in _The Running Injury Recovery Program_. Your _Self-Assessments_ will direct you to check off certain line-numbers on your _Course Map_. While you are doing your _WORKBOOK_ you should check off all of the lighter-shaded boxes (action lines) and the darker-shaded boxes (checkpoints) on your _Course Map_ in numerical order.

- All _Self-Assessments_ are numbered, starting with the Phase number. For example, _Self-Assessments 3A_ through _3H_ cover Phase Three.

- Almost all _Worksheets_ are part of a _Self-Assessment_ and are numbered for that _Self-Assessment_. For example, _Worksheet 2A1_ is in _Self-Assessment 2A_. The only _Worksheet_ that is not numbered is _Worksheet T: Training Plan for Phase Three Part Two_ which summarizes information from several other _Worksheets_.

- The _Log Forms_ that you fill in during your daily P.T. Time or Base Schedule are identified by letter rather than number. For example, you will use _Log Form C_ during Phase Two P.T. Time.

- Tables from _The Running Injury Recovery Program_ are also numbered by chapter. For example, _Table 3-1_ is the first table in Chapter 3.

- Tables in the _Self-Assessments_ are numbered for that _Self-Assessment_. For example, _Table 2A1_ is the first table in _Self-Assessment 2A_.

- Tables in the *Instructions for Log Forms* start with the letter of that *Log Form*. For example, *Table S1* is found in the *Instructions for Log Form S*.
- *Appendices* are also identified by letter. For example, you will refer to *Appendix A* when you start your *Self-Assessments*.

Q4: Can't you just tell me what to do?

- Each individual is different. Your *Recovery Program* is individualized for you and your specific running injury. You have to go through the process to create the best recovery program for your injury.

Q5: How long will it take for me to finish the entire Running Injury Recovery Program?

- The length of time will be different for each person, depending on their condition and injury.
- Typically, a simple injury with no Red Flags takes about two weeks. A simple injury with Red Flags takes about four weeks. A complex injury with no Red Flags takes about 14 weeks, and a complex injury with Red Flags takes about 16 weeks.

Q6: Do I have to do all these exercises?

- Yes. You must do all the exercises for your group and your injury as determined by your *Self-Assessments*.

Q7: Do I have to fill out all these Log Forms while I'm doing exercises?

- Do your best.
- Ask a friend, family member, or coach to help you.
- If you are on your own and can't stop to record every set, watch the clock, estimate your set times, and fill them in at the end of each exercise.
- If all else fails and you just can't cope with one of the *Log Forms*, then just do the exercises and use your best judgment when you are filling in your *Self-Assessments*.

Q8: Do I really have to fill out all these Self-Assessments?

- Yes.

Q9: What if my injury is in a "secondary injury region"?

- Follow the instructions for the primary region.

Q10: How do I get started?

- You must read all of the chapters in *The Running Injury Recovery Program* before you begin *The Running Injury Recovery Program WORKBOOK*.
- Read the Introduction to *The Running Injury Recovery Program WORKBOOK*, and print out your *Worksheets* and *Log Forms* from the website.
- Follow the Course Map. Start your *Workbook* at *Self-Assessment 1A* and follow the *Guidelines* for your treatment group.

Q11: How do I keep track of everything I have to do?

- Check off lines on your *Course Map* as you complete them.
- Follow the *Guidelines* for each phase.
- See *Table W-1: Time Management Schedules by Group.*

Q12: Where can I get more blank forms, information, and personalized help?

- Go to postinjuryrunning.com.

ABOUT THE AUTHOR

Bruce R. Wilk, P.T., O.C.S., has been writing and lecturing about running injury management around the world for more than thirty years, teaching specialized classes for running organizations, professional associations, medical schools, and the military. He received his degree in Physical Therapy from SUNY, and is certified in Manual Therapy and Orthopedic Physical Therapy. His primary practice is in Miami, Florida, where he is the director of Orthopedic Rehabilitation Specialists, Inc.. Wilk is also a lifelong runner and triathlete, Vice President of the Miami Runner's Club, and has worked with many racers as an RRCA certified running coach. Along with his wife, Sherry, he owns and operates a running specialty store called *The Runner's High*, which has become the center of Miami's running community.

www.ingramcontent.com/pod-product-compliance
Lightning Source LLC
Chambersburg PA
CBHW080323270326
41927CB00014B/3081